EMERGENCY MEDICINE

Emergency and Acute Medicine: Diagnosis and Management

Fifth edition

ANTHONY F.T. BROWN
MB ChB (Bristol), FRCP, FRCS(Edin), FACEM, FCEM

Associate Professor, Discipline of Anaesthesiology and Critical Care, School of Medicine, University of Queensland, Brisbane

Senior Staff Specialist, Department of Emergency Medicine, Royal Brisbane and Women's Hospital, Brisbane

Trained in the UK and currently working in Australia. Editor-in-Chief of *Emergency Medicine Australasia*. Senior Court of Examiners, Australasian College for Emergency Medicine (ACEM). Inaugural ACEM Teaching Excellence Award 2001.

MICHAEL D. CADOGAN
MA(Oxon), MB ChB (Edin), FACEM

Clinical Senior Lecturer, Faculty of Medicine, Dentistry and Health Sciences, University of Western Australia, Perth

Staff Specialist in Emergency Medicine, Department of Emergency Medicine, Sir Charles Gairdner Hospital, Perth

Trained in the UK and currently working in Australia. Expert in Medical Informatics. Winner, Gold Medal/Buchanan Prize, Australasian College for Emergency Medicine Fellowship Exam 2003

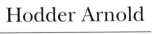

Hodder Arnold

A MEMBER OF THE HODDER HEADLINE GROUP

First published in Great Britain by Hodder Arnold
Fourth edition 2002
This fifth edition published in 2006 by
Hodder Arnold, an imprint of Hodder Education and a member of the Hodder Headline Group,
338 Euston Road, London NW1 3BH

http://www.hoddereducation.com

Distributed in the United States of America by
Oxford University Press Inc.,
198 Madison Avenue, New York, NY10016
Oxford is a registered trademark of Oxford University Press

British Library Cataloguing in Publication Data
A catalogue record for this book is available from the British Library

Library of Congress Cataloging-in-Publication Data
A catalog record for this book is available from the Library of Congress

ISBN-10: 0 340 92770 4
ISBN-13: 978 0 340 92770 0

1 2 3 4 5 6 7 8 9 10

Commissioning Editor: Philip Shaw
Project Editor: Heather Fyfe
Production Controller: Karen Tate
Cover Designer: Laura de Grasse

Typeset in 10/12pt Adobe Garamond by Dorchester Typesetting Group Ltd, Dorchester, Dorset
Printed and bound in Spain

What do you think about this book? Or any other Hodder Arnold title? Please send
your comments to www.hoddereducation.com

Dedication

To Regina, my beautiful and patient wife, for her encouragement and understanding. And to our wonderful children Edward and Lucy, who never cease to amaze and bring such joy and happiness, plus constantly reminding me what really matters.

A.F.T.B.

To my beautiful wife, Fiona, for her enduring patience, love and support; to William, Hamish and Olivia, for helping me to appreciate the importance of family and the necessity of life outside medicine.

M.D.C.

Contents

Dedication
Preface
Acknowledgements

Section VIII ORTHOPAEDIC EMERGENCIES

Section IX MUSCULOSKELETAL AND SOFT-TISSUE EMERGENCIES

Preface to the 5th Edition of
Emergency Medicine

Major changes have been made for this new edition in line with the modern delivery of emergency and acute medicine in front-line hospitals. The whole text has been completely revised, expanded and updated. A standardized approach to every condition has been followed by reformatting the text to maximize the ease of use and practical application of patient care at the bedside. Entire new sections have been added on acid–base, electrolyte and renal emergencies, infectious disease and foreign travel emergencies, toxicology emergencies, toxinology emergencies, and musculoskeletal and soft tissue emergencies.

Acute medicine is now covered in extensive detail to allow rapid, safe and appropriate care of those medical emergencies likely to be encountered on a typical 'on take' medical admitting call. In addition every conceivable emergency case in all other specialties is again included. The latest evidence-based information has been followed, such as the latest *2005 Resuscitation Guidelines*, and many new problems are described, from handling SARS and bird 'flu to neutropenia and acute renal failure. Finally, tips on how to be an excellent doctor and team player are added to emphasize the shared-care environment that emergency and acute medicine are practised in.

The text has been immeasurably improved by the addition of a second author, Mike Cadogan, who brings to it the logical approach and clarity of thought of an outstanding clinician. The text is still aimed directly at the house officer, senior resident, even junior registrar who is called to think and act quickly on their feet. Whether in a Foundation Programme, training SHO post, or service post, this book is aimed at making your life easier.

As acute hospitals fill up and inpatient beds are at a premium, it is essential that good emergency care is started at the front door. The book is written to give those patients the very best chance of quality care from the moment they arrive. We hope you find benefit from reading it, but more importantly that you enjoy then meeting the challenges this book prepares you for.

Anthony FT Brown
Michael D Cadogan
April 2006

Acknowledgements

Once again we are indebted to our emergency medicine colleagues for offering their usual helpful and astute suggestions for this new edition: Dr Mike Beckett, Dr Geoff Hughes, Dr Chris McLauchlan and Mr John Heyworth. Thank you all for sharing your expertise and knowledge so readily to keep this book in a constant cycle of change for the better.

Many thanks also to Dr Nicholas Evans and Dr Susannah Jackson (of Guys and St Thomas' Hospital, London) for reviewing and commenting on the drafts of the sections; and to Dr Peter Logan for expert help with CNBR information. In addition, particular thanks are due to Dr Joanna Koster, Editorial Director, for her tireless encouragement and advice over the years at Hodder Arnold Health Sciences, Dr Philip Shaw who took over the new edition, and to Heather Fyfe, Project Editor. We could not have asked for a more helpful, professional and efficient partnership.

Finally, the greatest debt is to Monique Cichocki, who typed the drafts with speed, accuracy and reliability, made every deadline, and remained calm and unruffled at all times.

This book would not have happened without all of your help. Thank you.

Tony Brown and Mike Cadogan

June 2006

GENERAL MEDICAL EMERGENCIES

CARDIOPULMONARY RESUSCITATION

DIAGNOSIS
(1) Sudden cardiac arrest causes over 60% of deaths from coronary heart disease in adults.
(2) Cardiopulmonary resuscitation (CPR) is required if a collapsed person is unconscious or unresponsive, not breathing, and has no pulse in a large artery such as the carotid or femoral, although the following may also be present:
(i) A brief tonic grand mal seizure.
(ii) Occasional (agonal) gasps.
(iii) Pallor or cyanosis.
(iv) Dilated pupils.

MANAGEMENT
(1) This is based on the European Resuscitation Council guidelines 2005 and the Australian Resuscitation Council guidelines 2006, derived from the International Liaison Committee on Resuscitation (ILCOR) 2005 International Consensus Conference.
(i) The first person on the scene stays with the patient and commences resuscitation, making a note of the time.
(ii) The second person summons help and organizes the arrival of equipment, then assists with the resuscitation.
(2) *Immediate actions*
The aim is to maintain oxygenation of the brain and myocardium until a stable cardiac output is achieved.
(i) Lay the patient flat on a hard surface such as a trolley. If the patient is on the floor and enough people are available, lift the patient onto a trolley to facilitate the resuscitation procedure.
(ii) Rapidly give a single, sharp pre-cordial thump in witnessed or monitored arrests, where the rhythm is ventricular fibrillation (VF) or pulseless ventricular tachycardia (VT), and a defibrillator is not handy.
(iii) Open the airway by tilting the head and lifting the chin if there is no response, to prevent the tongue from occluding the larynx ('head tilt, chin lift').
(iv) Look in the mouth for a foreign body or debris. Remove these with forceps or suction. Leave well-fitting dentures in place.

(v) Commence assisted ventilation.

(vi) Commence external cardiac massage.

(3) *Assisted ventilation*

(i) Look, listen and feel for no more than 10 seconds for normal breathing.

(ii) Start mouth-to-mouth/nose or mouth-to-mask respiration without delay if breathing is absent, using a pocket mask such as the Laerdal.

(iii) Use a bag–valve mask setup such as an Ambu or Laerdal bag with oxygen reservoir attached and face mask instead, if trained in the technique, after first inserting an oropharyngeal (Guedel) airway if necessary.

(iv) Check for leaks around the mask or convert to a two-person technique if the chest fails to inflate.

(iv) Consider possible obstruction of the upper airway if ventilation is still ineffective (see p. 47).

> **Warning:** adequate oxygenation is achieved by the above measures. Attempts at endotracheal intubation should only ever be made by doctors experienced in this technique.

(4) *External cardiac massage*

(i) Feel for a carotid or femoral pulse for no more than 10 seconds.

(ii) If absent, place the heel of one hand in the centre of the patient's chest. Place the heel of the other hand on top, interlocking the fingers.

(iii) Keeping the arms straight and applying a vertical compression force, depress the sternum 4–5 cm at a rate of about 100 compressions/min.

(iv) Do not apply pressure over the upper abdomen, lower end of sternum or the ribs, and take equal time for compression and for release.

(v) Perform 30 compressions to every 2 effective ventilations. This should create a palpable femoral pulse.

(vi) Change the person providing chest compressions every 2 min.

(vii) Use one or two hands to compress the chest in small children by approximately one third of its depth, at a rate of 100 compressions/min. In infants, use the tips of two fingers again at a rate of 100/min.

> ⓘ **Warning:** avoid using excessive or malpositioned force causing rib fractures, flail chest, liver lacerations, etc.

(5) *Defibrillation*
  (i) After confirming the diagnosis of cardiac arrest, give the patient an immediate 150–200-J shock when using a biphasic waveform defibrillator (all modern defibrillators are now biphasic).
      (a) give a 360-J shock if an older monophasic defibrillator is used.
  (ii) This is an emergency situation. Do not attach ECG electrodes just yet, but use a 'quick-look' paddle technique to assess the heart rhythm, as every 1 minute that passes increases mortality by 7–10% in the absence of bystander CPR.
  (iii) Rapidly shave excessive male chest hair, without delay. Place one self-adhesive defibrillation pad or conventional paddle to the right of the sternum below the clavicle, and the other adhesive pad or paddle in the mid-axillary line level with the V6 ECG electrode or female breast.
  (iv) Avoid positioning self-adhesive pads or paddles over ECG electrodes, medication patches, or implanted devices, e.g. pacemaker or automatic cardioverter defibrillator.
  (v) Then charge the pads or paddles once on the patient's chest.
  (vi) Ensure good electrical contact is made when applying manual paddles by using gel pads or electrode jelly (never use ultrasound or K-Y Jelly™). Apply firm pressure of 8-kg force in adults.
  (vii) Make sure that no one is touching the patient or bed. Give a '*Stand clear*' warning when the shock is about to be delivered.
  (viii) Deliver a shock if the initial rhythm is VF or pulseless VT.
(6) Connect the ECG monitor and observe one of four possible traces:
  (i) Shockable rhythms such as VF (see p. 5) or pulseless VT (see p. 5).
  (ii) Non-shockable rhythms such as asystole (see p. 8) and pulseless electrical activity (PEA) (see p. 8).

(7) Establish an initial intravenous (i.v.) line in the antecubital fossa.
   (i) Give at least 20 mL of normal saline to flush any drugs administered.
   (ii) Elevate the limb for 10–20 seconds to facilitate drug delivery to the central circulation.
(8) Establish a second intravenous line unless the cardiac resuscitation is rapidly successful.
   (i) Ideally, this line should be inserted into a central vein, either the external or internal jugular or the subclavian.
   (ii) The central line should be inserted only by a skilled doctor, because inadvertent arterial puncture, haemothorax or pneumothorax may invalidate further resuscitation attempts.
   (iii) Also, the central venous route poses additional serious hazards should thrombolytic therapy be indicated.
   (iv) All drugs are then given via this central line.
(9) *Endotracheal intubation*
   A skilled doctor with airway training may insert a cuffed endotracheal tube. This maintains airway patency, prevents regurgitation with inhalation of vomit or blood from the mouth or stomach, and allows lung ventilation without interrupting chest compressions.
   (i) Use an 8.5–9.5-mm diameter endotracheal tube in adult males and a 7.5–8.5-mm diameter tube in adult females.
   (ii) Pass the tube between the vocal cords under direct vision, using a curved-blade laryngoscope.
   (iii) Inflate the cuff, connect the oxygen supply, and check the correct position of the tube by observing bilateral chest expansion, auscultation or exhaled carbon dioxide detection. Tie the tube in place.
   (iv) Ventilate the lungs at 10 breaths/min, without now pausing for the chest compressions.
      (a) take care not to hyperventilate the patient at too fast a rate.
   (v) Never delay CPR to secure the airway except for a brief pause in chest compressions as the tube is passed between the vocal cords.
(10) Subsequent management depends on the cardiac rhythm and the patient's condition. Keep the ECG monitor attached to the patient at all times.
(11) Shockable rhythms: *ventricular fibrillation* (VF) or *pulseless ventricular tachycardia* (VT)

See Fig. 1.1 for a rapid overview of treatment.
(i) VF is asynchronous, chaotic ventricular depolarization and
      repolarization producing no cardiac output.

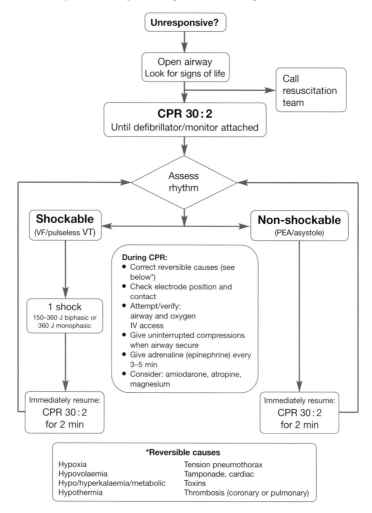

Figure 1.1 Advanced life support (ALS) cardiac arrest algorithm
ALS, advanced life support; CPR, cardiopulmonary resuscitation; IV, intravenous; J,
joules; PEA, pulseless electrical activity; VF, ventricular fibrillation; VT, ventricular
tachycardia. Reproduced with kind permission from European Resuscitation Council
(2005) European Resuscitation Council Guidelines for Resuscitation 2005. Section 4:
Adult advanced life support. *Resuscitation* **67(Suppl 1)**:S39–86.

(ii) Pulseless VT is a wide-complex, regular tachycardia associated with no clinically detectable cardiac output.

(iii) Give one DC shock if VF/VT is confirmed:
   (a) deliver 150–200 J if using a biphasic defibrillator
   (b) deliver 360 J if using an older monophasic defibrillator.

(iv) Immediately resume CPR, starting with chest compressions at a ratio of 30: 2, if the airway has not yet been secured.
   (a) do *not* delay CPR by reassessing the rhythm or feeling for a pulse
   (b) perform compressions at 100/min and ventilations at 10/min without interruption if the airway has been secured by now.

(v) Continue CPR for 2 min, then briefly pause to check the monitor.
   (a) if there is still VF/VT, give a second DC shock of 150–360 J biphasic or 360 J monophasic
   (b) immediately resume CPR after this shock.

(vi) Briefly pause after another 2 min of CPR to check the monitor:
   (a) give 10 mL of 1 in 10 000 adrenaline (epinephrine) (1 mg) if VF/VT persist, followed immediately by a third shock of 150–360 J biphasic or 360 J monophasic
   (b) resume CPR.

(vii) Analyse the rhythm again after another 2 min of CPR:
   (a) give a bolus of amiodarone 300 mg i.v. diluted in 5% dextrose to a volume of 20 mL if VF/VT persist
   (b) immediately deliver a fourth shock.

(12) Continue the drug–shock–CPR–rhythm check sequence.

(i) Again analyse the rhythm 2 min after giving the shock.

(ii) Palpate for a pulse if a non-shockable rhythm is now present with regular or narrow complexes.
   (a) resume CPR if the pulse is absent or difficult
   (b) begin post-resuscitation care when a pulse is felt, or the patient shows signs of life suggesting return of spontaneous circulation (ROSC). See p. 12.

(13) Irrespective of the arrest rhythm, give 1 in 10 000 adrenaline (epinephrine) 1 mg (10 mL) every 3–5 min until ROSC (see Fig. 1.1).

(i) This will be once every two loops of the algorithm.

(ii) Meanwhile continue providing CPR and make sure to change the person performing cardiac compressions every 2 min, to preserve optimum efficacy.

(14) During this period of CPR:

(i) If not already done:

(a) check the defibrillator pad or paddle position and contact

(b) attempt/verify the endotracheal tube position, and successful intravenous access.

(ii) Consider the following antiarrhythmics even though there are no data in support of them increasing survival to hospital discharge:

(a) *amiodarone* – give initial bolus of 300 mg i.v., which may be repeated once at a dose of 150 mg, and followed by an infusion of 900 mg over 24 hours for recurrent or refractory VF/VT

(b) *lignocaine (lidocaine)* – give initial bolus of 1 mg/kg i.v. if amiodarone is unavailable, followed by 0.5 mg/kg if necessary. Omit if amiodarone has been given

(c) *magnesium* – give 2 g (8 mmol or 4 mL) of 49.3% magnesium sulphate i.v., particularly in suspected hypomagnesaemia such as in patients on potassium-losing diuretics, torsades de pointes and digoxin toxicity.

(iii) Consider buffering agent:

(a) *8.4% sodium bicarbonate* – particular indications are for hyperkalaemia or tricyclic antidepressant overdose (see p. 116)

(b) give 50 mmol (50 mL) i.v., then as guided by arterial blood gases (ABGs).

(15) Non-shockable rhythms: *asystole* or *pulseless electrical activity*
See Fig. 1.1 for a rapid overview of treatment.

(i) Asystole is absence of any cardiac electrical activity.

(a) check appropriate ECG lead selection and gain setting. Never just rely on a gel pad–paddle combination to diagnose asystole

(b) make sure the ECG leads are not disconnected or broken by observing the cardiac compressions artefact on the ECG screen during CPR

(c) continue chest compressions and ventilation if there is any difficulty in differentiating from fine VF, in an attempt to 'coarsen' unsuspected VF.

(ii) Pulseless electrical activity (PEA) was formerly known as electromechanical dissociation (EMD). It is the presence of a

coordinated electrical rhythm without detectable cardiac output.
(iii) Survival is unlikely unless a reversible cause can be found and treated. See the '*4 Hs*' and the '*4 Ts*' below.
(iv) Asystole and PEA have a poor prognosis because defibrillation is of no use.
   (a) start CPR at a compression/ventilation (C/V) ratio of 30:2, unless the airway has been secured
   (b) give 1 in 10 000 adrenaline (epinephrine) 1 mg (10 mL) i.v.
   (c) give atropine 3 mg for asystole, or PEA with a rate of less than 60/min
   (d) recheck the rhythm after 2 min of CPR. If organized with a palpable pulse, begin post-resuscitation care
   (e) resume CPR immediately if asystole or PEA persist
   (f) continue CPR unless the rhythm changes to VF/VT (see above p. 5), and give 1 in 10 000 adrenaline (epinephrine) 1 mg (10 mL) every 3–5 min, i.e. every other loop of the algorithm in Fig. 1.1.

> ✓ **Tip:** if venous access is impossible, give adrenaline (epinephrine) 3 mg via the endotracheal tube, that is 30 mL of 1 in 10 000, or 3 mL of 1 in 1000 adrenaline (epinephrine) in at least 10 mL of sterile water and give up to 5 respirations.

(16) Potentially reversible causes: the *4 Hs* and the *4 Ts*
   Always look out for the following conditions, which may precipitate cardiorespiratory arrest or decrease the chances of successful resuscitation (see Fig. 1.1).
   (i) *Hypoxaemia.*
      (a) make sure maximal up to 100% oxygen is being delivered at 15 L/min
      (b) confirm ventilation at 500–600 mL tidal volume (6–7 mL/kg) is creating a visible rise and fall of both sides of the chest.
   (ii) *Hypovolaemia.*
      (a) severe blood loss following trauma, gastrointestinal haemorrhage, ruptured aortic aneurysm or ruptured ectopic pregnancy may cause cardiac arrest
      (b) always consider this in cases of unexplained cardiovascular collapse

    (c) get senior Emergency Department (ED) help, and search for the source of bleeding

    (d) give judicious fluid replacement and call the Surgical, Vascular, Obstetrics and Gynaecology team as appropriate.

(iii) *Hyper/hypokalaemia, hypocalcaemia, acidaemia and other metabolic disorders.*

    (a) rapidly check the potassium and calcium initially as suggested by the medical history, e.g. in renal failure (see p. 125)

    (b) give 10% calcium chloride 10 mL i.v. for hyperkalaemia, hypocalcaemia or calcium-channel blocking drug overdose

    (c) give a bolus of potassium 5 mmol i.v. for hypokalaemia.

(iv) *Hypothermia.*

    (a) check the core temperature with a low-reading thermometer particularly in any drowning incident (see p. 191)

    (b) moderate (30–32°C) or severe (under 30°C) hypothermia will require heroic measures such as active core re-warming with warmed pleural, peritoneal or gastric lavage, or even extracorporeal re-warming when the patient is in cardiac arrest (see p. 189)

    (c) get a senior ED doctor's help. Do not cease CPR until the temperature is at least 33°C or the team leader determines futility.

(v) *Tension pneumothorax.*

    (a) tension usually follows a traumatic rather than a spontaneous pneumothorax, particularly if positive-pressure ventilation is used

    (b) it results in extreme respiratory distress and circulatory collapse. It may follow attempts at central venous cannulation

    (c) the patient becomes increasingly breathless and cyanosed, and develops a tachycardia with hypotension

       – there is decreased chest expansion on the affected side, a hyper-resonant percussion note, and absent or diminished breath sounds

       – the trachea is displaced towards the other side, and the neck veins are usually distended

    (d) this is a life-threatening situation requiring immediate relief, without waiting for a CXR

(e) insert a wide-bore needle or cannula through the second intercostal space in the mid-clavicular line. This will be followed by a rush of air outwards

(f) insert an intercostal drain (see p. 44).

(vi) *Tamponade.*

(a) cardiac tamponade may follow trauma, usually penetrating, myocardial infarction, dissecting aneurysm or pericarditis

(b) there is hypotension, tachycardia, pulsus paradoxus and engorged neck veins that rise on inspiration (Kussmaul's sign). The heart sounds are quiet, the apex beat is impalpable, and PEA may ensue

(c) perform pericardiocentesis if the patient is *in extremis.* Insert a cardiac needle between the angle of the xiphisternum and the left costal margin at 45° to the horizontal, aiming for the left shoulder (see Fig. 1.2)

(d) sometimes aspirating as little as 50 mL restores the cardiac output, although immediate resuscitative thoracotomy is usually indicated in cases resulting from trauma (see p. 225).

(vii) *Toxins/poisons/drugs.*

(a) many substances cause cardiorespiratory arrest following accidental or deliberate ingestion, such as poisoning with tricyclic antidepressants (see p. 157), calcium-channel

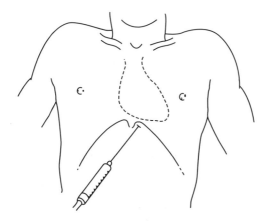

Figure 1.2 Pericardial aspiration

blocking drugs (see p. 166) or beta-blockers (see p. 166), and hydrofluoric acid burns (see p. 174)

(b) consider all these based on the history, recognize early, and treat supportively or with antidotes where available.

(viii) *Thromboembolism with mechanical circulatory obstruction.*

(a) perform external cardiac massage, which may break up a massive pulmonary embolus (PE), and give a fluid load of 20 mL/kg

(b) give thrombolysis such as alteplase (rt-PA) 100 mg i.v. if clinical suspicion is high and there are no absolute contraindications

(c) consider performing CPR for at least another 60–90 min before termination of the resuscitation.

(17) The prognosis is usually hopeless if the patient is still in asystole. However, consider pacing if P waves or any other electrical activity, such as severe bradycardia, is present with poor perfusion:

(i) Use an external (transcutaneous) pacemaker to maintain the cardiac output until a transvenous wire is inserted.

(ii) A temporary transvenous pacemaker wire should ideally be passed under X-ray guidance, but may be inserted blind via a central vein.

(18) *Post-resuscitation care*

It is important to continue effective CPR until the heartbeat is strong enough to produce a peripheral pulse.

(i) Check the ABG to exclude hypocarbia that causes cerebral vasoconstriction with decreased cerebral blood flow.

(a) adjust ventilation to aim for normocarbia with a $PaCO_2$ from 4.5 to 6 kPa (35–45 mmHg).

(ii) Insert a gastric tube to decompress the stomach.

(iii) Give 1 in 10 000 adrenaline (epinephrine) 100 µg (1 mL) i.v. if there is persistent hypotension, and treatable causes such as hypoxia, hypovolaemia, tension pneumothorax, etc. have been excluded, repeated to maintain a blood pressure equal to the patient's usual blood pressure, or at least a systolic blood pressure greater than 100 mmHg.

(a) give the adrenaline (epinephrine) and other vasoactive drugs as soon as possible via a dedicated central venous line.

(iv) Transfer the patient to the ICU or Coronary Care unit (CCU). Perform the following investigations but do not delay the transfer:

(a) CXR to look for correct positioning of the endotracheal tube, nasogastric tube and central line. Exclude a pneumothorax, pulmonary oedema and pulmonary collapse

(b) ABG if not already done

(c) serum sodium, potassium and glucose

(d) 12-lead ECG.

(v) Be aware of any local policy on induced cooling or mild therapeutic hypothermia following cardiac arrest.

(vi) Transfer the patient with a trained nurse and doctor in attendance. A portable cardiac monitor, defibrillator, oxygen and suction should be available on the trolley.

(19) *When to stop*

The decision to cease further attempts at resuscitation is difficult. Only the senior ED doctor should take this. Survival from cardiac arrest is greatest when:

(i) The event is witnessed.

(ii) A bystander starts resuscitation.

(iii) The heart arrests in VF or VT.

(iv) Defibrillation is carried out at an early stage, with successful cardioversion achieved in 2–3 min, and not more than 8 min.

> **Tip:** give special consideration to near-drowning, hypothermia and acute poisoning (especially with tricyclic antidepressants). Full recovery has followed in apparently hopeless cases (fixed dilated pupils, non-shockable rhythm) with resuscitation prolonged for several hours.

CHEST PAIN

DIFFERENTIAL DIAGNOSIS

Consider the life-threatening diagnoses first:

- Acute coronary syndromes, such as myocardial infarction or unstable angina
- Pulmonary embolus
- Aortic dissection

> (!) **Warning:** patients with these may present initially with a normal ECG and CXR, and therefore may have to be referred on clinical suspicion alone. Always attach a cardiac monitor and pulse oximeter to the patient, establish venous access and give 35% oxygen.

Other causes to consider include:
- Pericarditis
- Pleurisy
- Pneumonia
- Pneumothorax
- Abdominal – oesophagitis, oesophageal rupture, gall bladder disease, etc.
- Musculoskeletal and chest wall pain.

ACUTE CORONARY SYNDROME

The term acute coronary syndrome (ACS) encompasses the spectrum of patients presenting with chest pain or other symptoms due to myocardial ischaemia, ranging from ST elevation myocardial infarction (STEMI), non-ST elevation myocardial infarction (NSTEMI) to unstable angina pectoris (UA). The common pathophysiology of ACS is rupture or erosion of an atherosclerotic plaque.

ST ELEVATION MYOCARDIAL INFARCTION (STEMI)

DIAGNOSIS
(1) Predisposing factors include cigarette smoking, hypertension, diabetes, hypercholesterolaemia, male sex, increasing age and a positive family history.
(2) There may be a prior history of angina, myocardial infarction or heart failure, or alternatively the condition may arise *de novo*.
(3) 'Typical' pain is central, heavy, burning, crushing or tight retrosternal, usually lasting for several minutes or longer, is unrelieved by sublingual nitrates, and is associated with anxiety, dyspnoea, nausea and vomiting.
(4) The pain may radiate to the neck, jaw, one or both arms, the back and occasionally the epigastrium, or may present at these sites alone.
  (i) Atypical symptoms occur more frequently in diabetics, the

elderly and in females.

(5) The patient may be clammy, sweaty, breathless and pale. Or the patient may appear deceptively well.

(6) Alternatively, the patient may present with the complications of a cardiac arrhythmia, heart failure, hypotension, systemic embolism or collapse.

(7) Establish venous access with an intravenous cannula and attach a cardiac monitor and pulse oximeter to the patient.

(8) Send blood for FBC, coagulation profile, ELFTs, lipid profile and cardiac biomarker assays such as CK, CK-MB and cardiac troponin I (cTnI) or troponin T (cTnT).

  (i) Do not delay definitive management while awaiting a result.

  (ii) Cardiac biomarkers do not rise for 4 to 6 hours after symptom onset, so can be normal early on.

  (iii) Higher elevated troponin levels identify an increase in adverse outcome risk.

(9) ECG. Perform this within 10 min of patient arrival, and arrange for immediate review by a senior ED doctor.

  (i) Look for ST elevation in two or more contiguous leads.

  (ii) The greater the number of leads affected and the higher the ST segments, the higher the mortality.

  (iii) Inferior myocardial infarction causes changes in leads II, III and aVF.

  (iv) Anterior myocardial infarction causes changes in I, aVL and V1–V3 (anteroseptal) or V4–V6 (anterolateral).

  (v) True posterior myocardial infarction causes mirror-image changes of tall R waves and ST depression in leads V1–V4.

  (vi) Repeat the ECG after 5–10 min in symptomatic patients with an initial non-diagnostic ECG.

(10) Perform a CXR to look for pulmonary oedema, cardiomegaly and atelectasis. Request a portable X-ray in the Emergency Department, provided this does not delay definitive management.

MANAGEMENT

(1) Give high-dose 40–60% oxygen unless there is a prior history of obstructive airways disease, in which case give 28% oxygen. Aim for an oxygen saturation (SaO$_2$) over 94%.

(2) Give aspirin 150–300 mg orally unless contraindicated by known hypersensitivity.

  (i) Give clopidogrel 300 mg oral loading dose, then 75 mg orally once daily, if aspirin intolerant or in addition to aspirin if this is local policy.

(3) Maximize pain relief:

(i) Give glyceryl trinitrate (GTN) 150–300 µg sublingually, maintaining systolic BP above 100 mmHg and avoiding excessive hypotension.

(ii) Add morphine 2.5–5 mg i.v. with an antiemetic, e.g. metoclopramide 10 mg i.v. if pain persists.

(4) Reperfusion therapy:

Consider reperfusion therapy in consultation with the senior ED doctor. Aim to either commence thrombolysis within a maximum of 30 min of the patient's arrival in hospital, without delay by transferring to the CCU. Or arrange for percutaneous coronary intervention (PCI) if this is available in under 90 min (see later p. 17).

(i) *Thrombolysis.*

This is indicated within 12 hours of the onset of myocardial ischaemic pain in patients with STEMI, e.g. ECG evidence of ST elevation MI, with ST elevation of at least 1 mm in two contiguous limb leads or 2 mm in two contiguous pre-cordial leads, and for new bundle branch block, particularly left bundle branch block (LBBB).

(ii) *Absolute* contraindications to thrombolysis include:

(a) intracerebral or subarachnoid haemorrhage ever, intracranial neoplasm

(b) thrombotic stroke in previous 6 months

(c) active gastrointestinal bleeding in last month; major surgery or trauma in previous 3 weeks

(d) known bleeding diathesis

(e) aortic dissection (see p. 28).

(iii) *Relative* contraindications (thrombolysis may still be considered in those at highest risk of death, or with greatest net clinical benefit, such as a large anterior infarction presenting within 3 hours of symptom onset) include:

(a) oral anticoagulant therapy

(b) pregnancy within 1 week post partum

(c) non-compressible arterial puncture or central line

(d) refractory hypertension (systolic BP over 180 mmHg, diastolic BP over 110 mmHg)

(e) prolonged CPR over 10 min

        (f) infective endocarditis

        (g) severe hepatic or renal disease.

   (iv) Give tenecteplase (TNK) as the lytic agent of choice.

        (a) tenecteplase is chosen for its ease of administration and safety when given weight-based, its greater fibrin specificity and efficacy up to 12 hours

          – give tenecteplase 30 mg (for patients less than 60 kg) up to 50 mg (for patients 90 kg or over) as a single bolus over 10 seconds

        (b) use reteplase (r-PA) or alteplase (rt-PA) if tenecteplase is unavailable, in patients under 75 years presenting early with anterior myocardial infarction, or if the patient has ever had streptokinase before (except within the previous 5 days), or the patient is allergic

        (c) give reteplase 10 units as a bolus over no more than 2 min, followed after 30 min by a further 10 units bolus i.v.

        (d) or give a bolus of rt-PA 15 mg (15 mL), followed by an infusion of 0.75 mg/kg over 30 min (not to exceed 50 mg), then 0.5 mg/kg over 60 min (not to exceed 35 mg)

        (e) *plus* with all the above agents commence unfractionated heparin 5000 units i.v. as a bolus, followed by an infusion at 1000 units/h for patients over 80 kg, or 800 units/h for patients less than 80 kg

          – alternatively, give low-molecular-weight (LMW) heparin such as enoxaparin 30 mg i.v. immediately, then 1 mg/kg subcutaneously (s.c.) 12-hourly, but check your local policy.

   (v) Give streptokinase 1.5 million units over 45–60 min in 100 mL normal saline if the above agents are unavailable. The early infarct-related artery vessel patency rate is less than with the fibrin-specific agents.

        (a) continue ECG monitoring throughout for reperfusion arrhythmias

        (b) slow or stop the infusion if hypotension or rash occurs. Restart the infusion as soon as they have resolved

        (c) occasionally, severe hypotension and anaphylaxis may occur, requiring oxygen, adrenaline (epinephrine) and fluids, etc. (see p. 89).

(5) *Percutaneous coronary intervention (PCI)*

Organize coronary angioplasty as an alternative to thrombolysis, only if it is available locally in less than 90 min of patient arrival.

(i) It is superior to thrombolysis, particularly in a high-volume centre (over 75 procedures per operator per year).

(ii) It is preferred in cardiogenic shock, and if thrombolysis is contraindicated.

(iii) Give thrombolysis with tenecteplase if the PCI will take longer than 90 min to organize.

(6) Transfer the patient to the CCU (or catheter lab) following thrombolysis with a doctor and nurse escort, and resuscitation equipment and drugs available.

NON-ST ELEVATION MYOCARDIAL INFARCTION (NSTEMI), UNSTABLE ANGINA, AND NON-CARDIAC CHEST PAIN

DIAGNOSIS

(1) The predisposing factors and pathophysiology are the same as for STEMI (see p. 14).

(2) It is not possible from the character of the chest pain alone to accurately exclude ACS, *unless* a clear alternate cause for the pain is apparent (see Table 1.1).

(i) Unstable angina (UA) includes increasing severity or frequency of angina, angina at rest and angina for the first time or following a recent myocardial infarction.

(ii) Older patients, diabetics, chronic renal failure and female patients may present with less 'typical' ACS pain (see p. 14).

(iii) A stabbing, pleuritic, positional or palpation-induced pain is less characteristic of ACS, but does *not* exclude it.

(3) Establish venous access with an intravenous cannula, and attach a cardiac monitor and pulse oximeter to the patient.

(4) Send blood for FBC, coagulation profile, ELFTs, lipid profile and cardiac biomarkers, exactly as for STEMI.

(5) Perform an ECG within 10 min of patient arrival, with immediate review by a senior ED doctor.

(i) This may show ST depression, T-wave inversion or flattening, non-specific or transient changes.

(ii) Or the ECG may be normal.

MANAGEMENT

(1) Give aspirin 150–300 mg orally unless contraindicated by known hypersensitivity.

Table 1.1 Differential diagnosis of chest pain in patients presenting with possible acute coronary syndrome (ACS)

Diagnosis	Classic history	Physical examination	Diagnostic testing
Acute coronary syndrome (see p. 14)	Band-like, tight, or pressure pain with radiation to neck and arms, sweating, dyspnoea, cardiac risk factors	May be normal, or may have evidence of heart failure, hypotension	Cardiac biomarkers, ECG, possibly stress testing
Pulmonary embolus (see p. 22)	Sudden onset, pleuritic pain, dyspnoea, risks for venous thrombo-embolism	Tachycardia, tachypnoea, pleural rub, low-grade fever	CXR, V/Q scan, CTPA
Aortic dissection (see p. 28)	Sudden, sharp, tearing pain radiating to back, neurologic symptoms	Unequal pulses or BP, new murmur, bruits	CXR, echocardiogram, CT angiogram
Pericarditis (see p. 29)	Pleuritic, positional ache, worse lying down	Fever, pericardial rub, tachycardia	ECG, CXR, echocardiogram
Pneumonia (see p. 39)	Cough, fever, dyspnoea, pleuritic pain, malaise	Fever, hypoxia, tachypnoea, tachycardia, abnormal breath sounds	CXR, WCC
Pneumothorax (see p. 42)	Pleuritic pain, dyspnoea	Reduced breath sounds over hemithorax	CXR
Oesophageal rupture (Boerhaave's syndrome) (see p. 224)	Constant, severe retrosternal pain, dysphagia	Subcutaneous emphysema	CXR, CT chest

Continued on next page

Diagnosis	Classic history	Physical examination	Diagnostic testing
Gastrointestinal causes (see p. 50)	Burning, nocturnal pain, gastrointestinal symptoms	Abdominal tenderness, rebound or guarding	Lipase, AXR, ultrasound
Musculoskeletal causes (see p. 31)	Pain increased with movement or muscular activity	Chest-wall tenderness to palpation (may occur in ACS!)	Normal

ACS, acute coronary syndrome; AXR, abdominal X-ray; BP, blood pressure; CT, computerized tomography; CTPA, computerized tomography pulmonary angiogram; CXR, chest X-ray; ECG, electrocardiograph; V/Q, ventilation perfusion; WCC, white cell count.

(i) Give clopidogrel 300 mg oral loading dose, then 75 mg once daily if aspirin-intolerant, or in addition if this is local policy.

(2) Give GTN 150–300 µg sublingually, and add morphine 2.5–5 mg i.v. with an antiemetic, e.g. metoclopramide 10 mg i.v. if pain persists.

(3) Commence heparin for all UA patients and patients with ECG changes suspected of NSTEMI, without awaiting the first cardiac biomarker results.

   (i) Give LMW heparin such as enoxaparin 1 mg/kg s.c. or dalteparin 120 units/kg s.c. both 12-hourly.

   (ii) Or give unfractionated (UF) heparin 5000 units i.v. as a bolus, followed by an infusion at 1000 units/h for patients over 80 kg, or 800 units/h for patients weighing less.

     (a) UF heparin may be preferred in hospitals likely to offer coronary angioplasty (PCI) within 24–36 hours of symptom onset, so check your local policy

     (b) titrate the UF heparin infusion to an activated partial thromboplastin time (aPTT) of 50–70 seconds by 6 hours post infusion.

(4) Admit *all* patients.

The final diagnosis of NSTEMI (rise in troponin and CK-MB cardiac biomarkers), UA (smaller rise in troponin, normal CK-MB) or non-cardiac chest pain (normal cardiac biomarkers, normal ECGs, normal stress test) takes time to establish.

(i) Admit patients with '*high-risk*' features directly to the CCU. This includes any one or more of:

    (a) elevated troponin or CK-MB on arrival blood test, repetitive or prolonged chest pain over 10 min, diabetic patient or chronic kidney disease patient with estimated glomerular filtration rate of less than 60 mL/min and typical symptoms of ACS, associated syncope, symptoms or signs of heart failure (see p. 45), signs of new mitral incompetence (pansystolic murmur), PCI in the last six months or prior revascularization (CABG), haemodynamic instability or ECG changes.

(ii) Admit patients with '*intermediate-risk*' features under the Medical team, possibly to a shared Chest Pain Unit (CPU). This includes any one or more of:

    (a) chest pain or discomfort within the past 48 hours occurring at rest, or that was repetitive or prolonged (but currently resolved), age over 65 years, two or more risk factors of hypertension, family history, active smoking or hyperlipidaemia, and diabetic patient or chronic kidney disease patient with estimated glomerular filtration rate of less than 60 mL/min and atypical symptoms of ACS

        – lack of CCU beds may necessitate that all diabetic or chronic renal impairment patients are treated as intermediate-risk and are admitted to a general ward (rather than to CCU as high-risk when they have typical symptoms of ACS)

    (b) repeat the ECG and troponin plus CK-MB at 6–8 hours post arrival in the Emergency Department. Admit the patient to CCU if chest pain recurs, the ECG changes, or these cardiac biomarkers rise, as they are now a high-risk patient

    (c) meanwhile, arrange an immediate stress test such as an ECG exercise stress test (EST) if the ECG and the cardiac biomarkers remain normal and the pain has gone in intermediate-risk patients

    (d) only if this stress test is normal has ACS finally now been excluded and the patient may go home

    (e) local policy may be to arrange an outpatient stress test instead, when these are not available immediately. Make sure the general practitioner (GP) is kept informed.

> **(!) Warning:** *never* discharge *any* chest pain patient after a single normal troponin plus CK-MB test, as a second paired test plus repeat ECG at 6–8 hours post-arrival is mandatory, followed by some form of stress test to accurately rule out ACS.

VENOUS THROMBOEMBOLISM WITH PULMONARY EMBOLUS

DIAGNOSIS

(1) Venous thromboembolism (VTE) includes pulmonary embolus (PE) and deep venous thrombosis (DVT).

(2) Predisposing risk factors to VTE are best divided into acute provoking and chronic predisposing, and apply to both PE and DVT. See Table 1.2.

(3) A small PE causes sudden dyspnoea, pleuritic pain and possibly haemoptysis, with few physical signs. Look for a low-grade pyrexia (37.5 °C), tachypnoea over 20/min, tachycardia, and a pleural rub.

(4) A major PE causes dyspnoea, chest pain and light-headedness or collapse, followed by recovery. Look for cyanosis, tachycardia, hypotension, a parasternal heave, raised jugular venous pressure (JVP), and a loud delayed pulmonary second sound.

(5) Establish venous access with an intravenous cannula, send blood for FBC, coagulation profile, ELFTs, and attach a cardiac monitor and pulse oximeter to the patient.

   (i) Only request a D-dimer test after assessing the clinical pre-test probability to be low. See points (9) and (10) below.

(6) Consider a blood gas that will reflect hypocapnia from hyperventilation, and less commonly hypoxia, but may be normal in over 20% patients with PE.

   (i) Do *not* perform ABGs routinely, unless there is an unexplained low pulse oximeter reading on room air. They rarely help.

(7) Perform an ECG, mainly to exclude other diagnoses such as ACS or pericarditis.

   (i) It may show a tachycardia alone or possibly right axis deviation, right heart strain, right bundle branch block (RBBB) or atrial fibrillation (AF) in PE.

   (ii) The well-known 'S1Q3T3' pattern is neither sensitive nor specific for PE.

Table 1.2 Predisposing risk factors for venous thromboembolism (VTE)

Acute provoking factors
Hospitalization i.e. reduced mobility
Surgery, particularly abdominal, pelvic, leg
Trauma or fracture of lower limbs or pelvis
Immobilization (includes plaster cast)
Long haul travel – over 3000 miles or 5000 km
Recently commenced oestrogen therapy (e.g. within previous 2 weeks)
Intravascular device (e.g. venous catheter)

Chronic predisposing factors		
Inherited	Acquired	Inherited or acquired
Natural anticoagulant deficiency such as protein C, protein S, antithrombin III deficiency	Increasing age	High plasma homocysteine
Factor V Leiden	Obesity	High plasma coagulation factors VIII, IX, XI
Prothrombin G20210A mutation	Cancer (chemotherapy)	Antiphospholipid syndrome (anticardiolipin antibodies and lupus anticoagulant)
	Leg paralysis	
	Oestrogen therapy	
	Pregnancy or puerperium	
	Major medical illness[a]	
	Previous venous thromboembolism (DVT/PE)	

[a]Chronic cardiorespiratory disease, inflammatory bowel disease, nephritic syndrome, myeloproliferative disorders.
DVT, deep vein thrombosis; PE, pulmonary embolus.
Modified from Ho WK, Hankey GJ (2005) Venous thromboembolism: diagnosis and management of deep venous thrombosis. *Med J Aust* **182:**476–81.

Table 1.3 Estimation of the clinical pre-test probability for suspected pulmonary embolus (PE)

Feature	Score
Clinical signs and symptoms of DVT (minimum of leg swelling and pain with palpation of the deep veins. See p. 26)	3
Alternative diagnosis less likely than PE	3
Heart rate above 100 beats/min	1.5
Immobilization or surgery in previous 4 weeks	1.5
Previous DVT or PE	1.5
Haemoptysis	1
Cancer	1

Low pre-test probability = score < 2
Moderate pre-test probability = score 2–6
High pre-test probability = score > 6
DVT, deep venous thrombosis; PE, pulmonary embolus.
Modified from Wells PS, Anderson DR, Rodger M *et al.* (2001) Excluding pulmonary embolism at the bedside without diagnostic imaging: management of patients with suspected pulmonary embolism presenting to the emergency department by using a simple clinical model and D-dimer. *Ann Intern Med* **135:**98–107.

(8) Request a CXR, again mainly to exclude other diagnoses such as pneumonia or pneumothorax.
   (i) It may be normal in PE, or show a blunted costophrenic angle, raised hemidiaphragm, an area of infarction or linear atelectasis, or an area of oligaemia.

(9) Determine the clinical pre-test probability now *before* requesting any further diagnostic imaging. See Table 1.3.
   (i) A low pre-test probability on Wells' criteria has up to 3.6% probability of PE.
   (ii) A moderate pre-test probability has a 20.5% probability of PE, and a high pre-test probability a 66.7% probability of PE.

(10) Perform a D-dimer test only on a patient with a low pre-test probability.
   (i) Check with the laboratory which D-dimer test they use, and their test's reference ranges, in particular their normal cut-off range.
   (ii) Discharge the low pre-test probability patient if this D-dimer test is negative, i.e. there is no PE.

(11) Perform a high-speed, helical, multi-slice CT pulmonary angiogram (CTPA), if available, in all moderate or high pre-test probability patients, and in low pre-test probability patients with a positive D-dimer.

(12) Alternatively, start with a ventilation–perfusion isotope lung scan, the V/Q scan.

   (i)   This is preferred if the patient is allergic to contrast dye, has renal failure, possibly if the CXR is normal, or if CTPA is unavailable and according to local policy.

   (ii) Unfortunately, over half the results will not help, i.e. they are low or intermediate probability results, and *must* still be followed by further testing.

MANAGEMENT

(1) Give high-dose oxygen through a face mask. Aim for an oxygen saturation above 94%.

(2) Relieve pain if it is severe with morphine 5 mg i.v. and give an antiemetic such as metoclopramide 10 mg i.v.

(3) Commence heparin in intermediate or high pre-test probability patients, unless diagnostic imaging tests are imminently available, and contraindications such as active bleeding, thrombocytopenia, recent trauma, or cerebral haemorrhage are absent:

   (i)   Give LMW heparin such as enoxaparin 1 mg/kg s.c. or dalteparin s.c. according to body weight, both 12-hourly.

   (ii) Alternatively, give UF heparin 5000 units i.v. bolus, followed by 1000 units/h infusion.

       (a) this is preferred with a major PE, as a first dose bolus or according to local policy.

(4) Admit all patients with a confirmed PE under the Medical team, or if the test results are indeterminate.

   (i)   Arrange sequential testing with a V/Q scan then a CTPA or vice versa, plus or minus a lower-limb venous Doppler ultrasound to finally rule out the diagnosis.

   (ii) Commence heparin once a positive result is confirmed, if not already started.

(5) Get help from a senior ED doctor for any apparent major, life-threatening PE patient:

   (i)   Reserve thrombolysis with recombinant tissue plasminogen activator (rt-PA) 10 mg i.v. over 1–2 min, then 90 mg over 2 hours (or 1.5 mg/kg maximum if under 65 kg) for patients with a massive PE in shock, with acute right heart failure and systolic hypotension.

(ii) Involve the Intensive Care team early.

VENOUS THROMBOEMBOLISM WITH DEEP VEIN THROMBOSIS

DIAGNOSIS

(1) Predisposing risk factors are as for venous thromboembolism. Up to two thirds of patients have acute provoking factors (see Table 1.2).

(2) Typical symptoms include leg pain, swelling, tenderness and redness or discolouration.

Table 1.4 Estimation of the clinical pre-test probability for suspected deep venous thrombosis (DVT)

Clinical feature	Score
Active cancer (treatment ongoing or within 6 months or palliative)	1
Paralysis, paresis or recent plaster immobilization of the lower extremities	1
Recently bedridden for ≥ 3 days, or major surgery within the previous 12 weeks	1
Localized tenderness along the distribution of the deep venous system	1
Entire leg swollen	1
Calf swelling > 3 cm when compared with the asymptomatic leg (at 10 cm below the tibial tuberosity)	1
Pitting oedema: confined to the symptomatic leg	1
Collateral superficial veins (non-varicose)	1
Previously documented deep venous thrombosis	1
Alternative diagnosis as likely or greater than that of deep venous thrombosis	−2

In patients with symptoms in both legs, the more symptomatic leg is scored.
Low pre-test probability = score ≤ 0
Moderate pre-test probability = score 1–2
High pre-test probability = score ≥ 3
From Wells PS, Owen C, Doucette S et al. (2006) Does this patient have deep vein thrombosis? J Amer Med Assoc **295:**199–207.

(3) Examination may reveal unilateral oedema, warmth, superficial venous dilatation, increased limb girth or tenderness along the deep venous system.

    (i) Unfortunately, a similar picture is seen in cellulitis, musculoskeletal injury and varicose vein insufficiency.

    (ii) Homan's sign of pain on forced ankle dorsiflexion is unreliable, unhelpful and not indicated.

(4) Ask about any associated features of a concomitant PE (see p. 22), particularly in suspected proximal DVT above the knee.

(5) Exactly as with PE, determine the clinical pre-test probability of a DVT now *before* requesting diagnostic testing (see Table 1.4).

    (i) A low pre-test probability on Wells' criteria has up to a 5% probability of DVT.

    (ii) A moderate pre-test probability has a 17% probability of DVT, and a high pre-test probability has up to a 53% probability of DVT.

(6) Send blood for D-dimer only if the pre-test probability is low.

    (i) Discharge the patient if the D-dimer is negative, that is no DVT, providing alternative diagnoses do not require further care.

(7) Perform Doppler ultrasound on all moderate and high pre-test probability patients, and when the D-dimer test is positive.

MANAGEMENT

(1) Give the patient analgesia such as paracetamol 500 mg with codeine 8 mg two tablets orally q.d.s. or an anti-inflammatory such as a ibuprofen 200–400 mg orally t.d.s. or naproxen 250 mg orally t.d.s.

(2) Commence heparin if the diagnosis is confirmed.

    (i) Give LMW heparin such as enoxaparin 1 mg/kg s.c. 12-hourly or dalteparin according to body weight s.c. 12-hourly.

    (ii) Alternatively, give UF heparin 5000 units i.v. bolus followed by 1000 units/h infusion particularly for a large or extensive DVT, according to local policy.

(3) Refer all patients to the Medical team if the diagnosis is confirmed.

    (i) Some patients may be discharged for outpatient LMW heparin, or some even sent home without any treatment at all if the DVT is confined below the knee.

(ii) Organize a repeat US scan at 5–7 days in those not treated to exclude more proximal extension of the thrombosis. Check your local policy.

(4) Get senior ED doctor advice if the diagnosis is still indeterminate.

AORTIC DISSECTION

DIAGNOSIS

(1) Predisposed to by hypertension, Marfan syndrome, bicuspid aortic valve, coarctation or iatrogenic trauma.

(2) The onset is abrupt with sudden pain that is sharp or tearing, retrosternal, interscapular or lower in the back, migratory, and may be severe and resistant to opiates.

(3) Look for unequal or absent pulses, a difference of blood pressure in the arms, or the following complications of the dissection:
  (i) Myocardial ischaemia, aortic incompetence and haemopericardium with pericardial rub or cardiac tamponade (see p. 11).
  (ii) Dyspnoea, pleural rub or effusion.
  (iii) Altered consciousness, syncope, hemiplegia or paraplegia.
  (iv) Intestinal ischaemia or bowel infarction with abdominal pain and bloody diarrhoea.
  (v) Oliguria and haematuria.

(4) Establish venous access with a large-bore (14- or 16-gauge) intravenous cannula, and send blood for FBC, ELFTs, cardiac enzymes and group and cross-match. Attach a cardiac monitor and pulse oximeter to the patient.

(5) Perform an ECG, which may remain remarkably normal despite the severity of the pain, showing left ventricular hypertrophy and non-specific changes.

(6) Request a CXR that may show a widened mediastinum, blurred aortic knob and a left pleural effusion.

MANAGEMENT

(1) Give high-dose oxygen via a face mask. Aim for an oxygen saturation above 94%.

(2) Relieve the pain with morphine 5 mg i.v. and give an antiemetic.

(3) Reduce the systolic BP to below 110 mmHg using a labetalol infusion or sodium nitroprusside plus propranolol i.v. in

consultation with the senior ED doctor or Intensive Care team, when dissection is diagnosed or highly likely.

(4) Organize an urgent transoesophageal echocardiogram, helical CT scan or aortogram to confirm the diagnosis.

(5) Contact the cardiothoracic surgeons and arrange transfer without delay. Involve the Intensive Care team early.

PERICARDITIS

DIAGNOSIS

(1) This may be post-viral or follow a myocardial infarction, pericardiotomy, connective tissue disorder, uraemia, trauma, tuberculosis (TB) or a neoplasm.

(2) The pain is sharp, pleuritic, retrosternal and positional, relieved by sitting forward.

(3) Listen for a pericardial friction rub, best heard along the left sternal edge with the patient sitting forward, which may be transient or intermittent.

(4) Send blood for FBC, ELFTs, cardiac enzymes and viral serology. Attach a cardiac monitor and pulse oximeter to the patient.

(5) Perform an ECG that may show sinus tachycardia alone, widespread concave ST elevation or AF.

(6) Request a CXR which is usually normal, even if a pericardial effusion is present.

MANAGEMENT

(1) Give high-dose oxygen via a face mask. Aim for an oxygen saturation above 94%.

(2) Give the patient a non-steroidal anti-inflammatory analgesic such as ibuprofen 200–400 mg orally t.d.s. or naproxen 250 mg orally t.d.s.

(3) Refer the patient to the Medical team for bed rest and cardiac monitoring if there are widespread ECG changes or raised cardiac enzymes.

   (i) Arrange urgent echocardiography and pericardiocentesis for signs of cardiac tamponade, such as tachycardia, hypotension, pulsus paradoxus and a raised JVP that rises on inspiration, known as Kussmaul's sign (see p. 11).

PLEURISY

DIAGNOSIS

(1) Pleurisy or pleuritic pain occurs in association with pneumonia, pulmonary infarction from a PE, neoplasia, TB, connective tissue disorders, uraemia, or following trauma.

(2) It may also be due to viruses, especially enteroviruses, and may be mimicked by a pneumothorax or epidemic myalgia (Bornholm disease).

(3) The pain is sharp, knife-like, localized and exacerbated by moving, coughing or breathing, which tends to be shallow. Radiation to the shoulder or abdomen occurs with diaphragmatic involvement.

(4) Listen for a pleural rub, although this may be inaudible if pain limits deep breathing, and disappears as an effusion develops.

(5) Send ABGs if there are significant signs of pulmonary parenchymal disease. Perform an ECG which should be normal.

(6) Request a CXR that may reveal the underlying cause or may be quite normal.

MANAGEMENT

(1) Give the patient oxygen and a non-steroidal anti-inflammatory analgesic such as ibuprofen 200–400 mg orally t.d.s. or naproxen 250 mg orally t.d.s.

(2) Exclude a pulmonary embolus if there was sudden dyspnoea, tachypnoea and risk factors for thromboembolism. A PE is possible even with a normal CXR and ECG (see p. 22).

(3) Refer the patient to the Medical team for treatment of the underlying cause, or discuss with the senior ED doctor before discharging.

ABDOMINAL CAUSES OF CHEST PAIN

DIAGNOSIS AND MANAGEMENT

(1) *Oesophagitis*
   (i) This is suggested by burning retrosternal or epigastric pain, worse on stooping or recumbency, exacerbated by hot drinks or food, and relieved by antacids.
   (ii) It may mimic cardiac pain and may even be relieved by sublingual GTN, so consult the senior ED doctor.
      (a) admit the patient to rule out acute coronary syndrome if there is any doubt at all about the diagnosis.

(iii) Otherwise give an antacid or proton-pump inhibitor orally.
(2) *Oesophageal rupture.* See p. 224.
(3) *Acute cholecystitis, pancreatitis* and *peptic ulceration* may cause chest pain, but other diagnostic features should be present.

MUSCULOSKELETAL AND CHEST WALL PAIN

DIAGNOSIS AND MANAGEMENT

(1) Musculoskeletal disorders cause pain that is worse with movement and breathing. There may have been preceding strenuous exercise, a bout of coughing, or a history of minor trauma.
(2) Pain is localized on palpation and the ECG is normal. A CXR may show a fractured rib but is otherwise normal.
(3) Give the patient a non-steroidal anti-inflammatory analgesic such as ibuprofen 200–400 mg orally t.d.s., or naproxen 250 mg orally t.d.s. Refer back to the GP.
(4) Two specific causes are:
   (i) *Costochondritis (Tietze syndrome)*
      This causes localized pain and tenderness typically around the second costochondral junction. Prescribe ibuprofen 200–400 mg orally t.d.s., or naproxen 250 mg orally t.d.s. Refer the patient back to the GP.
   (ii) *Shingles*
      This causes pain localized to a dermatome, unaffected by breathing, associated with an area of hyperaesthesia preceding the characteristic rash.
      (a) give the patient (usually elderly) with severe pain a narcotic analgesic and aciclovir 800 mg orally five times a day for 7 days, or famciclovir 250 mg orally t.d.s. for 7 days, if seen within 72 hours of vesicle eruption
      (b) admit to a suitable isolation area if unable to be nursed at home.

CARDIAC ARRHYTHMIAS

DIAGNOSIS

(1) Cardiac rhythm disturbances include the bradycardias, tachycardias, atrial flutter and fibrillation, and the various degrees

of heart block.

(2) Exclude myocardial ischaemia from ACS as a priority (see p. 14).

(3) Consider other underlying precipitating factors for the arrhythmia such as hypoxia from any cause, hypovolaemia from blood or fluid loss, electrolyte disturbances particularly hyperkalaemia, thyroid disease, drug, alcohol or noxious gas toxicity whether inadvertent or deliberate, septicaemia, hypothermia, electrocution, or simple pain and fear.

(4) Ask the patient about palpitations, 'missed beats', breathlessness, chest pain, light-headedness and fatigue.

(5) Measure the temperature and vital signs and attach a cardiac monitor and pulse oximeter to the patient.

    (i) Abnormal vital signs including hypotension, confusion or associated features such as chest pain and breathlessness necessitate urgent management.

(6) Send blood for FBC, ELFTs, cardiac enzymes, coagulation profile, thyroid function and toxicology screen as indicated. Measure the ABGs if in respiratory distress.

(7) Perform an ECG. Systematically look at the following:

    (i) Rate: fast or slow; paroxysmal or continuous?

    (ii) Rhythm: regular, regularly irregular or irregularly irregular?

    (iii) P waves: present, absent and relationship to QRS complexes?

    (iv) PR interval: shortened less than 0.12 s or prolonged over 0.2 s?

    (v) QRS complexes: narrow or widened greater than 0.12 s?

    (vi) QTc interval (corrected for rate): normal or longer than 0.45 s?

    (vii) ST segment and T waves: elevated, depressed or inverted?

(8) Request a CXR and look for cardiomegaly or evidence of acute pulmonary oedema. See p. 45.

MANAGEMENT

This depends on the arrhythmia, cardiovascular stability and the presence of associated chest pain, breathlessness or confusion. See the European Resuscitation Guidelines for Resuscitation 2005.

> ✓ **Tip:** call the senior ED doctor immediately if the patient is hypotensive with a systolic BP less than 90 mmHg, breathless, confused or has chest pain.

(1) Give high-dose 40–60% oxygen unless there is a prior history of obstructive airways disease, in which case give 28% oxygen. Aim for an oxygen saturation over 94%.

(2) Give aspirin 150–300 mg orally if there is possible or probable ACS, unless contraindicated by known hypersensitivity.

(3) Provide pain relief if needed with GTN 150–300 µg sublingually for coronary ischaemic pain, or morphine 2.5–5 mg i.v. with an antiemetic, e.g. metoclopramide 10 mg i.v. for more severe pain, including non-ischaemic.

(4) Correct any electrolyte abnormality. See p. 114.

(5) *Bradycardia*

This may be sinus, junctional (nodal) or due to atrioventricular block:

(i) Give a bolus of atropine 0.5–0.6 mg i.v.

(ii) Repeat the atropine for sinus or junctional bradycardia if it persists, to a maximum of 3 mg i.v. total.

(iii) Consider the insertion of a temporary transvenous pacemaker wire by an expert, if the bradycardia persists with symptomatic second- or third-degree (complete) atrioventricular block, or the patient is unstable.

   (a) use an external (transcutaneous) pacemaker until X-ray guidance and the expert help are available.

(iv) Avoid excessive atropine or using an isoprenaline infusion immediately following an acute myocardial infarction, as this may provoke VF.

(6) *Tachycardia*

This may be sinus with normal preceding P waves, narrow-complex or broad-complex.

(i) Look urgently for and treat underlying causes such as hypoxia, hypovolaemia, fever, anaemia, pain, etc. if it is a definite sinus tachycardia.

(ii) Give a synchronized DC shock, if the patient is unstable with hypotension and a systolic BP less than 90 mmHg, is confused, has chest pain or heart failure.

   (a) start with 120–150 J biphasic or 200 J monophasic and repeat up to three times, with stepwise increases in joules

   (b) a senior doctor with airway experience must first give a short-acting general anaesthetic or intravenous midazolam in the conscious patient

   (c) give amiodarone 300 mg i.v. over 10–20 min if three attempts at synchronized DC cardioversion failed, then

repeat the DC shock and follow by an infusion of
amiodarone 900 mg over 24 hours.

(iii) *Broad-complex tachycardia.*

When regular this may be due to VT or supraventricular
tachycardia with aberrant conduction or block:

(a) give amiodarone 300 mg i.v. over 20–60 min if the patient
is stable, followed by an infusion of amiodarone 900 mg
over 24 hours

(b) consider AF with bundle branch block if the rhythm is
irregular, or AF with ventricular pre-excitation as in
Wolff–Parkinson–White syndrome:
– seek expert help if not already involved
– consider amiodarone 300 mg i.v. followed by an
infusion
– *avoid* adenosine, verapamil, digoxin and diltiazem, as
they block the AV node and may worsen pre-excited AF
leading to VT or even VF.

> ✓ **Tip:** frequent ventricular ectopic beats (VEBs) do not require
> treatment, unless they are multi-focal, in runs, or arrive on the T wave of
> the preceding complex.

(iv) *Narrow-complex tachycardia* or *supraventricular tachycardia*
(SVT).

When regular this may be one of the re-entry tachycardias or
atrial flutter with regular AV conduction (usually 2 to 1 block
if the rate is about 150/min).

(a) proceed directly to synchronized DC cardioversion if the
patient is shocked, unstable or deteriorating, starting at
70–120 J biphasic or 100 J monophasic, after a senior
doctor with airway experience has given a short-acting
anaesthetic

(b) use a vagal stimulus such as carotid sinus massage (CSM) if
stable and young with no carotid bruit or prior transient
ischaemic attack (TIA) or cerebrovascular accident (CVA)
– press firmly at the upper border of the thyroid cartilage
against the vertebral process with a circular motion
– or get the patient to perform a Valsalva manoeuvre

(c) give adenosine 6 mg rapidly over 2–5 seconds i.v. if CSM

fails, followed by 12 mg i.v. rapidly after 1–2 min, then a further 12 mg i.v. rapidly once more if still no response
- warn the patient to expect transient facial flushing, dyspnoea, chest discomfort and nausea from the adenosine

(d) alternatively, give verapamil 2.5–5 mg i.v. as a bolus over 30 seconds to 2 min. Verapamil may cause hypotension and bradycardia, particularly in elderly patients, who may be pre-treated with calcium gluconate 10 mL given slowly i.v. to prevent these

(e) *never* use verapamil after a beta-blocker, when digitalis toxicity is suspected, or if the patient has a wide complex tachycardia.

(v) *Irregular narrow-complex tachycardia* or *atrial fibrillation* (AF). Irregularly irregular narrow-complex tachycardia is usually AF or less frequently atrial flutter with variable AV block.

(a) proceed directly to synchronized DC cardioversion starting at 120–150 J biphasic or 200 J monophasic, if the patient is shocked, unstable or deteriorating. In patients on digoxin therapy, temporary transcutaneous pacing may be required as asystole may follow DC reversion

(b) otherwise try rhythm control, if the patient has been in the AF for less than 48 hours, with amiodarone 300 mg i.v. over 20–60 min, followed by an infusion of amiodarone 900 mg over 24 hours

(c) however, when the patient has been in AF for over 48 hours, or the time duration is unclear, rhythm control with drugs or elective DC reversion is contraindicated prior to full anticoagulation, due to the risk of clot embolization:
- attempt rate control only using an oral or intravenous beta-blocker, digoxin, diltiazem or magnesium. Seek senior ED doctor advice
- commence heparinization with LMW heparin such as enoxaparin 1 mg/kg s.c. or unfractionated UF heparin 5000 units i.v. as a bolus, followed by an infusion.

(vi) Admit all patients who required treatment to a monitored CCU bed.

THE BREATHLESS PATIENT

DIFFERENTIAL DIAGNOSIS

Consider the following, some of which were covered in the preceding section on chest pain:

- Acute asthma
- Community-acquired pneumonia (CAP)
- Chronic obstructive pulmonary disease (COPD)
- Pneumothorax
- Pulmonary embolus
- Pulmonary oedema
- Acute upper airway obstruction
- Metabolic causes, such as acidosis in diabetic ketosis or salicylate poisoning
- Respiratory muscle weakness from myasthenia gravis or Guillain–Barré syndrome

ACUTE ASTHMA

DIAGNOSIS

(1) Ascertain the precipitating factors in the present attack, its duration, treatment given including steroids and theophylline derivatives, and the response to treatment.

(2) Ask about previous attacks, hospital admissions, ventilation in an ICU, and the regular use of steroids.

(3) The highest risk categories for a severe attack are:
   (i) A recent acute attack within the last month, especially if the patient required steroids.
   (ii) The 'brittle' asthmatic prone to sudden catastrophic attacks or wide peak expiratory flow (PEF) variability.
   (iii) Any prior ICU admissions.
   (iv) Drug or alcohol abuse, mental illness, or non-compliance 'denial'.

(4) Assess the severity of the present attack by carefully examining the patient before any nebulizer therapy is given.
   (i) A *severe* attack is indicated by any one of the following:
      (a) inability to complete sentences in one breath
      (b) respiratory rate of 25 or more breaths/min
      (c) tachycardia of 110 or more beats/min

(d) peak expiratory flow or forced expiratory volume in 1 second (FEV_1) 33–50% or less of predicted or known best (see Fig. 1.3).

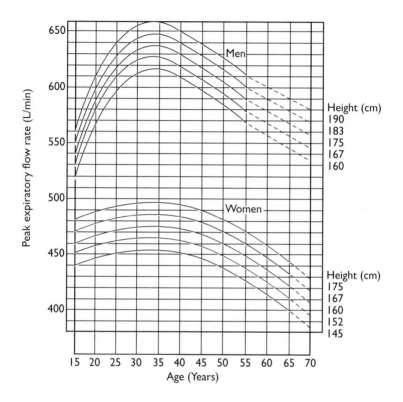

Figure 1.3 Predicted normal peak expiratory flow rates in adult men and women
Reproduced by kind permission of Clement Clark International Ltd.

(ii) A *life-threatening* attack is indicated by any one of the following:
   (a) PEF under 33% of predicted or best
   (b) silent chest, cyanosis or feeble respiratory effort
   (c) bradycardia, dysrhythmia or hypotension
   (d) exhaustion, confusion or coma

(e) oxygen saturation (SaO_2) less than 92%, PaO_2 less than 8 kPa (below 60 mmHg), normal $PaCO_2$ 4.6–6.0 kPa (34–45 mmHg), or worse a raised $PaCO_2$ (imminently fatal).

MANAGEMENT

(1) Commence high-dose 40–60% oxygen via a face mask. Maintain the oxygen saturation above 94%.

(2) Give salbutamol 5 mg via an oxygen-driven nebulizer, diluted with 3 mL normal saline.

(3) Add ipratropium (Atrovent™) 500 µg to a second dose of salbutamol 5 mg via the nebulizer if there is no response, or there is a severe attack.

(4) Involve the senior ED doctor if the patient is still wheezy, and perform the following:

    (i) Give prednisolone 50 mg orally or hydrocortisone 200 mg i.v. if unable to swallow.

    (ii) Repeat the salbutamol 5 mg via the nebulizer up to every 15–30 min, or even via continuous nebulization.

    (iii) Send blood for WCC, U&Es and blood sugar. Commence an i.v. infusion of normal saline for dehydration, with added potassium if low.

    (iv) Perform a CXR *only* when a pneumothorax, pneumomediastinum or an infection with consolidation is suspected, or the patient is deteriorating.

    (v) Take an ABG *only* if the patient is still not improving. ABG markers of a life-threatening attack are:

        (a) normal 4.6–6 kPa (34–45 mmHg), or high $PaCO_2$ (imminently fatal)

        (b) severe hypoxia with PaO_2 under 8 kPa (60 mmHg)

        (c) a low pH (or high hydrogen ion concentration)

        (d) also check potassium, which may be low.

(5) Call the ICU and/or the anaesthetist if the patient remains severe or has any life-threatening features.

    (i) Commence an i.v. bronchodilator under ECG control.

    (ii) Give salbutamol 250 µg i.v. over 10 min, followed by an infusion of 5 mg salbutamol in 500 mL of 5% dextrose, i.e. 10 µg/mL at 5 µg/min (30 mL/h or 0.5 mL/min) initially. Titrate up to response between 20 and 40 µg/min (120–240 mL/h).

(iii) Or consider a slow bolus of aminophylline 5 mg/kg over 20 min followed by an infusion of 500 mg aminophylline in 500 mL of 5% dextrose, i.e. 1 mg/mL at 0.5 mg/kg per hour (35 mL/h or 0.58 mL/min for a 70-kg patient).

(a) omit the bolus if the patient is already taking oral theophylline, and send blood for a theophylline level.

(6) Otherwise, admit the patient under the Medical team when stabilized with a PEF over 50%.

(7) Meanwhile, in the patient with a mild attack (PEF over 75% predicted) or a moderate attack (PEF 50–75% predicted) that improves with prednisolone and nebulizers to a PEF over 75%:

(i) Discharge if the GP can provide follow-up within 2 days and the patient has salbutamol and steroid inhalers (and knows how to use them), plus prednisolone 50 mg orally once daily reduced over 5 days.

(ii) Admit for overnight observation if there is any doubt about discharging the patient.

COMMUNITY-ACQUIRED PNEUMONIA (CAP)

DIAGNOSIS

(1) Common organisms include *Streptococcus pneumoniae* (over 50%), *Haemophilus influenzae* (especially in COPD), 'atypical' organisms such as *Legionella* spp., *Mycoplasma* and *Chlamydia* and viruses including influenza and chickenpox.

(i) Less common are *Staphylococcus aureus* (may follow the 'flu), Gram negatives (alcoholism) and *Coxiella* (Q fever).

(ii) Consider meliodosis in tropical areas due to *Burkholderia pseudomallei*, or in diabetics, alcoholism and chronic renal failure (CRF).

(iii) Finally remember TB, especially in alcoholism or social deprivation and also in HIV patients, who may also get *Pneumocystis carinii* pneumonia (PCP). See p. 137.

(2) Risk factors for community acquired pneumonia (CAP) include age over 50 years; smoking; coexisting chronic respiratory, cardiac, renal, cerebrovascular or hepatic disease; diabetes; alcoholism; neoplasia; nursing home residency; and immunosuppression.

(3) Fever, dyspnoea, productive cough, haemoptysis and pleuritic chest pain may occur.

(4) Less obvious presentations include septicaemia with shock, acute

confusional state particularly in the elderly, referred upper abdominal pain, or diarrhoea.

(5) Examine for signs of lobar infection, with a dull percussion note and bronchial breathing. Usually there are only localized moist crepitations with diminished breath sounds.

(6) Send blood for FBC, ELFTs, blood sugar and two sets of blood cultures, particularly if there is an intercurrent illness.
   (i) Only do an ABG when there are features of severe CAP (see below).

(7) Perform a CXR which may show diffuse shadowing unless there is lobar consolidation.

Look at the lateral, particularly for consolidation.

(8) Features of severe CAP include one or more of the following:
   (i) Respiratory rate $\geq$ 30/min.
   (ii) Systolic BP less than 90 mmHg or diastolic BP less than 60 mmHg.
   (iii) Confusion.
   (iv) FiO_2 more than 0.35 to maintain SaO_2 of more than 90%.
   (v) Multi-lobar CXR changes.
   (vi) Urea of more than 7 mmol/L or WCC less than 4×10^9/L or more than 30×10^9/L.
   (vii) Age $\geq$ 65 years.

MANAGEMENT

(1) Give the patient high-dose oxygen, unless there is a known history of obstructive airways disease (use 28%). Aim for an oxygen saturation above 92%.

(2) Start amoxicillin 500 mg to 1 g orally t.d.s. *plus* erythromycin 500 mg orally q.d.s. (or clarithromycin 500 mg orally b.d. or roxithromycin 300 mg orally once daily instead of the erythromycin).
   (i) Young, fit adults with single lobe involvement may be well enough to return home on the above treatment for 7–10 days.
   (ii) Inform the patient's GP by fax or a letter if the patient is discharged.

(3) Most patients will need admission to hospital and parenteral antibiotics such as ampicillin 1 g i.v. 6-hourly and clarithromycin 500 mg i.v. 12-hourly.
   (i) Refer to the Medical team.

(4) Refer patients with severe CAP to the ICU.

(i) Give ceftriaxone 2 g i.v. once daily or cefotaxime 1 g i.v. 8-hourly *plus* erythromycin 500 mg i.v. 6-hourly or clarithromycin 500 mg i.v. 12-hourly in these patients.

CHRONIC OBSTRUCTIVE PULMONARY DISEASE (COPD)

DIAGNOSIS

(1) Causes of chronic bronchitis with emphysema (COPD) include smoking, environmental pollution, occupational exposure such as silica, repeated or chronic lung infection, and alpha-1 antitrypsin deficiency.

(2) Productive cough, dyspnoea, wheeze and reduced exercise tolerance worsen with exacerbations, until end-stage disease when there is minimal variation.

   (i) Ask about normal daily exercise capacity and level of dependence.

   (ii) Enquire about current medication, home oxygen use, previous hospital admissions and associated cardiac disease.

(3) Exacerbations of COPD.

Consider the multiple possible causes from infection; bronchospasm; pneumothorax; pneumonia; right, left or biventricular heart failure; cardiac arrhythmia including AF; myocardial infarction; non-compliance with medication including steroid underdosing; iatrogenic response to excess sedatives or opiates or inadvertent beta-blockade; environmental allergens or weather change; to malignancy and a PE.

(4) Examine for fever, lip pursing, tachypnoea, tachycardia and wheeze. Also look for:

   (i) Cyanosis, ruddy complexion and signs of right heart failure due to cor pulmonale with raised JVP and peripheral oedema.

   (ii) Carbon dioxide retention causing headache, drowsiness, tremor and a bounding pulse.

(5) Establish venous access and send blood for FBC, ELFTs, glucose and two sets of blood cultures if pyrexial. Attach a cardiac monitor and pulse oximeter to the patient.

(6) Take an ABG if clearly unwell, to look for hypoxia PaO_2 less than 8 kPa (60 mmHg), hypercarbia $PaCO_2$ greater than 6 kPa (45 mmHg) and a raised bicarbonate indicating compensated respiratory acidosis.

(7) Perform an ECG and look for large P waves (P pulmonale), right

ventricular hypertrophy or strain (cor pulmonale), and signs of ischaemia with ST and T wave changes.

(8) Perform bedside lung function testing for PEF, FEV_1 and FVC to compare with previous respiratory function tests, and to follow the response to treatment.

(9) Request a CXR which may show hyperinflation, bullae, atelectasis, consolidation, pneumothorax, heart failure or a lung mass.

MANAGEMENT

(1) Commence controlled oxygen therapy initially at 28% via a Venturi mask if there is evidence of chronic carbon dioxide retention, with a raised $PaCO_2$ and bicarbonate. Aim for an oxygen saturation over 90%.
  (i) Otherwise give higher dose 40–60% oxygen via face mask to treat hypoxaemia. Watch for deterioration and a rising $PaCO_2$.

(2) Give salbutamol 5 mg via a nebulizer for bronchospasm as needed, and add ipratropium (Atrovent™) 500 µg to the initial nebulizer then 6-hourly.

(3) Give prednisolone 50 mg orally or hydrocortisone 200 mg i.v. if unable to swallow, for bronchospasm and if on long-term inhaled or oral steroid.

(4) Treat infection with amoxicillin 500 mg orally t.d.s. or doxycycline 100 mg orally b.d. then once daily.

(5) Consider frusemide (furosemide) 40 mg i.v. if heart failure is suspected.

(6) Admit under the Medical team.

(7) Call urgent senior ED doctor help if there is exhaustion, agitation or confusion; or a rising $PaCO_2$ and a falling pH. Involve the Intensive Care team.
  (i) Commence non-invasive ventilation (NIV) if there are trained and experienced staff to supervise.

PNEUMOTHORAX

DIAGNOSIS

(1) Spontaneous pneumothorax may occur in healthy people with no lung disease designated a 'primary' pneumothorax, particularly in tall, asthenic body types.
  (i) Or spontaneous pneumothorax may occur with chronic lung disease (CLD), and is then designated a 'secondary'

pneumothorax, in association with asthma, emphysema, fibrotic or bullous lung disease including cystic fibrosis and Marfan syndrome.

(ii) Finally, they occur more often in smokers, and may be related to both penetrating and blunt trauma (see p. 218 for traumatic pneumothorax).

(2) The pneumothorax may cause only slight dyspnoea and pleuritic chest pain in fit patients, even when the whole lung may be collapsed.

(i) 'Significant' dyspnoea means any deterioration in usual exercise tolerance.

(ii) Significant dyspnoea or breathlessness is common in a pneumothorax secondary to CLD.

(3) Look for reduced chest expansion on the affected side, increased resonance on percussion, and diminished breath sounds. Alternatively, lateralizing signs may be hard to confirm.

(4) Request a standard inspiratory CXR in all cases.

(i) Do not wait for this if there are signs of tension, but proceed immediately to insert a wide-bore cannula or intercostal drain (see p. 10).

(ii) Assess the size of the pneumothorax on the CXR:

(a) *small* is a visible rim of less than 2 cm

(b) *large* is a visible air rim 2 cm or more around all the lung edge, that represents over 50% of lung volume lost.

(iii) Expiratory CXRs are no longer routine.

MANAGEMENT

This is determined by the size of the pneumothorax (small or large), the presence of chronic lung disease (i.e. a primary or a secondary pneumothorax) and by the degree of dyspnoea (significant or not).

(1) No active management is indicated in patients with a small 'primary' pneumothorax less than 2 cm, with no CLD and no significant dyspnoea.

(i) Arrange follow-up by the GP for repeat CXR within 7 days.

(ii) Tell the patient to avoid heavy exertion or exercise, and to return immediately if they develop significant dyspnoea.

(iii) Advise them not to fly for at least 6 weeks after the CXR has returned to normal, and never to go scuba diving (unless they have had bilateral surgical pleurectomies).

(2) No active management may also be tried in patients with a small

pneumothorax less than 2 cm, with no significant dyspnoea, but with underlying lung disease, i.e. a 'secondary' pneumothorax.

(i) Admit for observation and give high-flow oxygen via a face mask, unless they have COPD in which case start at 28%.

(ii) Repeat the CXR after 6–12 hours and discharge after 24 hours only if they remain asymptomatic and the pneumothorax is not progressing. Arrange early respiratory or medical follow-up within 7 days.

(iii) Perform simple aspiration if there is any significant breathlessness, or enlargement of the air leak.

(3) *Simple aspiration (thoracocentesis)*
Perform this for a symptomatic primary pneumothorax (no CLD) with dyspnoea, whether large or small; and in a small secondary (with CLD) pneumothorax less than 2 cm with minimal breathlessness if aged under 50 years.

(i) Infiltrate local anaesthetic down to the pleura in the second intercostal space in the mid-clavicular line.

(ii) Insert a 16-gauge cannula into the pleural cavity, withdraw the needle, and connect to a 50-mL syringe with three-way tap. Alternatively use a proprietary chest aspiration kit, with special fenestrated cannula and one-way valve.

(iii) Aspirate air until resistance is felt, the patient coughs excessively, or more than 2500 mL is aspirated.

(iv) Repeat the CXR; if the lung has re-expanded, observe and repeat the CXR again after 6 hours:

(a) discharge patients with a primary pneumothorax if the lung remains expanded, and arrange follow-up with the GP and give discharge advice as above

(b) admit patients with CLD and a secondary pneumothorax overnight even if aspiration was successful, for further observation

(c) repeat aspiration may be tried with a primary pneumothorax if the lung has collapsed again (i.e. a failed aspiration), when less than 2500 mL was aspirated on the first attempt

(d) otherwise proceed directly to insertion of an intercostal drain, particularly for failed aspiration of a secondary pneumothorax.

(4) *Intercostal catheter (ICC) or tube thoracostomy*
This therefore is only indicated for:

(i) Tension pneumothorax following initial needle thoracocentesis (see p. 10).

(ii) Traumatic pneumothorax or haemothorax (see p. 218).

(iii) Failed simple aspiration, e.g. with more than just a small residual rim of air around the lung.

(iv) A secondary pneumothorax in a patient with CLD causing significant dyspnoea, or if aged over 50 years.

(v) Any pneumothorax prior to anaesthesia or positive-pressure ventilation.

(5) *Intercostal drain insertion*

(i) Insert the drain into the fifth intercostal space in the mid-axillary line after infiltration with local anaesthetic down to the pleura.

(ii) Use a scalpel blade to incise the skin and subcutaneous fat, followed by blunt dissection down to and through the parietal pleura.

(iii) Use a small size 16–20-French gauge drain directed apically for a simple pneumothorax, or a larger 28–32-French gauge directed basally for a haemothorax.

(iv) Slide the drain in gently with a pair of curved artery forceps having *removed* the trocar. Connect the drain to an underwater seal.

(v) Admit under the care of the Medical team.

PULMONARY EMBOLUS

See p. 22.

PULMONARY OEDEMA

DIAGNOSIS

(1) Pulmonary oedema is usually caused by left ventricular failure due to myocardial infarction, hypertension, an arrhythmia, valvular disease, myocarditis or fluid overload.

(2) Occasional non-cardiac causes include septicaemia, uraemia, head injury, intracranial haemorrhage, near drowning, and inhalation of smoke or noxious gases.

(3) The onset may be precipitate with breathlessness, cough, orthopnoea, paroxysmal nocturnal dyspnoea (PND) and dyspnoea at rest.

(4) The patient is clammy, distressed and prefers to sit upright. Look for wheeze, tachypnoea sometimes with pink froth, tachycardia, basal crepitations and a triple rhythm or gallop.

(5) Establish venous access and send blood for FBC, ELFTs and cardiac biomarkers, although they do not influence the initial management. Attach a cardiac monitor and pulse oximeter to the patient.

(6) Perform an ECG to look for acute ischaemia, arrhythmias and evidence of underlying cardiac disease.

(7) Request a CXR that shows engorged upper-lobe veins, a perihilar 'bats wing' haze, cardiomegaly, septal Kerley B lines, and small bilateral pleural effusions.

MANAGEMENT

(1) Sit the patient upright and give 40–60% oxygen, unless the patient is known to have chronic bronchitis, in which case 28% oxygen should be used. Aim for an oxygen saturation above 94%.

(2) Give GTN 150–300 μg sublingually, which may be repeated. Remove the tablet if excessive hypotension (systolic BP less than 100 mmHg) occurs.

(3) Give frusemide (furosemide) 40 mg i.v., or twice their usual oral daily dose i.v. if already on frusemide (furosemide).

(4) Get senior ED doctor help in refractory cases, repeat the frusemide (furosemide), and commence a GTN infusion, provided the patient is not hypotensive.
  (i) Add GTN 200 mg to 500 mL of 5% dextrose, i.e. 400 μg/mL, using a glass bottle and low-absorption polyethylene infusion set.
  (ii) Infuse initially at 1 mL/h, maintaining systolic BP above 100 mmHg. Progressively increase to 20 mL/h or more, avoiding hypotension.

(5) Commence mask continuous positive airways pressure (CPAP) respiratory support:
  (i) Use a dedicated, high-flow fresh gas circuit, tight-fitting mask and variable resistor valve, starting at 5–10 cmH$_2$O.
  (ii) A trained nurse must remain in attendance at all times, as some patients will not tolerate the mask.
  (iii) *Never* simply use wall oxygen with a black anaesthetic mask and head harness, as this will asphyxiate the patient.

(6) Morphine 0.5–2.5 mg i.v. with an antiemetic such as

metoclopramide 10 mg i.v. is rarely helpful, as it may further obtund the patient particularly if the patient is tired or has COPD.
(7) Admit the patient under the Medical team.

ACUTE UPPER AIRWAY OBSTRUCTION

DIAGNOSIS
(1) Acute upper airway obstruction may be due to croup, epiglottitis, choking on an inhaled foreign body, burns and smoke inhalation, angioedema, trauma, carcinoma or retropharyngeal abscess.
(2) There may be sudden wheeze, coughing, hoarseness or complete aphonia, with severe distress, ineffective respiratory efforts, stridor and cyanosis, followed by unconsciousness.
(3) Attach a cardiac monitor and pulse oximeter to the patient.

MANAGEMENT
This depends on the suspected cause.
(1) Sit the patient up and give 100% oxygen via a face mask. Aim for an oxygen saturation above 94%.
(2) *Inhalation of a foreign body*
  (i) Perform up to five back blows between the shoulder blades in adults and children over 1 year, using the heel of your hand with the victim leaning forwards or lying on the side.
  (ii) Perform up to five abdominal thrusts if this fails (Heimlich manoeuvre). Stand behind the patient, place your arms around the upper abdomen with your hands clasped between the umbilicus and xiphisternum, and give thrusts in and upwards to expel the obstruction.
  (iii) Continue alternating five back blows with five abdominal thrusts if the obstruction is still not relieved.
  (iv) Hold babies and infants up to 1 year head-down, and deliver up to five back blows with the heel of the free hand.
  (v) Perform up to five chest thrusts if this fails, using the same landmark as for cardiac compression, to dislodge foreign material in the airway.
  (vi) Attempt removal under direct vision if the foreign body is still present, using a laryngoscope and a pair of long-handled Magill forceps.
  (vii) *Cricothyrotomy.*
  Perform a cricothyrotomy if the patient is *in extremis*, and all

else has failed (see Fig. 1.4).

(a) extend the patient's neck and identify the cricothyroid membrane between the lower border of the thyroid cartilage and the upper border of the cricoid cartilage

(b) achieve rapid access by inserting a large-bore 14-gauge intravenous cannula through the cricothyroid membrane

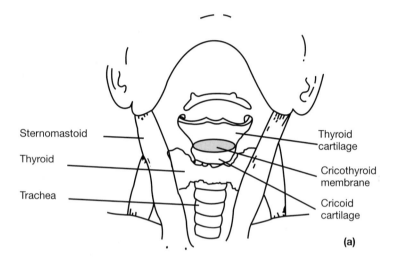

Sternomastoid

Thyroid

Trachea

Thyroid cartilage

Cricothyroid membrane

Cricoid cartilage

(a)

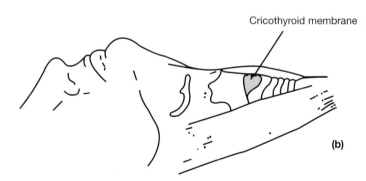

Cricothyroid membrane

(b)

Figure 1.4 Cricothyrotomy
The anatomical relationships of the cricothyroid membrane (a) anteroposterior view, and (b) oblique lateral view.

    (c) attach this to wall oxygen at 15 L/min using a Y-connector. Insufflate oxygen by intermittent occlusion of the open end of the Y-connector for 1 second in every 5 seconds

    (d) alternatively, make an incision through the cricothyroid membrane with a scalpel blade, and insert a 4–6-mm endotracheal tube (or small tracheostomy tube) and connect this to an Ambu or Laerdal bag and the oxygen supply.

(3) *Croup.* See p. 356.

A child with croup will have a barking cough, harsh stridor and hoarseness, and will be frightened and miserable but not systemically ill.

    (i) Give dexamethasone 0.15–0.3 mg/kg orally or i.m., nebulized budesonide 2 mg or prednisolone 1 mg/kg orally.

    (ii) Refer to the Paediatric team.

(4) *Epiglottitis.* See p. 357.

Inflammation of the epiglottis presents with sudden onset of fever, difficulty in breathing, soft inspiratory stridor, dysphagia and drooling. The child looks toxic, unwell and pale.

    (i) Do *not* examine further, i.e. no temperature, blood pressure, or X-ray. Do *not* attempt to visualize the throat.

    (ii) Leave the parent holding the child upright with an oxygen mask held near the child's face.

    (iii) Call for senior ED, paediatric, anaesthetic and ENT assistance immediately.

(5) *Smoke inhalation.* See p. 247.

    (i) Send blood for ABGs and a carboxyhaemoglobin level.

    (ii) Give 100% oxygen and nebulized salbutamol 5 mg, and refer to Intensive Care or Specialist Burns unit if there is an associated respiratory burn.

    (iii) Be prepared to intubate if gross laryngeal oedema occurs.

(6) *Angioedema with laryngeal oedema.* See p. 88.

    (i) Give high-dose oxygen and 1 in 1000 adrenaline (epinephrine) 0.3–0.5 mg (0.3–0.5 mL) intramuscularly (i.m.) into the thigh, repeated every 5 min as necessary.

    (ii) Change to adrenaline (epinephrine) 0.75–1.5 µg/kg i.v. if circulatory collapse occurs, i.e. 50–100 µg or 0.5–1.0 mL of 1 in 10 000 adrenaline (epinephrine), or 5–10 mL of 1 in 100 000 adrenaline (epinephrine) for a 70-kg patient, given slowly.

    (iii) Endotracheal intubation may still be required, performed by a skilled doctor with airway training, or even a cricothyrotomy.

UPPER GASTROINTESTINAL HAEMORRHAGE

DIAGNOSIS

(1) Causes of upper gastrointestinal haemorrhage include:
  (i) Peptic ulceration (over 40% of cases):
    (a) duodenal ulcer (DU)
    (b) gastric ulcer (GU) less common.
  (ii) Gastric erosions or gastritis:
    (a) post-alcohol
    (b) drug-induced (salicylates, non-steroidal anti-inflammatory drugs (NSAIDs), steroids).
  (iii) Mallory–Weiss tear (oesophageal tear following vomiting or retching).
  (iv) Bleeding oesophageal or gastric varices associated with portal hypertension (often due to alcoholic cirrhosis).
  (v) Reflux oesophagitis.
  (vi) Others, including gastric neoplasm, blood coagulation disorders, angiodysplasia and aorto-enteric fistula with a past history of an abdominal aortic aneurysm (AAA) repair.

(2) Mortality is 5–10% related to age over 60 years, comorbid disease, shock and coagulopathy.

(3) Patients can present in a variety of ways:
  (i) Haematemesis:
    (a) fresh red blood
    (b) altered blood 'coffee grounds'.
  (ii) Melaena.
  (iii) Collapse and shock.
  (iv) Syncope and postural hypotension.
  (v) Fatigue, dyspnoea, angina, etc.
  (vi) Haematochezia (bright red rectal bleeding).

(4) Examine for signs of chronic liver disease including jaundice, bruising, palmar erythema, clubbing, gynaecomastia, spider naevi, hepatomegaly and encephalopathy.
  (i) Examine for splenomegaly and ascites if portal hypertension is suspected.

(5) Establish venous access with a large-bore 14-gauge i.v. cannula, and attach a pulse oximeter and cardiac monitor to the patient.
  (i) Take blood for FBC, U&Es, blood sugar, LFTs, clotting studies including a prothrombin index (PTI) and cross-match

from 2–4 units of blood, according to the presumed aetiology and degree of shock.

MANAGEMENT

(1) Commence high-dose oxygen via a face mask. Maintain the oxygen saturation above 94%.

(2) Begin fluid replacement:
   (i) Start with normal saline 1–2 litres, aiming for a urine output of 0.5–1 mL/kg per hour.
   (ii) Give cross-matched blood when it is available if the patient is shocked, or if the bleeding is continuing.
   (iii) Use O-negative blood if the situation is desperate.

(3) Consider a proton-pump inhibitor if peptic ulcer disease is likely. Give omeprazole 40–80 mg i.v. followed by an infusion at 8 mg/h.
   (i) There is no supporting evidence for an H_2-antagonist.

(4) Give octreotide 50 μg i.v. then 50 μg/h if varices are known, or are likely from the presence of chronic liver disease and portal hypertension.

(5) Arrange for an urgent endoscopy, particularly in patients who continue to bleed, have suspected varices, remain unstable or are aged over 60 years. Contact the Intensive Care team.
   (i) Endoscopy will differentiate the cause of the bleeding and allow immediate thermal or injection therapy where appropriate, or banding for varices.

(6) Otherwise admit patients who have stopped bleeding and are haemodynamically stable under the Medical team, for endoscopy later.

Warning: inserting a central venous pressure (CVP) line in a hypotensive, shocked patient is difficult and dangerous. Leave it until initial transfusion is under way for a skilled doctor to perform.

DIABETIC COMA AND PRE-COMA

Hypoglycaemia rapidly produces coma in diabetics, compared with the slower onset of altered consciousness in diabetic ketoacidosis and hyper-glycaemic, hyperosmolar non-ketotic syndrome (HHNS).

DIABETIC KETOACIDOSIS (DKA)

DIAGNOSIS

(1) Diabetic ketoacidosis (DKA) may occur in a known diabetic, precipitated by infection, myocardial infarction, cerebral infarction, pancreatitis, trauma or inadequate insulin therapy, e.g. insulin stopped in an unwell diabetic patient 'because he was not eating'!

(2) Alternatively, it may arise *de novo* in an undiagnosed diabetic, heralded by polyuria, polydipsia, weight loss, lethargy, abdominal pain or coma.

(3) The predominant features arise from salt and water depletion and acidosis, hence there is dry skin, tachycardia, hypotension (especially postural) and deep sighing respirations (Kussmaul breathing).

   (i) The ketones may be detected on the breath as a sickly sweet, fruity smell.

(4) Establish venous access and send blood urgently for FBC, ELFTs, blood glucose and blood cultures if infection is suspected. Attach a cardiac monitor and pulse oximeter to the patient.

(5) Take blood for ABGs and organize an ECG, CXR and an MSU.

   (i) Look at the ECG for an early indication of critical hyperkalaemia with peaked T waves, QRS widening, then absent P waves and finally a 'sine wave' trace (see p. 115).

> **Tip:** *every* patient who presents with abdominal pain, vomiting or thirst must have urine tested for sugar and ketones.

MANAGEMENT

(1) Give high-dose oxygen via a face mask and aim for an oxygen saturation above 94%.

(2) Start an i.v. infusion and run in normal saline 500 mL to 1 litre, followed by a further 500 mL/h for the next 4 hours if the diagnosis is confirmed.

   (i) Continue the i.v. normal saline resuscitation until the blood sugar is 15 mmol/L or less, then change to 5% dextrose but continue the insulin infusion.

   (ii) Aim to replace the fluid deficit steadily over the first 24 hours.

(3) Commence short-acting soluble insulin therapy.

   (i) Give soluble insulin 10 units i.v. immediately.

   (ii) Start an insulin infusion.

Add 50 units soluble insulin to 50 mL normal saline, i.e. 1 unit/mL, and run at 5 units/h or 5 mL/h via an infusion pump.

(4) Add potassium to the i.v. fluid when the plasma K level is known. This should be within 30 min:

   (i) Potassium is less than 3.0 mmol/L – give potassium chloride (KCl) 40 mmol/h (3 g KCl). *Must* give via an infusion pump.

   (ii) Potassium is 3.0–4.0 mmol/L – give 26.8 mmol KCl/h (2 g KCl).

   (iii) Potassium is 4.0–5.0 mmol/L – give 20 mmol KCl/h (1.5 g KCl).

   (iv) Potassium is 5.0–6.0 mmol/L – give 13.4 mmol KCl/h (1 g KCl).

   (v) Stop the potassium if:

     (a) the patient is anuric

     (b) the serum level is over 6.0 mmol/L

     (c) the ECG shows peaked T waves or QRS complex widening.

(5) Refer the patient to the Medical team or ICU. Remember to have looked for any underlying precipitating factor(s) for the DKA.

(6) Do *not* give i.v. sodium bicarbonate except on the advice of the senior ED doctor.

   (i) It may be considered if the pH remains below 7.0, particularly with circulatory failure.

HYPERGLYCAEMIC, HYPEROSMOLAR NON-KETOTIC SYNDROME (HHNS)

DIAGNOSIS

(1) Hyperglycaemic, hyperosmolar non-ketotic syndrome is more common in the elderly, non-insulin-dependent patient, with a more gradual onset than DKA.

(2) It may be precipitated by infection, myocardial infarction, a stroke or by thiazide diuretic use and steroids.

(3) The patient presents with an altered level of consciousness, profound dehydration and may develop seizures or focal neurological signs. Mortality is 20–40%, compared to DKA where it is under 5% in younger patients.

(4) Blood glucose and serum osmolarity tend to be higher than in DKA. The osmolarity usually exceeds 350 mOsmol/L.

   (i) Estimate the osmolarity by 2(Na + K) + urea + glucose (all units in mmol/L).

MANAGEMENT

(1) This is comparable to DKA (see p. 52).

(2) Give i.v. normal saline or half-normal saline if the serum sodium exceeds 150 mmol/L, at a similar or slower rate to DKA. Beware of over-rapid rehydration causing pulmonary oedema.

(3) Use a slower insulin infusion rate of 2–3 units/h. Lower potassium replacement rates are also usually required than in DKA.

(4) Commence prophylactic heparin, either unfractionated (UF) heparin 5000 units i.v. bolus then an infusion at 1000 units/h, or LMW heparin such as enoxaparin 1.5 mg/kg per day, assuming there is no active bleeding, particularly intracerebral.

THE PATIENT WITH AN ALTERED CONSCIOUS LEVEL

Patients with an altered conscious level frequently present to the Emergency Department. Although history taking is compromised, a methodical, careful approach is essential.

The following categories are covered, though they do overlap:

- The collapsed or unconscious patient
- The confused patient
- Alcohol-related medical problems
- The patient with an altered conscious level and smelling of alcohol
- Alcohol withdrawal

THE COLLAPSED OR UNCONSCIOUS PATIENT

The aim is to resuscitate the patient and treat urgent precipitating conditions while a picture of the situation is built up. The definitive diagnosis may not be made in the Emergency Department.

MANAGEMENT

(1) Manage the patient in a monitored resuscitation area, and call the senior ED doctor immediately.

   (i) Clear obstructing material using a tongue depressor or laryngoscope blade if the patient is unconscious with a noisy airway, and remove broken dentures, vomit or blood with a Yankauer sucker.

    (ii) Improve airway opening using head tilt, chin lift and jaw thrust.

        (a) open the airway with the jaw thrust only in trauma cases, avoiding movement of the neck.

    (iii) Insert an oropharyngeal airway and give high-dose oxygen via a face mask. Attach a cardiac monitor and pulse oximeter to the patient and aim for an oxygen saturation above 94%.

(2) Commence cardiopulmonary resuscitation if no pulse is felt (see p. 2).

(3) An airway-skilled doctor should now insert an endotracheal tube if there is a reduced or absent gag reflex and an unprotected airway, using a rapid sequence induction technique.

Rapid sequence induction (RSI) intubation

    (i)   Use an i.v. induction agent such as thiopentone (thiopental) 0.5–5 mg/kg, etomidate 0.3 mg/kg, or midazolam 0.1 mg/kg plus fentanyl 2.5–5 μg/kg *after* pre-oxygenation ideally for 3 min.

    (ii) Follow with a muscle relaxant, usually suxamethonium 1.5 mg/kg, applying cricoid pressure as muscle tone is lost.

    (iii) Insert the endotracheal tube under direct vision, visualizing its passage through the vocal cords, and inflate the cuff.

    (iv) Confirm correct tube placement using capnography to measure end-tidal carbon dioxide ($ETCO_2$) and release cricoid pressure when happy with tube position.

    (v) Tie the tube in place and carefully monitor the patient as a CXR is arranged.

    (vi) Use in-line manual stabilization of the neck in trauma cases (see p. 205).

> **(!)** **Warning:** *never* attempt RSI unless you have been trained. Use a bag–valve mask technique instead, while waiting for help.

(4) Otherwise:

    (i)   Apply a semi-rigid collar if there is any suggestion of face, head or neck trauma, before moving the patient.

    (ii) Remove all the patient's clothing, but keep covered.

(5) Insert an i.v. cannula and take blood for FBC, coagulation profile, blood sugar, ELFTs, blood culture and drug screen for salicylate and paracetamol if not already done.

    (i)   Perform ABGs, recording the amount of oxygen being delivered (FiO_2).

    (ii) Give 50% dextrose 50 mL i.v. if the blood glucose test strip is low.

        (a)   remember dextrose i.v. can precipitate Wernicke's encephalopathy in alcoholic or malnourished patients, who require thiamine 100 mg i.v. immediately.

(6) Record the temperature (if 35 °C, repeat with a low-reading thermometer to exclude hypothermia), pulse, blood pressure, and the pupil size and reaction.

    (i)   Consider naloxone 0.4–2 mg i.v. if there are pinpoint pupils with hypoventilation to reverse narcotic poisoning, but beware of precipitating an acute withdrawal reaction.

(7) Consider other critical conditions requiring immediate action:

    (i)   *Tension pneumothorax.*

        (a)   this usually follows trauma, especially if positive-pressure ventilation is being given

        (b)   insert a large-bore cannula or intercostal drain without waiting for an X-ray (see p. 10).

    (ii) *Cardiac arrhythmia.*

        (a)   treat as necessary after recording a formal 12-lead ECG (see p. 31).

    (iii) *Exsanguination.*

        (a)   bleeding may be obvious, or concealed coming from the gastrointestinal tract, an aortic aneurysm or a ruptured ectopic pregnancy

        (b)   cross-match blood, give i.v. fluids, and refer the patient for an urgent surgical opinion.

    (iv) *Anaphylaxis.*

        (a)   this may follow drug therapy, food ingestion, or an insect sting

        (b)   give 1 in 1000 adrenaline (epinephrine) 0.3–0.5 mg (0.3–0.5 mL) i.m. repeated as necessary every 5 min

        (c)   give 1 in 10 000 or 1 in 100 000 adrenaline (epinephrine) 0.75–1.5 μg/kg if there is circulatory collapse, i.e. 50–100 μg or 0.5–1.0 mL of 1 in 10 000, 5–10 mL of 1 in 100 000 adrenaline (epinephrine), slowly i.v. for a 70-kg patient (see p. 89).

(v) *Extradural haemorrhage.*
   (a) this may follow even trivial trauma; look for a local bruise on the scalp, for instance in the temporoparietal area over the middle meningeal artery territory
   (b) watch for deterioration in the level of consciousness, ultimately with the development of Cheyne–Stokes breathing and a unilateral fixed, dilated pupil
   (c) call an airway-skilled doctor to pass a cuffed endotracheal tube if one is not already in place
   (d) arrange an urgent head CT scan, and refer the patient immediately to the Neurosurgical team, before critical mass lesion signs develop.

DIAGNOSIS
(1) The patient's cardiorespiratory status should have been stabilized by this stage, bloods sent, an IDC and a nasogastric tube placed, and an ECG and CXR performed. Now focus on the underlying cause. The most common causes of an unconscious patient are:
   (i) Poisoning (accidental or deliberate, including alcohol, CO).
   (ii) Hypoglycaemia.
   (iii) Post-ictal state.
   (iv) Stroke.
   (v) Head injury.
   (vi) Subarachnoid haemorrhage.
   (vii) Respiratory failure.
   (viii) Hypotension, including cardiac arrhythmia or myocardial infarction.
(2) Less common causes of an unconscious patient are:
   (i) Meningitis or encephalitis.
   (ii) Hepatic or renal failure.
   (iii) Septicaemia.
   (iv) Subdural haematoma.
   (v) Hyperglycaemia (DKA or HHNS).
   (vi) Hypothermia or hyperthermia.
(3) Rare causes of an unconscious patient are:
   (i) Cerebral space-occupying lesion.
   (ii) Hyponatraemia or hypercalcaemia.
   (iii) Myxoedema.
   (iv) Addison's disease.
   (v) Hypertensive encephalopathy.

(4) Finally, in those who have recently been abroad, consider:
  (i) Cerebral malaria.
  (ii) Typhus, yellow fever, trypanosomiasis and typhoid.
  (iii) Severe acute respiratory syndrome (SARS) or avian influenza (bird 'flu).
(5) These four lists may seem daunting, but aim to build up a picture of the events as follows.
(6) History:
  (i) Any clues from relatives, passers-by or ambulance crew?
  (ii) Witnessed fit, trauma, alcohol or drug ingestion?
  (iii) Prior medical or surgical conditions?
  (iv) Known drug therapy or abuse?
  (v) Recent travel abroad?
(7) Further examination:
  (i) Search the clothing for a diabetic card, steroid card or outpatient card.
  (ii) Look particularly for signs of trauma, needle puncture marks, or petechiae on the skin.
  (iii) Reassess the vital signs, including the temperature. Exclude any neck stiffness.
  (iv) Examine the front of the chest, feel the abdomen and examine the back, inspect the perineum and perform a rectal examination.
  (v) Reassess the neurological state, including the level of consciousness using the Glasgow coma scale (GCS) score (see p. 237), the pupil responses, eye movements and fundi. Assess the muscle power, tone and reflexes including the plantar responses.
(8) Perform:
  (i) Lateral cervical spine X-ray, CXR and pelvic X-ray in trauma (see p. 208).
  (ii) Head CT scan if intracranial pathology is suspected or cannot be excluded, which is frequently the case.
(9) Refer the patient to the Medical (or Surgical) team, or ICU if they are not already involved, having treated any urgent conditions and built up a list of the likely causes of unconsciousness.

THE CONFUSED PATIENT

'Confusion' should be reserved to describe a state of clouding of consciousness or disturbed awareness, which may fluctuate.

DIAGNOSIS

(1) There is a spectrum of confusional states between the following two pictures, which may overlap:

    (i) Usually abrupt onset of difficulty maintaining attention, irritability, emotional lability and illusions.

    (ii) Delirium with disorientation in time and place, impaired memory, restlessness, visual, olfactory or tactile hallucinations and poor comprehension.

(2) Causes of confusion.

    (i) Hypoxia:

        (a) chest infection, pulmonary embolus, cardiac failure

        (b) respiratory depression from drugs or muscle disorders, e.g. myasthenia gravis or muscular dystrophy

        (c) head injury or chest injury.

    (ii) Drugs:

        (a) intoxication or withdrawal from alcohol, LSD, cocaine and amphetamines

        (b) side effects (especially in the elderly) of analgesics, anticonvulsants, digoxin, psychotropics, anticholinergics and antiparkinsonian drugs such as benzhexol (trihexyphenidyl) and levodopa.

    (iii) Cerebral:

        (a) traumatic head injury

        (b) post-ictal state, complex partial (temporal lobe) seizures

        (c) cerebrovascular accident, subarachnoid haemorrhage

        (d) meningitis, encephalitis

        (e) space-occupying lesion, e.g. tumour, abscess or haematoma

        (f) hypertensive encephalopathy

        (g) SLE.

    (iv) Metabolic:

        (a) respiratory, cardiac, renal or liver failure

        (b) electrolyte disorder, such as hyponatraemia, hypernatraemia or hypercalcaemia

        (c) vitamin deficiency, e.g. thiamine (Wernicke's encephalopathy), nicotinic acid or B_{12}

        (d) acute intermittent porphyria.

    (v) Endocrine:

        (a) hypoglycaemia or hyperglycaemia

        (b) thyrotoxicosis, myxoedema, Cushing syndrome, steroids, Addison's disease.

Table 1.5 Mini-Mental State Examination (MMSE)

Cognition tested			Score
Orientation (10 points)			
1.	What is the date?		1
	What is the day?		1
	What is the month?		1
	What is the year?		1
	What is the season?		1
2.	What is the name of this building?		1
	What floor of the building are we on?		1
	What city are we in?		1
	What state are we in?		1
	What country are we in?		1
Registration (3 points)			
3.	I am going to name three objects. After I have said them I want you to repeat them. Remember what they are because I am going to ask you to name them in a few minutes. Apple. Table. Penny. *(Code the first attempt and then repeat the answers until the patient learns all three)*	Apple	1
		Table	1
		Penny	1
Attention and calculation (5 points max)			
4.	*Either:* Can you subtract 7 from 100, and then subtract 7 from the answer you get and keep subtracting until I tell you to stop?	93	1
		86	1
		79	1
		72	1
		65	1
5.	*Or:* I'm going to spell a word forwards and I want you to spell it backwards. The word is W-O-R-L-D. Now you spell it backwards *(Repeat if necessary)*	D	1
		L	1
		R	1
		O	1
		W	1
Recall (3 points)			
6.	Now what were the three objects I asked you to remember?	Apple	1
		Table	1
		Penny	1

Language (9 points)		
7.	What is this called? *(Show wristwatch)*	1
	What is this called? *(Show pencil)*	1
8.	I'd like you to repeat a phrase after me: No ifs ands or buts	1
9.	Read the words on the bottom of this page and do what it says	Closes eyes	1
10.	*(Read the full statement below before handing the respondent a piece of paper. Do not repeat or coach)* I'm going to give you a piece of paper. What I want you to do is take the paper in your right hand, fold it in half and put the paper on your lap.	Takes with right hand	1
		Folds in half	1
		Puts on lap	1
11.	Write a complete sentence on this piece of paper. The sentence should have a subject, verb and make sense. Spelling and grammatical errors are OK		1
12.	Here is a drawing. Please copy the drawing on the same piece of paper *(Hand the respondent a drawing of two intersecting pentagons)*	Correct if two five-sided pentagons intersect to make a four-sided figure	1
Total score (out of 30)		

CLOSE YOUR EYES

A score of 20 or less indicates cognitive impairment.
Higher scores are expected in the well-educated, and lower scores in the elderly, the uneducated, and the mentally impaired.
From Folstein MF, Folstein SE, McHugh PR (1975) Mini-Mental State. A practical method for grading the cognitive state of patients for the clinician. *J Psychiatr Res* **12:**189–98.

    (vi) Septicaemia, e.g. urinary tract, biliary, meningococcaemia or malaria.

    (viii) Faecal impaction and urinary retention in the elderly (*rarely* the sole cause).

(3) Build up a picture of which condition or conditions are responsible from a detailed history and examination.

    (i) Document a formal Mini-Mental State Examination (MMSE). See Table 1.5.

    (ii) This records cognitive impairment by assessing orientation, attention and calculation, immediate and short-term recall, language, and ability to follow simple verbal and written commands.

    (a) a score of 20 or less suggests cognitive impairment, and the possibility of an organic cause.

(4) Record the vital signs including temperature, pulse, blood pressure and GCS score.

    (i) *Any* abnormality of the vital signs should be assumed to have an organic cause until proven otherwise.

(5) Always exclude hypoglycaemia, and perform some or all of the following investigations based on the suspected aetiology:

    (i) FBC, coagulation profile.

    (ii) U&Es, blood sugar, calcium, liver function tests, thyroid function tests, drug screen.

    (iii) ABGs.

    (iv) Blood cultures, MSU.

    (v) ECG, CXR.

    (vi) CT brain scan.

    (vii) Lumbar puncture.

MANAGEMENT

(1) Admit all patients under the appropriate specialist team.

(2) Avoid the temptation to simply sedate the confused patient, without looking carefully for the underlying cause first.

ALCOHOL-RELATED MEDICAL PROBLEMS

Alcohol is causally related to all types of trauma, including motor vehicle crashes, incidents in the home, deliberate self-harm, assaults, drownings, child abuse, and falls in the elderly. It also predisposes to a variety of medical conditions, and sudden reductions in intake cause withdrawal problems.

MEASUREMENT OF ALCOHOL LEVEL

- Various methods are available, including a breath test, a urine test, and a blood level test. None is admissible in a court of law, unless special forensic kits are used under police direction (see p. 463).

- The British legal limit for driving is a blood alcohol level below 80 mg%. Intoxication is marked above a level of 150 mg%, and coma usually occurs above a level of 300 mg%.

- The Australian legal limits vary from 0.05 to 0.08 g/100 mL, according to the State or Territory.

THE PATIENT WITH AN ALTERED CONSCIOUS LEVEL AND SMELLING OF ALCOHOL

DIAGNOSIS AND MANAGEMENT

Never assume that a confused, obtunded or unconscious patient smelling of alcohol is simply 'drunk' until you have excluded *all* of the following:

(1) *Hypoglycaemia*
- (i) Check a blood sugar, and give 50% dextrose 50 mL i.v. if it is low.
- (ii) This may precipitate worsening of the confusion due to Wernicke's encephalopathy, associated with alcohol abuse and malnutrition causing confusion, ataxia, nystagmus, and bilateral lateral rectus palsy.
  - (a) give thiamine 100 mg i.v. immediately. This should be routine in the malnourished, and in suspected alcoholism.

(2) *Head injury*
- (i) Always remember the possibility of an extradural or subdural haematoma.
- (ii) Commence neurological observations and perform a CT head scan if confusion persists or there is a deteriorating conscious level (see p. 54).
  - (a) a skull X-ray is a possibility only in the absence of a CT scan and may show a fracture, but if normal it does *not* exclude intracranial injury.

(3) *Other general medical problems*
- (i) Epileptic seizure.
- (ii) Acute poisoning.
- (iii) Meningitis, chest infection, etc.
- (iv) Cerebral haemorrhage.
- (v) Rib fracture, wrist fracture, abdominal trauma.
- (vi) Hypothermia.

(4) *An acute condition more prevalent in alcoholics*
- (i) Aspiration or pneumococcal pneumonia, TB.
- (ii) Cardiac arrhythmia, cardiomyopathy.
- (iii) Gastrointestinal haemorrhage.
- (iv) Pancreatitis.
- (v) Liver failure.
- (vi) Hypokalaemia, hypomagnesaemia, hypocalcaemia.
- (vii) Renal failure.
- (viii) Lactic acidosis.

(ix) Ketoacidosis.

(x) Withdrawal seizures or delirium tremens.

(xi) Wernicke's encephalopathy.

(5) Thus, many patients will require admission to exclude the above conditions. If in doubt, always admit for observation and do not discharge until sober, safe and medically well.

ALCOHOL WITHDRAWAL

This is caused by an absolute or relative decrease in the usual intake of alcohol through lack of funds or by detention in hospital or by the police.

DIAGNOSIS AND MANAGEMENT

Two conditions are recognized: the alcohol withdrawal syndrome, and the progression to delirium tremens.

(1) *Alcohol withdrawal syndrome*

(i) This is common, occurring within 12 hours of abstinence and lasting a few days. It is characterized by agitation, irritability, fine tremor, sweats and tachycardia.

(ii) Commence diazepam 10–20 mg orally 2–6-hourly until the patient is comfortable, plus thiamine 100 mg i.v. or i.m. once daily.

(iii) Control seizures with lorazepam 0.07 mg/kg up to 4 mg i.v., or diazepam 0.1–0.2 mg/kg up to 20 mg i.v., or midazolam 0.05–0.1 mg/kg up to 10 mg i.v., after excluding hypoglycaemia.

(iv) Refer the patient to the Medical team.

(2) *Delirium tremens*

(i) This is uncommon, occurring 72 hours after abstinence. There is clouding of consciousness, terrifying visual hallucinations, gross tremor, autonomic hyperactivity with tachycardia and cardiac arrhythmias, dilated pupils, fever, sweating, dehydration, and grand mal seizures that may be prolonged (status epilepticus).

(ii) Delirium tremens is a medical emergency.

(a) control seizures with lorazepam, diazepam or midazolam i.v. (see doses above)

(b) exclude other causes of status epilepticus such as head injury and meningitis (see p. 69).

(iii) Replace fluid and electrolyte losses, avoiding excessive normal saline in liver failure. Give thiamine 100 mg i.v. once daily.

(iv) Refer all patients immediately to the ICU.

> (!) **Warning:** never dispense chlomethiazole capsules or a benzodiazepine supply in the Emergency Department to take home. They are reserved for inpatient detoxification programmes only.

ACUTE NEUROLOGICAL CONDITIONS

The following neurological conditions frequently present to the Emergency Department:

- Syncope (faint)
- Seizure (fit)
- Generalized convulsive status epilepticus
- TIA
- Stroke

Headache is covered separately on page 75.

SYNCOPE

DIAGNOSIS

(1) Syncope or a 'faint' is the transient loss of consciousness due to reduced cerebral perfusion, usually with a rapid onset associated with blurred vision, dizziness, sweating and loss of postural tone, followed by spontaneous and full recovery.

(i) A brief tonic–clonic seizure may follow if cerebral perfusion remains impaired.

(2) Faints may be difficult to distinguish from seizures or acute vertigo, so an eye-witness account is vital. Always interview ambulance crew or accompanying adults.

(3) Causes vary from benign to imminently life threatening. The aim is to always exclude the most serious conditions such as cardiac or haemorrhage:

(i) Cardiac:

(a) arrhythmia, either a tachycardia or a bradycardia, Stokes–Adams attack

(b) myocardial infarction

(c) stenotic valve lesion (especially aortic stenosis)

(d) hypertrophic cardiomyopathy

(e) drug toxicity or side effect
- calcium-channel or beta-blocker
- prolonged QT from sotalol, tricyclics, erythromycin, etc.

(ii) Vascular:

(a) carotid sinus hypersensitivity

(b) pulmonary embolism.

(iii) Haemorrhage or fluid loss:

(a) haematemesis and melaena

(b) concealed haemorrhage (such as an abdominal aortic aneurysm or ectopic pregnancy)

(c) vomiting and or diarrhoea, with dehydration.

(iv) Neurological:

(a) subarachnoid haemorrhage

(b) vertebrobasilar insufficiency.

(v) Postural (orthostatic) hypotension:

(a) diabetes, hypoadrenalism (Addison's)

(b) Parkinson's disease, and autonomic failure

(c) drugs:
- antihypertensives, e.g. ACE inhibitors, prazosin
- diuretics
- nitrates
- levodopa
- phenothiazines
- tricyclic antidepressants.

(vi) Cough, micturition or defecation syncope.

(vii) Vasovagal (neurocardiogenic) – 'simple' faint, triggered by heat, pain or emotion. Do *not* diagnose if over 45 years.

(viii) Hypoglycaemia (relative).

(4) Examine carefully all patients, looking for hypotension (including postural), a cardiac lesion, an abdominal mass or tenderness, and focal neurological signs.

(5) Check the blood glucose test strip for hypoglycaemia, and perform an ECG.

(6) Request other investigations only as indicated such as FBC, U&Es, cardiac biomarkers, pregnancy test, CXR and CT scan.

MANAGEMENT

(1) Refer the patient to the Medical (or Surgical) team for admission as appropriate.

    (i) Be sure to include any patient with a history of heart failure or ventricular arrhythmias, an abnormal ECG or if aged over 75 years.

(2) Refer other patients with no clear inciting history, a normal examination and a normal ECG for outpatient follow-up if no immediately life-threatening cause for syncope is found.

    (i) A 24-hour ambulatory ECG (Holter monitor) may help, particularly in unexplained recurrent syncope.

(3) Inform the GP by fax or letter if the patient is discharged and arrange early follow-up.

SEIZURE (FIT)

DIAGNOSIS

(1) An eye-witness account is crucial to establish the true diagnosis. Helpful indicators of an epileptic seizure having occurred, rather than a faint, fall or episode of vertigo, are:

    (i) Bitten tongue, urinary incontinence.

    (ii) Preceding aura or proceeding drowsiness.

    (iii) Known epilepsy.

(2) The most common causes of seizures in known epileptics are:

    (i) Not taking their medication or rarely medication toxicity.

    (ii) Alcohol abuse, either excess or withdrawal.

    (iii) Intercurrent infection (remember meningitis).

    (iv) Head injury.

    (v) Hypoglycaemia.

(3) *Never* diagnose new-onset 'epilepsy' in non-epileptic patients presenting with a first seizure or a sporadic seizure, until all the following 'acute symptomatic' causes of a secondary seizure are excluded:

    (i) Hypoglycaemia.

    (ii) Head injury.

    (iii) Hypoxia.

    (iv) Infection – especially meningitis, encephalitis, cerebral abscess, HIV or a febrile seizure in a child.

    (v) Acute poisoning, e.g. alcohol, tricyclic antidepressants,

anticholinergics, theophylline, cocaine, amphetamine, and isoniazid.
(vi) Drug withdrawal, e.g. alcohol, benzodiazepine, narcotics, cocaine.
(vii) Intracranial pathology:
  (a) space-occupying lesion
  (b) cerebral ischaemia
  (c) subarachnoid or intracerebral haemorrhage.
(viii) Hyponatraemia, hypocalcaemia, uraemia and eclampsia.

> **Warning:** exclude the above same 'acute symptomatic' causes of grand mal seizures in a patient presenting with generalized convulsive status epilepticus (see p. 69).

(4) Check a blood glucose test strip.
  (i) Give 50% dextrose 50 mL i.v. if it is low, after taking blood for a laboratory glucose estimation, or give glucagon 1 mg i.m. when venous access is impossible.
(5) Insert an i.v. cannula and take blood for FBC, U&Es, LFTs, drug and alcohol screen and blood cultures.
  (i) Proceed to ABGs, ECG, CXR, and CT head scan as indicated clinically, and attach a cardiac monitor and pulse oximeter to the patient.
  (ii) Send urgent anticonvulsant levels if the patient is on treatment.

MANAGEMENT
(1) Give high-dose oxygen via a face mask. Aim for an oxygen saturation above 94%.
(2) Do not attempt to wedge the mouth open. Make sure the head is protected from harm and turn the patient semi-prone.
(3) Give lorazepam 0.07 mg/kg up to 4 mg i.v., diazepam 0.1–0.2 mg/kg up to 20 mg i.v. or midazolam 0.05–0.1 mg/kg up to 10 mg i.v. if the patient is having a seizure, or if the seizure recurs.
(4) Refer the following patients for admission to the Medical team:
  (i) Suspected underlying cause such as meningitis, tumour, etc.
  (ii) A seizure exceeding 5 min, or recurrent seizures, especially if there is no full recovery between them.

(iii) Residual focal CNS signs.

(iv) Seizure following a head injury (refer to the surgeons).

(5) Discharge home a previously known epileptic if:

(i) A rapid, full recovery is made.

(ii) The seizure lasted less than 5 min and was not associated with trauma either before or during the seizure.

(iii) There are no residual focal CNS signs and the level of consciousness is normal.

(iv) Their usual medication is adequate and being taken.

(v) There is an adult to accompany the patient.

(6) In addition, discharge home a patient under 40 years with a non-focal first seizure, with no serious underlying cause found (having considered the causes listed under point (3) on p. 67), and who makes a full recovery without focal neurology.

(i) Discuss discharge with the senior ED doctor.

(ii) Perform a CT head scan first, or organize within the next day or two.

(iii) Organize an Outpatient EEG and Medical clinic review.

(iv) Advise the patient not to drive, operate machinery, supervise children swimming, or bath a baby alone etc. until seen by the specialist. Record this advice in writing in the notes.

(7) Always inform the GP by fax or letter on discharging the patient, and if the patient was referred to the Medical or Neurology clinic for follow-up.

GENERALIZED CONVULSIVE STATUS EPILEPTICUS

DIAGNOSIS

(1) Generalized convulsive, grand mal, major motor or tonic–clonic status epilepticus is defined as two or more grand mal seizures without full recovery of consciousness in between, or recurrent grand mal seizures for more than 5–10 min.

(2) Over 50% patients have no prior history of seizures.

(i) Thus it is essential to look for any of the underlying 'acute symptomatic' causes listed under point (3) on p. 67.

(ii) Therefore, perform all the tests mentioned under point (5) on p. 68, once the seizures have been terminated.

(3) Attach a cardiac monitor and pulse oximeter to the patient on arrival.

MANAGEMENT

(1) Give the patient oxygen via a face mask, and aim for an oxygen saturation above 94%.

(2) Check the blood sugar:
   (i) Give 50% dextrose 50 mL i.v. if it is low.
   (ii) Give thiamine 100 mg i.v. in addition if chronic alcoholism or malnutrition is likely, to avoid precipitating Wernicke's encephalopathy.

(3) Give lorazepam 0.07 mg/kg up to 4 mg i.v., or diazepam 0.1–0.2 mg/kg up to 20 mg i.v., or midazolam 0.05–0.1 mg/kg up to 10 mg i.v.
   (i) Beware of causing respiratory depression, bradycardia and hypotension, especially in the elderly.

(4) Get senior ED doctor help if the patient is still having a seizure:
   (i) Repeat the lorazepam, diazepam or midazolam i.v. until seizures cease.
   (ii) Then give phenytoin 15–17 mg/kg i.v. no faster than 50 mg/min by slow bolus, or preferably as an infusion in 250 mL normal saline (never in dextrose) over 30 min under ECG monitoring.
   (iii) Or give the pro-drug fosphenytoin at an equivalent dose but faster rate.

(5) Other drugs that may be used include phenobarbitone (phenobarbital) 10–20 mg/kg i.v. no faster than 100 mg/min, and clonazepam 0.5–2 mg i.v.
   (i) By now, make sure the ICU team is involved if seizures continue.
   (ii) All patients require medical admission.

(6) Occasionally, if i.v. access is impossible, give:
   (i) Rectal diazepam, especially in children, using parenteral diazepam solution 0.5 mg/kg given through a small syringe (see p. 369) or midazolam 0.5 mg/kg p.r. or via the buccal route.
   (ii) Paraldehyde 0.4 mL/kg rectally diluted 1 in 1 with olive oil or normal saline if the seizure persists.

(7) Consider the following underlying reasons when a patient fails to regain consciousness, despite the seizures stopping:
   (i) Medical consequences of the seizures:
      (a) hypoxia
      (b) hypo- or hyperglycaemia
      (c) hypotension

(d) hyperpyrexia

(e) cerebral oedema

(f) lactic acidosis

(g) iatrogenic over-sedation.

(ii) Progression of the underlying disease process:

(a) meningitis or encephalitis

(b) head injury e.g. extradural or subdural

(c) cerebral hypoxia

(d) drug toxicity e.g. theophylline.

(iii) Subtle generalized convulsive status epilepticus.

(iv) Non-convulsive status epilepticus:

(a) complex–partial (temporal lobe) seizures

(b) petit mal status.

TRANSIENT ISCHAEMIC ATTACK

DIAGNOSIS

(1) Transient ischaemic attacks (TIAs) are episodes of sudden transient focal neurological deficit, maximal at the outset and lasting for less than 24 hours, usually less than 10 min.

(i) They may recur and are important in that they are in a continuum that can progress to a reversible ischaemic neurologic deficit (RIND) lasting over 24 hours, or to a full-blown stroke.

(ii) Thus they herald a major ischaemic stroke or other serious vascular event in 12% of patients by 1 month, often within the first 1–7 days.

(2) The causes may be considered in three groups.

(i) Embolic:

(a) cardiac – post-myocardial infarction, AF, mitral stenosis, valve prostheses

(b) extracranial vessels – carotid stenosis, narrowed vertebral artery.

(ii) Reduced cerebral perfusion:

(a) hypotension from hypovolaemia, drugs or a cardiac arrhythmia

(b) hypertension (especially in hypertensive encephalopathy)

(c) polycythaemia, paraproteinaemia, or a hypercoagulable state such as protein C, protein S or antithrombin III deficiency, and with antiphospholipid antibodies

      (d) vasculitis, e.g. temporal arteritis, SLE, polyarteritis nodosa, or syphilis.

  (iii) Lack of nutrients:

      (a) anaemia

      (b) hypoglycaemia.

(3) TIAs present clinically as:

  (i) Carotid territory dysfunction causing hemiparesis, hemianaesthesia, homonymous hemianopia, dysphasia, dysarthria and amaurosis fugax (transitory monocular blindness).

  (ii) Vertebrobasilar territory dysfunction (posterior circulation) causing combinations of bilateral limb paresis, crossed sensory symptoms, diplopia, nystagmus, ataxia, vertigo and cortical blindness.

(4) Examine the pulse rhythm, heart sounds, blood pressure (in both arms and postural), listen for carotid bruits and perform a full neurological assessment.

(5) Check a bedside blood glucose test strip. Send blood for FBC, ESR, coagulation profile, blood sugar, ELFTs and a lipid profile in all patients.

(6) Perform an ECG and request a CXR.

(7) Arrange an urgent CT brain scan to differentiate haemorrhage from infarction, and to look for a structural, non-vascular lesion.

(8) Organize a duplex carotid ultrasound for a suspected carotid territory ischaemic event as soon as possible, certainly within the week.

MANAGEMENT

(1) Deciding who to admit can be difficult. Refer the patient for Medical admission if:

  (i) The ECG is abnormal, and a cardiac embolic source is suspected.

  (ii) TIAs are recurring over a period of hours or progress in severity and intensity (known as crescendo TIAs).

  (iii) A severe transient neurological deficit occurred or there are residual neurological findings.

  (iv) A significant systemic disorder is suspected.

  (v) The patient is a newly diagnosed hypertensive, or has a diastolic BP over 110 mmHg.

  (vi) Carotid territory disease is suspected in a younger patient, particularly if the patient has risk factors for atherosclerosis (see under *Acute Coronary Syndrome* for these on p. 14).

(2) Otherwise, commence low-dose aspirin 300 mg immediately then 75–150 mg once daily if complete recovery has occurred, and refer the patient to Medical or Neurology outpatients within 7 days.
   (i) Inform the GP by fax and by letter.

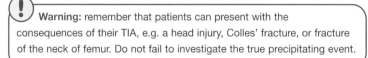

Warning: remember that patients can present with the consequences of their TIA, e.g. a head injury, Colles' fracture, or fracture of the neck of femur. Do not fail to investigate the true precipitating event.

STROKE

These are due to a vascular disturbance producing a focal neurological deficit for over 24 hours.

DIAGNOSIS

(1) The causes include:
   (i) Cerebral ischaemia or infarction (80%):
      (a) cerebral thrombosis from atherosclerosis, hypertension or rarely arteritis, etc.
      (b) cerebral embolism from AF, post-myocardial infarction, mitral stenosis or from atheromatous plaques in a neck vessel
      (c) hypotension causing cerebral hypoperfusion.
   (ii) Cerebral haemorrhage (20%):
      (a) intracerebral haemorrhage associated with hypertension or rarely intracranial tumour and bleeding disorders including anticoagulation
      (b) subarachnoid haemorrhage from ruptured berry aneurysm or arteriovenous malformation.
(2) Presentation may give a clue to aetiology.
   (i) Cerebral thrombosis is often preceded by a TIA and the neurological deficit usually progresses gradually. Headache and loss of consciousness are uncommon.
   (ii) Cerebral embolism causes a sudden, complete neurological deficit.
   (iii) Intracerebral haemorrhage causes sudden onset of headache, vomiting, stupor or coma with a rapidly progressive neurological deficit.
   (iv) Subarachnoid haemorrhage is heralded by:
      (a) sudden, severe '*worst headache ever*', sometimes following

exertion, associated with meningism, i.e. stiff neck, photophobia, vomiting and Kernig's sign (see p. 77)

(b) confusion or lethargy, which are common, or focal neurological deficit and coma, which are rare and serious.

(3) Record the vital signs, including the temperature, pulse, blood pressure and respiratory rate.

(4) Perform a careful neurological examination, recording any progression of symptoms and signs.

(5) Gain i.v. access and send blood for FBC, ESR, coagulation profile, ELFTs and blood sugar. Attach a cardiac monitor and pulse oximeter to the patient, and catheterize the bladder.

(6) Obtain an ECG and CXR, and arrange an urgent CT head scan. This CT scan may initially be normal with a cerebral infarct.

MANAGEMENT

(1) This is essentially supportive. Make certain a bedside blood glucose test strip has been done and give 50% dextrose 50 mL i.v. if it is low.

(2) If the patient is unconscious:

(i) Open the airway by tilting the head and lifting the chin, insert an oropharyngeal airway, give high-dose oxygen via a face mask and pass a nasogastric tube.

(ii) Place the patient in the left lateral position. Get senior ED doctor help.

(iii) Consider endotracheal intubation if there is respiratory depression, deteriorating neurological status and/or signs of raised intracranial pressure. Discuss this with the Intensive Care team.

(3) Otherwise, commence oxygen, and aim for an oxygen saturation above 94%.

(4) Refer the patient to the Medical team or Stroke Unit for admission and definitive management.

(i) *Avoid* the temptation to treat acutely raised blood pressure unless aortic dissection (see p. 28) or hypertensive encephalopathy (see p. 79) are suspected.

(5) Seek an urgent neurosurgical opinion for a cerebellar stroke presenting with headache, dizziness, vertigo, truncal or limb ataxia, gaze palsy and a diagnostic CT brain scan.

HEADACHE

DIFFERENTIAL DIAGNOSIS

Consider the serious or life-threatening diagnoses first:

- Meningitis
- Subarachnoid haemorrhage
- Space-occupying lesion
- Temporal arteritis
- Acute narrow-angle glaucoma
- Hypertensive encephalopathy

The majority, however, will be due to:

- Migraine
- Tension or muscle contraction headache
- Post-traumatic headache
- Disease in other cranial structures

The history is vital as physical signs may be minimal or lacking, even in the serious group. A new headache or a change in quality of a usual one must be evaluated carefully, especially in the elderly.

MENINGITIS

DIAGNOSIS

(1) Causes include meningococcus, *Streptococcus pneumoniae*, *Listeria monocytogenes* (infants under 3 months, adults over 55 years, and in alcoholism, cancer or immunosuppression), viruses and *Cryptococcus neoformans* and TB (immunosuppression). *Haemophilus influenzae* is now becoming rare following vaccination programs.

(2) Prodromal malaise followed by generalized headache, fever and vomiting occur, with altered mental status with irritability and drowsiness progressing to confusion or coma.

(3) Pyrexia, photophobia and neck stiffness are found. Localized cranial nerve palsies or seizures may occur.

(4) Eliciting signs of meningeal irritation is rarely positive (less than 10%):

   (i) Kernig's sign: pain and spasm in the hamstrings on attempted knee extension, with a flexed hip.

   (ii) Brudzinski's sign: involuntary flexion of both hips and knees on passive neck flexion.

(5) Always consider meningitis in the confused elderly, sick neonate, in generalized convulsive status epilepticus, and in coma of unknown cause.

(6) A petechial rash, impaired consciousness and meningism are classic features of meningococcal septicaemia, but these are relatively late signs. Therefore:
   (i) Look out for the earlier signs of possible meningococcal septicaemia (meningococcaemia) such as muscle pain including leg pains, abnormal skin colour with pallor or mottling, and cold hands and feet.
   (ii) Also rigors, vomiting, headache or abdominal pain and the rapid evolution of the illness within 24 hours.
   (iii) Progression to shock and obtundation indicate fulminant meningococcal disease.

(7) Gain i.v. access and send blood for FBC, coagulation profile, ELFTs, blood sugar, viral studies and two sets of blood cultures.

(8) Attach a cardiac monitor and pulse oximeter to the patient, and perform a CXR.

MANAGEMENT

(1) Give the patient oxygen and commence a normal saline infusion.

(2) Seek immediate senior ED doctor help.
   (i) Give ceftriaxone 2 g i.v. then 12-hourly, or cefotaxime 2 g i.v. then 6-hourly, plus benzylpenicillin 2.4 g i.v. or ampicillin 2 g i.v. (for *Listeria*), as soon as the diagnosis of meningitis is suspected.
   (ii) Give dexamethasone 10 mg i.v. then 6-hourly at the same time, if bacterial meningitis is strongly suspected, particularly when ill or obtunded.

(3) Then perform a CT scan, especially if there are focal neurological signs, papilloedema or mental obtundation.
   (i) Even if this CT scan is normal, a lumbar puncture should be delayed until these signs improve.

(4) Otherwise, consider LP, without CT if there are no focal neurological signs and the patient has a normal mental state.

(5) Admit the patient under the Medical team, or to the ICU if haemodynamically unstable or altered mental status.

SUBARACHNOID HAEMORRHAGE

DIAGNOSIS

(1) The majority of cases are associated with a ruptured berry aneurysm, in patients who may have a family history, hypertension, polycystic kidneys or coarctation of the aorta.

    (i) The remainder are due to an arteriovenous malformation, or rarely coagulopathy and vasculitis.

(2) Ask about any prodromal episodes of headache or diplopia due to 'warning leaks'. These may precede a sudden, severe '*worst headache ever*', sometimes following exertion.

(3) Lethargy, nausea, vomiting and meningism with photophobia and neck stiffness occur, although fever is usually absent or is low-grade.

    (i) A IIIrd nerve oculomotor palsy suggests bleeding from a posterior communicating artery aneurysm.

(4) Less typical presentations include acute confusion, transient loss of consciousness with recovery or coma, when a stiff neck and subhyaloid (pre-retinal) haemorrhages are useful diagnostic pointers on examination.

(5) Gain i.v. access and send blood for FBC, coagulation profile, U&Es, blood sugar and a group and hold. Attach a cardiac monitor and pulse oximeter to the patient.

(6) Perform an ECG and request a CXR.

MANAGEMENT

(1) Give the patient oxygen and nurse head upwards. Aim for an oxygen saturation above 94%.

(2) Give lorazepam 0.07 mg/kg up to 4 mg i.v., or diazepam 0.1–0.2 mg/kg up to 20 mg i.v., or midazolam 0.05–0.1 mg/kg up to 10 mg i.v. for seizures or severe agitation.

(3) Give paracetamol 500 mg and codeine phosphate 8 mg two tablets orally or rarely morphine 2.5–5 mg i.v. for pain relief, with an antiemetic such as metoclopramide 10 mg i.v.

(4) Arrange a CT head scan urgently to confirm the diagnosis.

(5) Proceed to perform a lumbar puncture if the CT brain scan is negative or unavailable, provided that 8–10 hours ideally have passed since headache onset and there are no focal neurological signs or papilloedema.

    (i) Always request xanthochromia studies by spectrophotometry of the CSF to differentiate a traumatic tap (absent) from a true subarachnoid haemorrhage (positive).

(6) Refer the patient to the Medical team or Neurosurgical unit.
    (i) Consider nimodipine 60 mg orally 4-hourly or an infusion at 1 mg/h, increased to 2 mg/h after 2 hours if the blood pressure is stable, when the diagnosis is confirmed and after specialist consultation.

SPACE-OCCUPYING LESION

DIAGNOSIS

(1) Causes include an intracranial haematoma, cerebral tumour, or cerebral abscess.

(2) The headaches become progressively more frequent and severe, worse in the mornings and exacerbated by coughing, bending or straining.

(3) Vomiting without nausea occurs, and focal neurological signs develop, ranging from subtle personality changes, ataxia, and visual problems to cranial nerve palsies, hemiparesis and seizures.

(4) Papilloedema may be seen, with loss of venous pulsation and blurring of the disc margin with filling in of the optic cup as the earliest signs on fundoscopy.

(5) Perform a CXR to look for a primary tumour and arrange an immediate CT head scan.

MANAGEMENT

(1) Give oxygen, and treat seizures with lorazepam 0.07 mg/kg up to 4 mg i.v., or diazepam 0.1–0.2 mg/kg up to 20 mg i.v., or midazolam 0.05–0.1 mg/kg up to 10 mg i.v.

(2) Refer a patient with an extradural or subdural haematoma to the Neurosurgical team.

(3) Otherwise refer the patient to the Medical team for full investigation.

TEMPORAL ARTERITIS

DIAGNOSIS

(1) This occurs in patients over 50 years, with relentless, diffuse or bitemporal headache often associated with a history of malaise, weight loss and myalgia.
    (i) Occasionally there is pain on chewing (jaw claudication).
    (ii) Polymyalgia rheumatica (PMR) with shoulder girdle weakness

and discomfort coexists in 30% of patients.

(2) Look for localized scalp tenderness, hyperaesthesia and decreased temporal arterial pulsation.

(3) Send blood for an urgent ESR (one of the few times this is really necessary in the Emergency Department!).

(4) The immediate danger is sudden visual loss due to ophthalmic artery involvement, which may affect both eyes if steroid treatment is delayed.

(1) Commence prednisolone 60 mg orally if the ESR is raised, or not available immediately.

(2) Refer the patient to the Medical or Ophthalmology team for admission for urgent temporal artery biopsy and continued high-dose steroid therapy.

ACUTE NARROW-ANGLE GLAUCOMA

See p. 429.

HYPERTENSIVE ENCEPHALOPATHY

(1) This is due to an acute accelerated or malignant hypertensive crisis, causing severe hypertension (diastolic over 140 mmHg), headache, confusion, vomiting, and blurred vision.

   (i) Look for retinal haemorrhages, exudates or papilloedema on fundoscopy.

(2) Focal neurological signs, seizures and coma may develop later.

(3) Gain i.v. access and send blood for FBC, ELFTs and blood sugar. Attach a cardiac monitor and pulse oximeter to the patient.

(4) Perform an ECG and request a CXR.

(5) Examine an MSU for proteinuria and send it for microscopy to look for evidence of renal disease, with casts or abnormal urinary red blood cells (greater than 70% dysmorphic).

(1) Give the patient oxygen, and aim for an oxygen saturation above 94%.

(2) Get senior ED doctor help and take expert advice.

(i) Aim to initially reduce mean arterial pressure (MAP) by 25% or aim for a diastolic BP of 100–110 mmHg within the first 24 hours.

(ii) Use oral treatment with labetalol 100 mg, atenolol 100 mg or long-acting nifedipine 20–30 mg.

(iii) Sodium nitroprusside 0.25–10 μg/kg per min i.v. with intra-arterial blood pressure monitoring is rarely indicated.

(3) Refer the patient to the Medical team for blood pressure control and to observe for the complications of heart failure, aortic dissection, intracranial haemorrhage and renal impairment (cause or effect).

MIGRAINE

DIAGNOSIS

(1) 'Common' migraine or migraine without aura is diagnosed by a history of at least five attacks that:
   (i) Last 4–72 hours if untreated.
   (ii) Have at least two of the following headache characteristics:
      (a) unilateral
      (b) pulsating or throbbing
      (c) moderate to severe
      (d) aggravated by movement.
   (iii) Have at least one associated symptom of:
      (a) nausea and/or vomiting
      (b) photophobia
      (c) phonophobia.

(2) 'Classic' migraine, or migraine with aura, is less common and has similar features to those above, plus a history of at least two attacks that:
   (i) Have a typical aura:
      (a) fully reversible visual, sensory or speech symptoms (or mixed), but not motor
      (b) visual can be uni- or bilateral flashing lights, zig-zag lines (teichopsia), fortification spectra and a central scotoma
      (c) symptoms develop over 5 min, or each symptom lasts ≥ 5 min but less than 60 min.
   (ii) Headache precedes, accompanies, or follows the aura within 60 min, although up to 40% can have an aura with no headache.

(iii) Or that have a less typical aura:
  (a) hemiplegic
  (b) ophthalmoplegic
  (c) basilar (ataxia, vertigo, tinnitus, nystagmus, diplopia, confusion).

MANAGEMENT

(1) Nurse the patient in a darkened room, give oxygen by face mask and an oral analgesic such as aspirin 300 mg two or three tables, ibuprofen 200 mg two or three tablets, or paracetamol 500 mg and codeine phosphate 8 mg two tablets.

(2) Give an antiemetic with antidopaminergic effects, such as metoclopramide 10–20 mg i.v.

(3) Give chlorpromazine 0.2 mg/kg i.v. if the above fail, with a fluid bolus of normal saline 10 mL/kg.

(4) Or consider a triptan such as sumatriptan 6 mg s.c. for resistant headache:
  (i) Side effects of tingling, heat and flushing may occur, or rarely chest pain and tightness.
  (ii) Sumatriptan is contraindicated in known coronary artery disease, previous myocardial infarction, and in patients with possible unrecognized coronary artery disease, such as men over 40 years or post-menopausal women, with CAD risk factors.
  (iii) Sumatriptan is also contraindicated within 24 hours of ergotamine-containing therapy.

(5) Discharge the patient back to the GP, after a discussion of precipitating factors such as fatigue, alcohol, caffeine, hunger, etc. that might then be avoided.

TENSION (MUSCLE CONTRACTION) HEADACHE

DIAGNOSIS

(1) Women are more commonly affected by muscle contraction headaches associated with stress but lacking any prodrome.

(2) The pain comes on gradually, and is bilateral, mild to moderate, dull, constant and band-like.

(3) Mild nausea, phonophobia and photophobia can occur, but are usually absent and vomiting is rare. Headaches often become chronic.

MANAGEMENT
(1) Give the patient an analgesic such as paracetamol 500 mg and codeine phosphate 8 mg two tablets orally 6-hourly.
(2) Reassure the patient and discharge back to the care of the GP.

POST-TRAUMATIC HEADACHE

DIAGNOSIS
(1) Headache following head injury may begin immediately or after a few days, and is present in up to 30% of patients at 6 weeks after mild concussion.
(2) Inability to concentrate, irritability, dizziness, insomnia and even depression may develop, known as the 'post-concussion syndrome'.
(3) Request an urgent CT head scan if there is persistent worsening of headache, recurrent vomiting, clouding of consciousness, or focal neurological signs, to exclude a subdural haematoma.

MANAGEMENT
(1) Treatment is supportive including analgesics, rest, and reassurance that complete recovery is the rule.
(2) Refer the patient back to the GP, as symptoms may persist for up to 1 year.
(3) Discuss patients with an abnormal CT scan with the neurosurgeons.

DISEASE IN OTHER CRANIAL STRUCTURES

DIAGNOSIS AND MANAGEMENT
(1) Iritis (see p. 428), otitis media (see p. 405), sinusitis or dental caries may all present with headache.
(2) Treatment is aimed at the underlying condition.

ACUTE ARTHROPATHY

Acute joint pain in the Emergency Department may be divided into three main types:
- Acute monoarthropathy
- Acute polyarthropathy
- Periarticular swellings

ACUTE MONOARTHROPATHY

DIFFERENTIAL DIAGNOSIS

It is important to distinguish between:
- Septic arthritis
- Trauma and haemarthrosis
- Gout or pseudogout

and occasionally:
- Rheumatoid arthritis
- Osteoarthritis

though these last two are more commonly polyarticular.

SEPTIC ARTHRITIS

DIAGNOSIS

(1) This may occur with penetrating trauma, which may be trivial (such as a rose thorn) or following arthrocentesis.

(2) Most cases, however, develop from haematogenous spread predisposed to by rheumatoid arthritis, osteoarthritis particularly in the elderly, i.v. drug abuse, diabetes mellitus, immunosuppression, disseminated gonococcal or meningococcal infection and sickle cell disease, often from *Salmonella*.

(3) Check temperature, pulse and blood pressure. There is localized joint pain, warmth, erythema and severely restricted movement, with a less precipitate onset than with gout.

(4) Send blood for two sets of blood cultures, FBC, ESR and CRP.

(5) Request an X-ray which will initially be normal, but subsequently may show destruction of bone with loss of the joint space.

(6) Or arrange an ultrasound scan, which is most helpful in demonstrating an effusion in joints such as the hip (see p. 373), or even a CT scan for the sternoclavicular joint.

MANAGEMENT

(1) Give an analgesic such as paracetamol 500 mg and codeine phosphate 8 mg two tablets orally.

(2) Refer the patient immediately to the Orthopaedic team for joint aspiration under sterile conditions, rest, i.v. antibiotics, and repeated operative drainage.

   (i) Joint aspiration should yield turbid, yellow fluid with a polymorph WCC greater than 50 000/mL, and fluid culture is positive in over 50%.

TRAUMATIC ARTHRITIS

DIAGNOSIS

(1) Severe joint pain is usually associated with obvious trauma, although occasionally the trauma is mild or even forgotten.

(2) Haemarthroses may also occur spontaneously in haemophilia A, haemophilia B (Christmas disease) or severe von Willebrand disease.

(3) Request an X-ray, although it may not always demonstrate an obvious fracture but may show only a joint effusion or periosteal elevation as supporting evidence of the fracture (e.g. scaphoid or radial head).

(4) Arrange joint aspiration performed by a senior ED doctor to look for a haemorrhagic joint effusion, with fat globules floating on the surface in cases of intra-articular fracture, if there is doubt about the diagnosis.

  (i) Also perform joint aspiration when septic arthritis cannot be excluded, or refer the patient directly to the Orthopaedic team.

MANAGEMENT

(1) Give analgesia and refer the patient to the Orthopaedic team as necessary. Management varies according to the joint involved (see *Section VIII Orthopaedic Emergencies*).

(2) Give factor VIII to a patient with known haemophilia A or von Willebrand's, and factor IX to a known haemophilia B patient.

  (i) Organize this as rapidly as possible in consultation with the Haematology team.

GOUTY ARTHRITIS

DIAGNOSIS

(1) Gout is much more common in men, and predisposed to by thiazide diuretic therapy, renal failure, myeloproliferative disease (especially following treatment), and dietary excess, alcohol, and trauma.

(2) It is commonest in the metatarsophalangeal joint of the great toe or knee, sometimes with a precipitate onset waking the patient from sleep.

(3) Chronic cases may be associated with gouty tophi on the ear and around the joints, polyarthropathy and recurrent acute attacks.

(4) The patient may be mildly pyrexial with a red, shiny 'angry' joint.

(5) Send blood for FBC, ELFTs, and ESR plus CRP if septic arthritis is as likely.
  (i) The laboratory blood result may show a mild leucocytosis, with a raised uric acid level (over 0.4 mmol/L), but the serum uric acid may be normal in up to 40% of acute attacks.
(6) Definitive diagnosis is by joint aspiration and polarizing light microscopy showing strongly negative birefringent crystals.
  (i) Joint aspiration yields cloudy yellow fluid, with a WCC of 2000–50 000/mL. Polarizing microscopy is diagnostic.

MANAGEMENT

(1) Give the patient an NSAID in a known relapsing case, or if there is strong clinical suspicion of gout, such as ibuprofen 600 mg orally once, then 200–400 mg orally t.d.s. or naproxen 500 mg orally, followed by 250 mg orally t.d.s.
  (i) Give colchicine 1 mg orally then 0.5 mg orally up to 4-hourly or diarrhoea occurs, if the patient has heart failure, or cannot take NSAIDs due to intolerance or asthma.
(2) Refer the patient back to the GP or to Medical outpatients.
(3) Refer the patient immediately to the Orthopaedic team for joint aspiration if septic arthritis cannot be excluded (see p. 83).

PSEUDOGOUT

(1) This is much less common than gout, typically affecting the knee or wrist, and is associated with diabetes, osteoarthritis, hyperparathyroidism, haemochromatosis and many other rare conditions.
(2) X-ray may show chondrocalcinosis, and joint aspiration shows weakly positive birefringent crystals under polarizing light microscopy.
(3) Treatment is as for acute gout, with referral back to the GP or to Medical outpatients for follow-up.

ACUTE POLYARTHROPATHY

DIAGNOSIS

(1) There are many causes, including:
  (i) Rheumatoid arthritis.
  (ii) Osteoarthritis.

    (iii) SLE.

    (iv) Psoriatic arthritis.

    (v) Ankylosing spondylitis.

    (vi) Reiter syndrome.

    (vii) Viral illness, e.g. hepatitis B, rubella, parvovirus B_{19}, and HIV.

    (viii) Serum sickness.

    (ix) Ulcerative colitis, Crohn's disease, gonococcus (early bacteraemic phase), Behçet's disease, and Lyme disease.

(2) Send blood for FBC, ESR, ELFTs, uric acid, rheumatoid factor, ANA and DNA antibodies.

(3) Request X-rays of the affected joints.

MANAGEMENT

(1) Refer to the Medical team for admission, bed rest, drug treatment and definitive diagnosis if the patient is systemically unwell.

(2) Otherwise, commence an NSAID analgesic such as ibuprofen 200–400 mg orally t.d.s. or naproxen 250 mg orally t.d.s. and refer the patient to Medical or Rheumatology outpatients.

RHEUMATOID ARTHRITIS

DIAGNOSIS

(1) This occasionally presents as a monoarthritis, though usually it causes a symmetrical polyarthritis affecting the metacarpophalangeal and proximal interphalangeal joints in particular, with morning stiffness.

    (i) Other joints affected include the elbows, wrists, hips and knees.

(2) Systemic involvement may occur with malaise, weight loss, fever, myalgia, nodules, pleurisy, pericarditis, splenomegaly, episcleritis and pancytopenia.

(3) Check FBC, ESR, rheumatoid factor, ANA and DNA antibodies.

(4) X-rays initially show soft-tissue swelling only and juxta-articular osteoporosis, followed by joint deformity.

MANAGEMENT

(1) Refer the patient to the Medical team for admission if systemically unwell.

(2) Refer the patient to the Orthopaedic team if septic arthritis cannot be excluded, remembering that rheumatoid arthritis actually predisposes to septic arthritis.

(3) Otherwise commence a non-steroidal anti-inflammatory analgesic such as ibuprofen 200–400 mg orally t.d.s. or naproxen 250 mg orally t.d.s. and refer the patient to Medical outpatients or the GP.

OSTEOARTHRITIS

DIAGNOSIS
(1) This usually presents as a polyarthritis of insidious onset, typically affecting the distal interphalangeal joints, hips and knees with pain on movement, but no systemic features.
(2) However, occasionally an acute monoarthritis exacerbation may be seen associated with marked joint crepitus.
(3) Request an X-ray that may show loss of joint space, osteophyte formation, and bony cysts.

MANAGEMENT
(1) Refer the patient to the Orthopaedic team if septic arthritis cannot be excluded.
(2) Otherwise, give the patient an NSAID analgesic and return to the care of the GP.

PERIARTICULAR SWELLINGS

See pp. 330–334 in *Section IX Musculoskeletal and Soft-Tissue Emergencies*.

ALLERGIC OR IMMUNOLOGICAL CONDITIONS

The following immunological conditions may present, ranging from those that are socially inconvenient to imminently life-threatening:
- Urticaria (hives)
- Angioedema
- Anaphylaxis

URTICARIA (HIVES)

DIAGNOSIS
(1) There are many immunological and non-immune causes, including:

(i) Foods – shellfish, eggs, nuts, strawberries, chocolate, food dyes or preservatives.

(ii) Drugs – penicillin, sulphonamide, aspirin, NSAIDs, codeine, morphine.

(iii) Insect stings, animals, parasitic infections including nematodes (in children).

(iv) Physical – cold, heat, sun, pressure, exercise.

(v) Systemic illness – malignancy including Hodgkin's lymphoma, vasculitis, viruses such as hepatitis A or Epstein–Barr virus (EBV) and serum sickness.

(vi) Idiopathic (over 90% of chronic cases).

(2) Itchy, oedematous, transient skin swellings are seen, which may occur in crops lasting several hours.

MANAGEMENT

(1) Give the patient a less sedating H_1 histamine antagonist such as loratadine 10 mg orally b.d. This is minimally sedating, unlike chlorphenamine.

(i) Refractory cases may respond to the addition of an H_2 histamine antagonist such as ranitidine 150 mg orally b.d.

(2) Attempt to identify the likely cause from the recent history. Most reactions occur within minutes but may be delayed for up to 24 h.

(3) Observe for any multi-system involvement suggesting progression to anaphylaxis (see later p. 89).

ANGIOEDEMA

DIAGNOSIS

(1) This is an urticarial reaction involving the deep tissues of the face, eyelids, lips, tongue, and occasionally the larynx, often without pruritus.

(2) The causes are as for urticaria, especially ACE inhibitors, aspirin, or a bee sting.

(3) It may cause facial, lip and tongue swelling, progressing to laryngeal oedema with hoarseness, dysphagia, dysphonia and stridor.

(4) Attach a cardiac monitor and pulse oximeter to the patient.

(5) A rare autosomal dominant hereditary form is due to C1 esterase inhibitor deficiency. A family history of attacks without urticaria, often following minor trauma, and recurrent abdominal pain are suggestive.

MANAGEMENT

(1) Commence high-dose oxygen aiming for an oxygen saturation above 94%.

(2) Give 1 in 1000 adrenaline (epinephrine) 0.3–0.5 mg (0.3–0.5 mL) i.m. into the thigh, repeated as necessary.

    (i) If rapid deterioration occurs, change to 1 in 10 000 or 1 in 100 000 adrenaline (epinephrine) 0.75– 1.5 µg/kg i.v.; i.e. 50–100 µg or 0.5–1.0 mL of 1 in 10 000 or 5–10 mL of 1 in 100 000 adrenaline (epinephrine) over 5 min i.v. The ECG *must* be monitored.

    (ii) Give 1 in 1000 adrenaline (epinephrine) 2–4 mg (2–4 mL) nebulized whilst preparing the i.v. adrenaline (epinephrine).

(3) Call the senior ED doctor urgently and be prepared to intubate if airway obstruction persists.

(4) Give H_1 and H_2 blockers and steroids, only when cardiorespiratory stability has been achieved (see below p. 91).

(5) Hereditary angioedema responds poorly to adrenaline (epinephrine). Give urgent C1 esterase inhibitor i.v. or fresh frozen plasma.

(6) Admit the patient when stable for 6–8 hours observation, as late deterioration may occur in up to 5% (known as biphasic anaphylaxis).

ANAPHYLAXIS

DIAGNOSIS

(1) Allergic anaphylaxis is an immunological, IgE-mediated multisystem reaction that may rapidly follow drug ingestion, particularly parenteral penicillin, a bee or wasp sting, or food such as nuts and seafood.

    (i) Non-allergic anaphylaxis (previously termed an anaphylactoid reaction) is a clinically identical reaction most commonly following radio-contrast media or aspirin or NSAID exposure, which is not triggered by IgE antibody.

(2) Respiratory manifestations:

    (i) Laryngeal oedema, hoarseness and stridor.

    (ii) Cough and bronchospasm (wheeze).

    (iii) Rhinitis and conjunctivitis.

(3) Cardiovascular manifestations:

    (i) Tachycardia, occasionally bradycardia.

    (ii) Hypotension, with massive vasodilation.
    (iii) Collapse with loss of consciousness.
(4) Other manifestations:
    (i) Gastrointestinal:
        (a) abdominal cramps or pain
        (b) vomiting
        (c) diarrhoea.
    (ii) Cutaneous:
        (a) erythema
        (b) local or widespread urticaria
        (c) pruritus
        (d) angioedema.
    (iii) Miscellaneous:
        (a) headache
        (b) joint pains and back pain.
(5) Attach a cardiac monitor and pulse oximeter to the patient.

MANAGEMENT

(1) Give high-dose oxygen via a face mask aiming for an oxygen saturation above 94%, and place the patient supine.
(2) *Laryngeal oedema and wheeze*
    (i) Give 1 in 1000 adrenaline (epinephrine) 0.3–0.5 mg (0.3–0.5 mL) i.m. immediately into the thigh.
    (ii) If rapid deterioration occurs, change to 1 in 10 000 or 1 in 100 000 adrenaline (epinephrine) 0.75–1.5 µg/kg i.v.; i.e. 50–100 µg or 0.5–1.0 mL of 1 in 10 000, or 5–10 mL of 1 in 100 000 adrenaline (epinephrine) over 5 min i.v. The ECG *must* be monitored.
    (iii) Give 1 in 1000 adrenaline (epinephrine) 2–4 mg (2–4 mL) nebulized in oxygen while preparing the i.v. adrenaline (epinephrine).
    (iv) Give hydrocortisone 200 mg i.v.
        (a) consider aminophylline 5 mg/kg i.v. over 20 min for persistent wheeze (provided the patient is not already taking oral theophylline).
(3) *Shock and circulatory collapse*
    (i) Give 1 in 1000 adrenaline (epinephrine) 0.3–0.5 mg (0.3–0.5 mL) i.m. immediately into the thigh, repeated every 5–10 min until improvement occurs.
    (ii) Give a bolus of normal saline 20 mL/kg i.v.

    (iii) If rapid deterioration occurs, change to 1 in 10 000 or 1 in
           100 000 adrenaline (epinephrine) 0.75–1.5 µg/kg i.v.; i.e.
           50–100 µg or 0.5–1.0 mL of 1 in 10 000, or 5–10 mL of 1 in
           100 000 adrenaline (epinephrine) over 5 min i.v. The ECG
           must be monitored.

(4) Second-line measures *after* achieving cardiorespiratory stability
    include:

    (i) Promethazine 12.5–25 mg i.v. or chlorphenamine 10–20 mg
        slowly i.v. plus ranitidine 50 mg i.v.

    (ii) Hydrocortisone 200 mg i.v. (if not given already).

    (iii) Glucagon 1–2 mg i.v. repeated as necessary, for patients on
        beta-blockers resistant to the above treatment.

(5) Admit all patients receiving adrenaline (epinephrine) for 6–8 hours
    observation as late deterioration may occur in up to 5%, known as
    biphasic anaphylaxis.

    (i) Discharge home on prednisolone 50 mg once daily,
        promethazine 10 mg t.d.s. or chlorphenamine 4 mg q.d.s. plus
        ranitidine 150 mg b.d., all orally for 3 days.

    (ii) Inform the GP by fax or letter.

    (iii) Refer all significant or recurrent attacks to the Allergy clinic,
        especially if the cause is unavoidable or unknown.

SKIN DISORDERS

The vast majority of skin disorders are managed by GPs and the
Dermatology Department. Some patients may present as emergencies
with blistering, itching or purpuric conditions. Exanthematous diseases
are common in children and young adults, and malignant melanoma
particularly in Australia.

BLISTERING (VESICOBULLOUS) CONDITIONS

DIAGNOSIS

(1) Common causes:

    (i) Viral:

        (a) herpes zoster

        (b) herpes simplex.

    (ii) Impetigo.

(iii) Scabies.

(iv) Insect bites and papular urticaria.

(v) Bullous eczema and pompholyx.

(vi) Drugs – sulphonamides, penicillin, barbiturates.

(2) Less common causes:

(i) Erythema multiforme major ('target lesions' rash, plus one mucous membrane involved) or erythema multiforme minor (1–2 cm 'target lesions' only):

(a) mycoplasma pneumonia

(b) herpes simplex

(c) drugs – sulphur and penicillins

(d) idiopathic (50%).

(ii) Stevens–Johnson syndrome and toxic epidermal necrolysis (epidermal detachment with mucosal erosions):

(a) drugs such as anticonvulsants, sulphonamides, NSAIDs and penicillins.

(iii) Staphylococcal scalded-skin syndrome (children).

(iv) Dermatitis herpetiformis (gluten sensitivity).

(v) Pemphigus and pemphigoid.

(vi) Porphyria cutanea tarda.

(3) Rare causes: congenital – epidermolysis bullosa.

MANAGEMENT

(1) Refer patients with widespread or potentially life-threatening blistering immediately to the Dermatology team or Medical team.

(i) This should include any patient with Stevens–Johnson syndrome, toxic epidermal necrolysis (TEN), staphylococcal scalded-skin syndrome, pemphigus and pemphigoid, who may die from intercurrent infection and multi-organ failure.

(2) Otherwise give symptomatic treatment including:

(i) Antihistamine orally such as promethazine 10 mg t.d.s. or chlorphenamine 4 mg q.d.s. if there is associated pruritus, with a warning about drowsiness.

(ii) Antibiotics orally such as flucloxacillin 500 mg q.d.s. for secondary staphylococcal infection in herpes zoster, impetigo, insect bites and eczema, or erythromycin 500 mg q.d.s. for patients allergic to penicillin.

(iii) Parasiticidal preparation for scabies (see p. 94).

(iv) Antiviral agent orally such as aciclovir 200 mg five times a day for 5 days for severe herpes simplex, or 800 mg five times a day or famciclovir 250 mg t.d.s. for 7 days for severe herpes zoster.

(v) Topical steroid antiseptic such as 0.1% betamethasone with 3% clioquinol cream t.d.s. for papular urticaria and bullous eczema.

(3) Return the patient to the care of their GP.

PRURITUS (ITCHING CONDITIONS)

DIAGNOSIS

(1) Causes of pruritus with skin disease:
   (i) Scabies, pediculosis, insect bites, parasites (roundworm).
   (ii) Eczema.
   (iii) Contact dermatitis.
   (iv) Urticaria.
   (v) Lichen planus.
   (vi) Pityriasis rosea ('herald' patch).
   (vii) Dermatitis herpetiformis (with gluten sensitivity).
   (viii) Drugs, which may cause any of the conditions (ii)–(vi) above.

(2) Causes of pruritus without skin disease:
   (i) Hepatobiliary – jaundice, including primary biliary cirrhosis.
   (ii) Chronic renal failure.
   (iii) Haematological:
      (a) lymphoma
      (b) polycythaemia rubra vera.
   (iv) Endocrine:
      (a) myxoedema
      (b) thyrotoxicosis.
   (v) Carcinoma:
      (a) lung
      (b) stomach.
   (vi) Drugs.

(3) Take a general medical history, and ask about medications.

MANAGEMENT

(1) Refer patients unable to sleep with intractable pruritus to the Dermatology team or Medical team.

(2) Otherwise give symptomatic treatment including:
   (i) Antipruritic drug orally:

  (a) promethazine 10 mg t.d.s. or chlorphenamine 4 mg q.d.s. with a warning about drowsiness.
  (ii) For scabies:
  (a) scabies is suggested by itch worse at night that does not involve the head, a close partner affected, and finding burrows (often excoriated) in interdigital webs, around the genitalia, or on the nipples
  (b) treat the patient and close contacts with 5% permethrin aqueous lotion over the whole body including the face and hair, washed off after 8–24 hours; all clothes should also be washed
  (c) explain to the patient that although itching may persist, it is no longer contagious
  (d) advise the patient to attend a Genitourinary Medicine clinic to exclude an associated sexually transmitted disease if the scabies follows casual sex.
  (iii) For urticaria, see p. 87.
  (iv) Cease any recent drug therapy considered causal, including non-prescription drugs.
(4) Return the patient to the care of their GP.

PURPURIC CONDITIONS

DIAGNOSIS
(1) Petechiae and purpura are non-blanching, cutaneous bleeding that may be non-palpable or palpable.
(2) Causes of non-palpable purpura include:
  (i) Thrombocytopenia with splenomegaly:
  (a) normal marrow:
      – liver disease with portal hypertension
      – myeloproliferative disorders
      – lymphoproliferative disorders
      – hypersplenism.
  (b) abnormal marrow:
      – leukaemia
      – lymphoma
      – myeloid metaplasia.
  (ii) Thrombocytopenia without splenomegaly:
  (a) normal marrow:

- immune: idiopathic thrombocytopenic purpura (ITP), drugs, infections including HIV
- non-immune: vasculitis, sepsis, disseminated intravascular coagulation (DIC), haemolytic–uraemic syndrome (HUS), thrombotic thrombocytopenic purpura (TTP).

  (b) abnormal marrow:
- cytotoxics
- aplasia, fibrosis or infiltration
- alcohol, thiazides.

(iii) Non-thrombocytopenic:
  (a) cutaneous disorders:
- trauma, sun
- steroids, old age.

  (b) systemic disorders:
- uraemia
- von Willebrand's disease
- scurvy, amyloid.

(3) Causes of palpable purpura include:
  (i) Vasculitis:
    (a) polyarteritis nodosa
    (b) leucocytoclastic (allergic), Henoch–Schönlein purpura.

  (ii) Emboli:
    (a) meningococcaemia
    (b) gonococcaemia
    (c) other infections: Staphylococcus, Rickettsia (Rocky Mountain spotted fever), enteroviruses.

(4) Ask about any drugs taken, systemic symptoms, bleeding tendency, travel history, alcohol use and known HIV disease.

(5) Check the temperature, pulse, blood pressure, SaO_2 and examine for hepatosplenomegaly and lymphadenopathy. Perform a urinalysis for casts.

(6) Send blood for FBC and film, coagulation profile, ELFTs and blood cultures according to the likely aetiology.

MANAGEMENT

(1) Management is of the underlying cause.

(2) This is urgent for meningococcaemia with ceftriaxone 2 g i.v. and for Rocky Mountain spotted fever with doxycycline.

Table 1.6 Common exanthematous diseases

Disease	Incubation period (days)	Prodrome	Rash	Other features and infectivity
Chickenpox	10–20	None	Macules, papules, vesicles and pustules of differing ages	Infective until all vesicles are crusted over (usually 6 days after last crop)
Fifth disease (erythema infectiosum)	7–10	Fever, malaise	Raised red 'slapped cheeks', diffuse maculopapular	Transient arthralgia, then relapsing rash; infective *before* onset of rash. Fetal abnormality
Glandular fever	5–14	Fever, sore throat, malaise	Transient maculopapular (rare); itchy drug rash with ampicillin (common)	Tonsillar exudate, cervical lymphadenopathy; hepatosplenomegaly; infective for many months by close physical contact
Measles	9–14	3 days of cough, cold, conjunctivitis	Red, confluent, maculopapular; lasts 7–11 days	Koplik's spots; cough predominates; may be quite ill; infective for 5 days after rash appears
Rubella	14–21	None	Pink, maculopapular, discrete; lasts 3–5 days	Occipital and pre-auricular lymphadenopathy; infective until rash disappears. Fetal abnormality
Scarlet fever	2–5	1–2 days of sore throat, fever, vomiting	Minute, red punctuate papules; last 7 days	Unwell; circumoral pallor; 'strawberry tongue'; infective until negative throat swabs following penicillin

EXANTHEMATOUS DISEASES

DIAGNOSIS

(1) Exanthems are generalized erythematous, often blanching, maculopapular eruptions, secondary to viral or bacterial infection.

  (i) Some have 'classic' clinical presentations such as chickenpox, fifth disease, glandular fever, measles, rubella and scarlet fever (see Table 1.6).

  (ii) Others are non-specific rashes, secondary to enteroviruses or respiratory viruses.

(2) Ask about recent known contacts, particularly at childcare or in school, as well as any constitutional symptoms such as fever and malaise.

(3) Most are diagnosed on clinical features, but serology for antibody titres may aid confirmation, particularly when there is concern following contact with a pregnant person.

MANAGEMENT

(1) Give symptomatic treatment, or phenoxymethylpenicillin 250–500 mg orally q.d.s. for 10 days in the case of streptococcal scarlet fever.

(2) Isolate the patient at home until non-infectious.

  (i) Rarely admission is indicated in the immunosuppressed, or patients with severe systemic features.

(3) Discuss pregnant contacts of a rubella or fifth disease patient with an infectious disease specialist or obstetrician.

MALIGNANT MELANOMA

The incidence of malignant melanoma has doubled in many countries over the last decade.

DIAGNOSIS AND MANAGEMENT

(1) Look for the following suspicious signs when a malignant melanoma is possible:

  (i) Major signs:

    (a) change in size, e.g. an increase in size of a new or pre-existing cutaneous lesion

    (b) change in shape, especially an irregular outline

    (c) change in colour.

(ii) Minor signs:
  (a) inflammation
  (b) crusting or bleeding
  (c) sensory changes, including mild itch
  (d) diameter 7 mm or more.

(2) Refer a patient with a pigmented lesion with any major sign urgently to the Dermatology team.

(3) Also refer a patient with a pigmented lesion and a minor sign, although less than 50% will have a melanoma.

(4) Remember that the most common sites for melanoma are on the back and on the legs.

THE ELDERLY PATIENT

(1) An increasing number of patients over the age of 65 years attend Emergency Departments and pose unique problems of their own.

(2) These problems begin in the waiting area, where old people may become frightened or confused due to their inability to see, hear or move easily, and understand instructions.

(3) Always consider particular factors before discharging an elderly patient. Ask yourself the following:
  (i) Can the patient walk safely with or without a stick?
  (ii) Can the patient understand new or existing medication?
  (iii) Can the patient get home safely and easily?
  (iv) Once home, can the patient cope with dressing, washing, using the toilet, shopping, cooking, cleaning or relaxing?
  (v) Can relatives or friends cope any more?

(4) Do *not* discharge the patient until seeking help from the following people if the answer to any of the above questions is '*No*'. If necessary, keep the patient in overnight to facilitate arrangements:
  (i) General practitioner:
    (a) the key person to coordinate the care of the patient at home
    (b) always contact by fax as well as by letter.
  (ii) Social worker (hospital- or community-based), who can offer:
    (a) home help
    (b) 'meals on wheels'
    (c) lunch and recreational clubs

(d) voluntary visiting services
(e) laundry service
(f) chiropody service
(g) home adaptation service
(h) emergency accommodation.
(iii) District or community nursing service: this includes an evening and night-time nursing service.
(iv) Health visitor.
(v) Domiciliary physiotherapist or occupational therapist.

DISORDERED BEHAVIOUR IN THE ELDERLY

A breakdown in a patient's normal, socially acceptable behaviour can be classified into three broad categories:
- Delirium – an acute organic brain syndrome
- Dementia – a progressive intellectual decline
- Depression – pathological, unrelenting and disabling low mood

DIAGNOSIS
(1) *Delirium*
   (i) This includes clouding of consciousness, inattention and failure of recent memory.
   (ii) It results in an acute or fluctuating confusional state with recent memory loss, associated with aggressive, restless behaviour and non-auditory hallucinations. It is often worse at night.
   (iii) Causes are many, including:
      (a) infection – pneumonia, urinary tract infection (UTI), cholecystitis, septicaemia
      (b) hypoxia – respiratory disease, heart failure, anaemia
      (c) cerebral ischaemia – TIA, stroke
      (d) cerebral lesion – haematoma, tumour, infection
      (e) iatrogenic – many drugs (remember poisoning, both accidental and deliberate), alcohol
      (f) vitamin deficiency – including thiamine, nicotinic acid, B_{12}
      (g) metabolic – including dehydration, electrolyte imbalance, hypoglycaemia or hyperglycaemia and thyroid disease
      (h) pain, cold, urinary retention, faecal impaction.

(2) *Dementia*
- (i) This includes disorientation in place, time and person, abnormal or antisocial behaviour, short-term memory loss, loss of intellect, and loss of insight. There is no clouding of consciousness.
- (ii) The causes are many, although a definitive new diagnosis is seldom made in the Emergency Department.
- (iii) However, look for and exclude the causes listed in (1) (iii) above if a known demented patient is brought into the Emergency Department with recent deterioration.

(3) *Depression*
- (i) This includes difficulty in sleeping, demanding, anxious or withdrawn behaviour, hypochondriasis, a loss of self-interest and a sense of futility.
- (ii) Suicide is a risk, particularly if the patient lives alone and is physically incapacitated, or has made previous attempts at suicide.

MANAGEMENT
(1) Delirium and decompensated dementia require hospital admission (do not simply sedate).
(2) Depression and a high suicide risk require urgent referral to a psychiatrist and possible hospital admission.

FALLS IN THE ELDERLY

DIAGNOSIS
Always consider the underlying cause and then the result, following a fall in the elderly:
(1) The cause of the fall:
- (i) Accidental:
  - (a) obstacles in the home, such as a trailing flex, the edge of a carpet, poor lighting, or no handrails
  - (b) inappropriate footwear.
- (ii) Musculoskeletal:
  - (a) arthritis
  - (b) obesity
  - (c) weakness
  - (d) physical inactivity.

(iii) Visual failure:
    (a) cataracts
    (b) senile macular degeneration
    (c) glaucoma.

(iv) Sedating drugs:
    (a) benzodiazepines
    (b) antihistamines
    (c) psychotropics
    (d) alcohol.

(v) Postural hypotension:
    (a) occult bleeding
    (b) autonomic failure
    (c) drug-induced.

(vi) Syncopal episode:
    (a) cardiac arrhythmia, infarction, heart block
    (b) vertebrobasilar insufficiency.

(vii) Cerebral disorder:
    (a) Parkinson's disease
    (b) ataxia
    (c) seizure
    (d) stroke.

(viii) Balance disorder:
    (a) inner ear disease
    (b) impaired proprioception.

(2) The result of the fall:

(i) Fracture:
    (a) Colles'
    (b) neck of femur or pelvis
    (c) skull
    (d) ribs
    (e) neck of humerus.

(ii) Hypothermia.

(iii) Rhabdomyolysis, pressure sores.

(iv) Hypostatic pneumonia.

(v) Fear, loss of confidence and independence, loss of mobility.

(3) All falls in the elderly, particularly if recurrent, must be diagnosed correctly, otherwise ultimately a fatal event will occur.

MANAGEMENT
(1) Refer the patient to the Medical or Geriatric team for admission if acute care is needed, or if there is any doubt about their ability to cope at home.
(2) Otherwise, refer to outpatients, physiotherapy, occupational therapy or social services and liaise closely with the GP.

FURTHER READING

American Heart Association (2005) Guidelines for cardiopulmonary resuscitation and emergency cardiovascular care. *Circulation* **112**:IV-1–211.

American Heart Association. http://www.circulationaha.org/ (CPR and ECC guidelines).

Australian Resuscitation Council (2006) Australian Resuscitation Council Guidelines 2006. *Emerg Med Australas* **18**:322-71

Australian Resuscitation Council. http://www.resus.org.au/ (resuscitation guidelines 2006).

British Infection Society. http://www.britishinfectionsociety.org/ (meningitis and meninogococcaemia).

British Society of Gastroenterology. http://www.bsg.org.uk/ (gastrointestinal bleeding).

British Thoracic Society. http://www.brit-thoracic.org.uk/ (pulmonary embolus, pneumonia, chronic obstructive pulmonary disease and pneumothorax).

DEY® (affiliate of Merck KGaA). http://www.anaphylaxis.com/ (anaphylaxis information).

European Resuscitation Council (2005) Guidelines for Resuscitation. *Resuscitation* **67**(**Suppl 1**):S1–190.

European Resuscitation Council. http://www.erc.edu/ (CPR and ECC guidelines).

Meningitis Research Foundation. http://www.meningitis.org/ (meningitis and septicaemia).

National Electronic Library for Health, NHS UK. http://www.nelh.nhs.uk/.

National Heart Foundation of Australia, Cardiac Society of Australia and New Zealand (2006) Guidelines for the management of acute coronary syndrome 2006. *Med J Aust* **184**:S1–S30.

National Institute for Health and Clinical Excellence, NHS UK. http://www.nice.org.uk/.

National Institute of Clinical Studies (Australia). http://www.nicsl.com.au/.

Resuscitation Council UK. http://www.resus.org.uk/ (resuscitation guidelines 2005).

Rothwell P, Warlow C (2005) Timing of TIAs preceding stroke. *Neurology* **64**:817–20.

Scottish Intercollegiate Guidelines Network. http://www.sign.ac.uk/.

Thompson M, Ninis M, Perera R (2006) Clinical recognition of meningococcal disease in children and adolescents. *Lancet* **367**:397–403.

ACID–BASE, ELECTROLYTE AND RENAL EMERGENCIES

ACID–BASE DISTURBANCES

ARTERIAL BLOOD GAS INTERPRETATION

Blood gas analysis provides information regarding potential primary and compensatory processes that affect the body's acid–base buffering system.

Acidosis is an abnormal process that increases the serum hydrogen ion concentration, lowers the pH, and results in *acidaemia*. *Alkalosis* is an abnormal process with decrease in the hydrogen ion concentration, resulting in *alkalaemia*.

(1) Blood gas analysis is used to:
  (i) Determine the adequacy of oxygenation and ventilation.
  (ii) Assess the respiratory function.
  (iii) Determine the acid–base balance.
(2) Interpret the arterial blood gas result in a stepwise manner as follows (see Table 2.1):
  (i) Determine the adequacy of oxygenation (PaO_2):
    (a) normal range 10.6–13.3 kPa (80–100 mmHg)
    (b) this provides direct evidence of hypoxaemia.
  (ii) Review the pH or hydrogen ion status:
    (a) normal range pH 7.35–7.45 (H^+ 35–45 nmol/L)
    (b) *acidaemia* is a pH < 7.35 (H^+ > 45 nmol/L)
    (c) *alkalaemia* is a pH > 7.45 (H^+ < 35 nmol/L).
  (iii) Determine the respiratory component ($PaCO_2$):
    (a) normal range 4.7–6.0 kPa (35–45 mmHg)
    (b) $PaCO_2$ > 6.0 kPa (45 mmHg)
      – acidaemia indicates a primary respiratory acidosis
      – alkalaemia indicates respiratory compensation for a metabolic alkalosis.
    (c) $PaCO_2$ < 4.7 kPa (35 mmHg)
      – alkalaemia indicates a primary respiratory alkalosis
      – acidaemia indicates respiratory compensation for a metabolic acidosis.
  (iv) Determine the metabolic component (bicarbonate, HCO_3):
    (a) HCO_3 normal range 22–26 mmol/L
    (b) HCO_3 < 22 mmol/L
      – acidaemia indicates a primary metabolic acidosis

- alkalaemia indicates renal compensation for a respiratory alkalosis.

   (c) HCO_3 > 26 mmol/L

- alkalaemia indicates a primary metabolic alkalosis
- acidaemia indicates renal compensation for a respiratory acidosis.

(3) This approach determines most primary disturbances of acid–base and the associated renal or respiratory compensatory changes.

(4) Remember:

   (i) Renal or respiratory compensation is always a secondary process and really should not be described in terms of an 'acidosis' or 'alkalosis':

      (a) thus in the presence of metabolic acidaemia, consider the respiratory compensation as 'compensatory hyperventilation' rather than a 'secondary respiratory alkalosis'.

Table 2.1 Determining the likely acid–base disorder from the pH, $PaCO_2$ and HCO_3

pH	$PaCO_2$	HCO_3	Acid–base disorder
↓	N	↓	**Primary metabolic acidosis**
↓	↓	↓	Metabolic acidosis with respiratory compensation
↓	↑	N	**Primary respiratory acidosis**
↓	↑	↑	Respiratory acidosis with renal compensation
↓	↑	↓	**Mixed metabolic and respiratory acidosis**
↑	↓	N	**Primary respiratory alkalosis**
↑	↓	↓	Respiratory alkalosis with renal compensation
↑	N	↑	**Primary metabolic alkalosis**
↑	↑	↑	Metabolic alkalosis with respiratory compensation
↑	↓	↑	**Mixed metabolic and respiratory alkalosis**

Note: respiratory compensation occurs rapidly by changes in $PaCO_2$. Renal compensation occurs more slowly by changes in HCO_3.

(ii) Chronic compensation returns the pH value towards normal, but overcompensation never occurs.

(iii) The presence of a normal pH with abnormal HCO_3 and $PaCO_2$ suggests both primary respiratory *and* metabolic processes are present:

    (a) pH normal: $PaCO_2$ > 6.0 kPa, HCO_3 > 26 mmol/L
       – dual primary process involving a primary respiratory acidosis and a primary metabolic alkalosis

    (b) pH normal: $PaCO_2$ < 4.7 kPa, HCO_3 < 22 mmol/L
       – dual primary process involving a primary respiratory alkalosis and a primary metabolic acidosis.

(5) Alternatively use an acid–base nomogram to plot and read off the interpretation of the arterial blood gas abnormality (see Fig. 2.1)

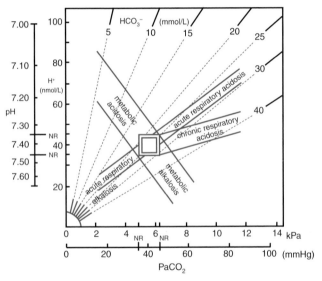

Figure 2.1 Acid–base nomogram for plotting interpretation of the arterial blood gas (NR is normal range)

METABOLIC ACIDOSIS

DIAGNOSIS

(1) An abnormal process or condition leading to the increase of fixed acids in the blood, best determined by a fall in plasma bicarbonate to less than 22 mmol/L.

(2) Metabolic acidosis may be associated with a high, normal, or low anion gap.

    (i) The anion gap is calculated from the equation
$[Na^+] - ([Cl^-] + [HCO_3^-])$ with all units in mmol/L.

    (ii) A normal anion gap is 8–16.

(3) Causes of a high anion gap metabolic acidosis (anion gap greater than 16) include:

    (i) Increased acid production:

        (a) ketoacidosis, e.g. diabetic, alcoholic, starvation

        (b) lactic acidosis (serum lactate more than 2.5 mmol/L):

           – type A: impaired tissue perfusion in cardiac arrest, shock, hypoxia, sepsis

           – type B: impaired carbohydrate metabolism in hepatic or renal failure, lymphoma, pancreatitis and drugs such as metformin.

    (ii) Decreased acid excretion, as in renal failure.

    (iii) Exogenous acid ingestion:

        (a) ethanol, methanol, ethylene glycol, iron, cyanide and salicylates.

(4) Causes of a normal anion gap metabolic acidosis (anion gap 8–16) include:

    (i) Renal:

        (a) renal tubular acidosis

        (b) carbonic anhydrase inhibitors.

    (ii) Gastrointestinal:

        (a) severe diarrhoea

        (b) small bowel fistula

        (c) drainage of pancreatic or biliary secretions.

    (iii) Other:

        (a) administration of synthetic amino acid solutions, ammonium chloride

        (b) recovery from ketoacidosis.

(5) The body compensates to reduce the acid load by hyperventilation. The expected compensatory reduction in $PaCO_2$ may be calculated (see Table 2.2):

    (i) The acidosis is partially compensated if the $PaCO_2$ value is higher than predicted.

    (ii) A primary respiratory alkalosis coexists if the $PaCO_2$ value is lower than predicted.

Table 2.2 Predicting the expected compensatory changes in $PaCO_2$ and HCO_3

	Metabolic acidosis	Metabolic alkalosis
Predicted $PaCO_2$ (kPa)	$0.2 \times [HCO_3] + 1$ kPa $(+/- 0.25)$	$\dfrac{[HCO_3]}{10} + 2.5$ kPa $(+/- 0.7)$
Predicted $PaCO_2$ (mmHg)	$1.5 \times [HCO_3] + 8$ mmHg $(+/- 2)$	$0.7 \times [HCO_3] + 20$ mmHg $(+/- 5)$

	Respiratory acidosis		Respiratory alkalosis	
	Acute	**Chronic**	**Acute**	**Chronic**
Predicted HCO_3 (kPa)	$24 + (PaCO_2 - 5.33) \times 0.75$	$24 + (PaCO_2 - 5.33) \times 3$	$24 - (5.33 - PaCO_2) \times 1.5$	$24 - (5.33 - PaCO_2) \times 3.75$
Predicted HCO_3 (mmHg)	$24 + \dfrac{PaCO_2 - 40}{10}$	$24 + \left(\dfrac{PaCO_2 - 40}{10}\right) \times 4$	$24 - \left(\dfrac{40 - PaCO_2}{10}\right) \times 2$	$24 - \left(\dfrac{40 - PaCO_2}{10}\right) \times 5$

(6) There are few specific clinical features in acute metabolic acidosis other than hyperventilation with Kussmaul breathing.

(7) U&Es confirm a primary fall in plasma bicarbonate below 22 mmol/L and usually an associated rise in plasma potassium.

MANAGEMENT

(1) Provide supportive treatment with oxygen, i.v. fluids and treat symptomatic hyperkalaemia (see p. 115).

(2) Correct any reversible underlying disorders:
   (i) Administer fluid and insulin, and replace potassium in diabetic ketoacidosis.
   (ii) Restore adequate intravascular volume to improve peripheral perfusion in lactic acidosis.

(3) Refer the patient to the Medical team. Dialysis will be necessary for renal failure, and severe salicylate or methanol poisoning.

METABOLIC ALKALOSIS

DIAGNOSIS

(1) An abnormal process or condition leading to a serum bicarbonate level of more than 28 mmol/L.

(2) Causes include:
   (i) Addition of base to extracellular fluid:

(a) recovery from organic acidosis secondary to metabolism of lactate and acetate

(b) milk-alkali syndrome

(c) massive blood transfusion (metabolism of citrate).

(ii) Chloride depletion:

(a) loss of gastric acid from vomiting or gastric aspiration

(b) diuretics.

(iii) Potassium depletion:

(a) primary (Conn's) and secondary hyperaldosteronism

(b) Cushing or Bartter syndromes

(c) severe hypokalaemia.

(iv) Other:

(a) laxative abuse

(b) severe hypoalbuminaemia.

(3) The body compensates to reduce the bicarbonate load by hypoventilation. The expected compensatory rise in $PaCO_2$ may be calculated (see Table 2.2).

(i) This effect can be profound. Compensatory arterial $PaCO_2$ levels as high as 11.5 kPa (86 mmHg) have been recorded.

(ii) However, this compensatory $PaCO_2$ elevation is variable:

(a) pain or hypoxia cause the respiratory rate to rise and the $PaCO_2$ to fall, thus worsening the alkalosis.

(4) There are few specific clinical features other than hypoventilation. Symptoms relating to associated hypocalcaemia and hypokalaemia may be present.

MANAGEMENT

(1) Give high-flow oxygen to reduce complications associated with hypoventilation. Try to avoid hyperventilation as this worsens the alkalaemia.

(2) Correct any reversible underlying disorder.

(3) Administer normal saline at 500 mL/h i.v to replace lost chloride, restore intravascular volume, and enhance renal bicarbonate excretion.

(4) Replace potassium with potassium chloride 10–20 mmol/h i.v. if the potassium is low.

(5) Consider the use of acetazolamide 250 mg orally to increase the rate of bicarbonate elimination.

RESPIRATORY ACIDOSIS

DIAGNOSIS

(1) A primary acid–base disorder associated with respiratory failure, inadequate alveolar ventilation and an arterial $PaCO_2$ greater than 6.0 kPa (45 mmHg).

(2) Causes include:
    (i) Loss of central respiratory drive:
        (a) drugs, e.g. opiates, sedatives, anaesthetic agents
        (b) cerebral trauma, tumour, haemorrhage, and stroke.
    (ii) Neuromuscular disorders:
        (a) Guillain–Barré syndrome, myasthenia gravis
        (b) toxins, e.g. organophosphates and snake venoms.
    (iii) Respiratory compromise:
        (a) chronic obstructive pulmonary disease (COPD), critical asthma, restrictive lung disease
        (b) pulmonary oedema, aspiration, pneumonia
        (c) upper airway obstruction and laryngospasm
        (d) thoracic trauma, pneumothorax, diaphragm splinting
        (e) high thoracic or cervical spine trauma
        (f) morbid obesity.

(3) Clinical manifestations of respiratory acidosis are secondary to the hypercapnia. Look for the following:
    (i) The patient is usually warm, flushed, sweaty and tachycardic with 'bounding' peripheral pulses, from cardiovascular stimulation.
    (ii) Acute confusion, mental obtundation, somnolence and occasionally focal neurological signs from increased cerebral blood flow, cerebral vasodilation and raised intracranial pressure.

(4) The body compensates to reduce acidaemia by minimizing the excretion of bicarbonate by the kidneys. However, this renal compensatory response is slow.
    (i) There is no time for any significant renal compensatory response in acute respiratory acidosis.
    (ii) The kidneys are able to retain bicarbonate in chronic respiratory acidosis lasting over a few days, so plasma bicarbonate levels rise and the pH returns towards normal.
    (iii) The expected compensatory rise in plasma bicarbonate in acute and chronic respiratory acidosis may be calculated (see Table 2.2).

MANAGEMENT

(1) Give oxygen and commence assisted ventilation by bag–mask ventilation. Call for senior ED doctor help and prepare for emergency endotracheal intubation.

(2) Correct any reversible underlying disorder, e.g. naloxone for opiate poisoning.

> **Warning:** the pulse oximeter may record a normal oxygen saturation in a patient receiving supplemental oxygen, despite the presence of dangerous hypoventilation.

RESPIRATORY ALKALOSIS

DIAGNOSIS

(1) A primary acid–base disturbance, associated with increased alveolar ventilation and an arterial $PaCO_2$ of less than 4.7 kPa (35 mmHg).

(2) Causes include:
   (i) Asthma, pneumonia, pulmonary embolus, pulmonary oedema, and pulmonary fibrosis (mediated by intrapulmonary receptors).
   (ii) Hypoxia (mediated by peripheral chemoreceptors).
   (iii) Centrally-induced hyperventilation secondary to respiratory centre stimulation:
      (a) head injury, stroke
      (b) pain, fear, stress, psychogenic, voluntary
      (c) fever (cytokines), pregnancy (progesterone), thyrotoxicosis, liver disease
      (d) drugs:, e.g. salicylate poisoning.
   (iv) Iatrogenic from excessive artificial ventilation.

(3) Clinical manifestations are secondary to hypocapnia, hypokalaemia and hypocalcaemia. Look for the specific effects of hypocapnia:
   (i) Circumoral paraesthesia, carpopedal spasm and tetany from neuromuscular irritability.
   (ii) Light headedness and confusion from cerebral vasoconstriction (usually adapts in 6–8 hours).
   (iii) Cardiac arrhythmias and decreased myocardial contractility.

(4) The body compensates to reduce alkalaemia by excreting or buffering bicarbonate ions.
   (i) A moderate compensatory response via a non-renal-mediated buffering process can reduce plasma bicarbonate levels to 18–20 mmol/L in acute respiratory alkalosis within hours.

(ii) The kidneys increase the rate of bicarbonate excretion in chronic respiratory alkalosis, and reduce serum bicarbonate levels to as low as 12–15 mmol/L returning the pH towards normal.

    (a) this renal compensatory response is slow. The maximal effect takes 2–3 days to occur.

(iii) The expected compensatory fall in plasma bicarbonate in acute and chronic respiratory alkalosis may be calculated (see Table 2.2).

MANAGEMENT

(1) Give oxygen to treat any coexistent hypoxia.

(2) Look for and correct any reversible underlying disorder.

(3) Never diagnose 'hysterical' hyperventilation until subtle presentations of pneumonia, pulmonary embolism (PE), pneumothorax, fever, etc., have been actively excluded.

(4) Otherwise if no significant underlying cause for hyperventilation is likely, reassure the patient and ask them to re-breathe into a paper bag.

ELECTROLYTE DISORDERS

Electrolyte disturbances are commonly associated with cardiovascular emergencies and may cause cardiac arrhythmias and cardiopulmonary arrest. Prompt recognition and immediate treatment of electrolyte disorders can prevent cardiac arrest.

POTASSIUM DISORDERS

Extracellular potassium levels are strictly regulated between 3.5 and 5.0 mmol/L and may be affected by many processes including serum pH. As pH rises, serum potassium falls as potassium is shifted intracellularly; when serum pH decreases, serum potassium increases as intracellular potassium shifts into the vascular space. The potassium gradient across the cellular membrane is essential to maintain excitability of nerve and muscle cells, including the myocardium.

HYPERKALAEMIA

DIAGNOSIS

(1) This is the most common electrolyte disturbance associated with cardiac arrest.

(2) Causes include:

    (i) Increased potassium intake:

        (a) oral or i.v. potassium supplements and transfusion of stored blood.

    (ii) Increased production:

        (a) rhabdomyolysis, tumour lysis syndrome

        (b) burns, ischaemia, haemolysis

        (c) intense physical activity.

    (iii) Decreased renal excretion:

        (a) acute and chronic renal failure

        (b) Addison's disease, hypoaldosteronism

        (c) drugs, e.g. potassium-sparing diuretics, ACE inhibitors, non-steroidal anti-inflammatory drugs (NSAIDs).

    (iv) Transcellular compartmental shift:

        (a) acidosis (metabolic or respiratory)

        (b) hyperglycaemia

        (c) digoxin poisoning, suxamethonium.

    (v) Fictitious:

        (a) haemolyzed specimen, thrombocytosis and massive leucocytosis.

(3) The risk of adverse events associated with hyperkalaemia increases with serum concentration levels. The severity of hyperkalaemia may be defined by serum potassium levels:

    (i) Mild hyperkalaemia: potassium more than 5 mmol/L.

    (ii) Moderate hyperkalaemia: potassium 6–7 mmol/L.

    (iii) Severe hyperkalaemia: potassium more than 7 mmol/L.

(4) Patients may present with weakness, ascending paralysis, loss of deep tendon reflexes, and respiratory failure.

(5) Gain i.v. access and attach an ECG monitor and pulse oximeter to the patient.

(6) Look for the characteristic ECG changes that are usually progressive and determined by the absolute serum potassium, as well as its rate of increase:

    (i) Tall, peaked (tented) T waves.

    (ii) Prolonged PR interval with flattened P waves.

(iii) ST segment depression.

(iv) QRS widening, absent P waves and sinusoidal wave pattern.

(v) Ventricular tachycardia and cardiac arrest from ventricular fibrillation, pulseless electrical activity (PEA) or asystole.

> ✓ **Tip:** consider hyperkalaemia in all patients with an arrhythmia or cardiac arrest.

MANAGEMENT

(1) Give high-flow oxygen via face mask. Cease any exogenous sources of potassium supplementation.

(2) *Severe hyperkalaemia* (more than 7 mmol/L) or hyperkalaemia with life-threatening ECG changes.

Provide immediate cardioprotection to prevent cardiac arrest:

(i) Give 10% calcium chloride 10 mL i.v. over 2–5 min, repeated until the ECG and cardiac output normalize.

(a) this does not lower the potassium level, but antagonizes the deleterious effects of hyperkalaemia on the myocardium, reducing the risk of ventricular fibrillation (onset of protection in 1–3 min).

(ii) Use the other therapies outlined below to shift potassium into the cells, and eliminate potassium from the body.

(3) *Moderate hyperkalaemia* (6–7 mmol/L).

Shift potassium intracellularly with:

(i) 50% dextrose 50 mL i.v. with 10 units of soluble insulin over 20 min (onset of action 15 min, with maximal effect within 1 hour).

(a) beware more rapid delivery of the 50% dextrose with the insulin as it may paradoxically release intracellular potassium due to its hypertonicity

(b) give the soluble insulin alone in hyperglycaemic patients with a blood sugar of more than 12 mmol/L (i.e. without the dextrose).

(ii) Salbutamol 5–10 mg nebulized. Several doses may be required (onset of action 15 min).

(iii) 8.4% sodium bicarbonate 50 mL i.v. over 5 min, provided there is no danger of fluid overload, as it contains 50 mmol sodium.

(a) less effective as a sole agent, but works well in combination with salbutamol and dextrose/insulin (onset of action 15–30 min).

(4) *Mild hyperkalaemia* (5.5–6.0 mmol/L).
   Remove potassium from the body with:
   (i) Frusemide (furosemide) 40–80 mg i.v. (onset of action with diuresis, provided not anuric).
   (ii) Potassium-exchange resin: calcium resonium 30 g orally or by enema (onset of action 1–3 hours after administration).

(5) Refer the patient to the Medical team, and according to the potassium level and underlying cause, organize urgent haemodialysis or peritoneal dialysis as needed, particularly in known renal failure.

HYPOKALAEMIA

DIAGNOSIS

(1) Hypokalaemia is associated with an increased incidence of cardiac arrhythmias especially in those patients with pre-existing heart disease.

(2) Causes include:
   (i) Inadequate intake of potassium, e.g. alcoholism, starvation.
   (ii) Abnormal gastrointestinal losses from vomiting, diarrhoea and laxative abuse.
   (iii) Abnormal renal losses:
      (a) Cushing, Conn and Bartter syndromes
      (b) ectopic adrenocorticotrophic hormone (ACTH) production
      (c) drugs, e.g. diuretics and steroids
      (d) hypomagnesaemia.
   (iv) Compartmental shift:
      (a) metabolic alkalosis
      (b) insulin
      (c) drugs, e.g. salbutamol, terbutaline, aminophylline.

(3) Hypokalaemia occurs when serum potassium level is less than 3.5 mmol/L and is defined as severe if the serum potassium is less than 2.5 mmol/L.

(4) Look for weakness, fatigue, leg cramps and constipation.
   (i) Polydipsia, polyuria, rhabdomyolysis, ascending paralysis and respiratory compromise may develop as the potassium level falls.

(5) Gain i.v. access and attach an ECG monitor. Non-specific ECG changes include:

(i) Flat or inverted T waves, prominent U waves.

(ii) Prolonged PR interval.

(iii) Ventricular arrhythmias, including torsades de pointes.

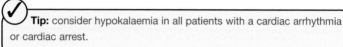

Tip: consider hypokalaemia in all patients with a cardiac arrhythmia or cardiac arrest.

MANAGEMENT

(1) Replace potassium immediately in the following situations:

    (i) Serum potassium below 3.0 mmol/L.

    (ii) Serum potassium 3.0–3.5 mmol/L in patients with chronic heart failure or cardiac arrhythmias, particularly if on digoxin or following myocardial infarction.

(2) Give potassium 10–20 mmol/h i.v. under ECG control using a fluid infusion device, but do *not* exceed 40 mmol/h.

(3) Give magnesium sulphate 10 mmol (2.5 g) diluted in 100 mL normal saline over 30–45 min in severe or intractable hypokalaemia, because magnesium enhances potassium uptake and helps maintain intracellular potassium levels.

(4) Change to oral supplements or maintenance i.v. replacement when the serum potassium is above 3.5 mmol/L.

(5) Refer the patient to the Medical team as necessary for treatment of the underlying condition.

SODIUM DISORDERS

Sodium is the most common intravascular cation. It has a major influence on serum osmolality and determines the volume of the extracellular fluid.

HYPERNATRAEMIA

DIAGNOSIS

(1) Hypernatraemia is defined as a serum sodium level of more than 145–150 mmol/L.

(2) Causes include:

    (i) Decreased fluid intake with normal fluid loss:

        (a) disordered thirst perception, e.g. hypothalamic lesion

        (b) inability to communicate water needs, e.g. CVA, infants and intubated patients.

(ii) Hypotonic fluid loss, with water loss in excess of salt loss:
    (a) skin loss from excessive sweating in hot climates and dermal burns
    (b) gastrointestinal loss from diarrhoea and vomiting
    (c) renal loss from impaired salt-concentrating ability, e.g. diabetes insipidus, osmotic diuretic agents, hyperglycaemia, hypercalcaemia, chronic renal disease.

(iii) Increased salt load:
    (a) hyperaldosteronism or Cushing syndrome
    (b) ingestion of seawater, salt tablets, or administration of sodium bicarbonate and hypertonic saline.

(3) Symptoms and signs of hypernatraemia are progressive and directly related to the serum osmolality and sodium levels. Look for:
    (i) Increased thirst, weakness, lethargy and irritability.
    (ii) Altered mental status, ataxia, tremor and focal neurological signs.
    (iii) Seizures and coma.

(4) Assess the underlying volume status. Look at the skin turgor, jugular venous pressure (JVP), measure lying and sitting blood pressures, listen for basal crackles.

(5) Send blood for FBC, U&Es, LFTs, and serum osmolality.

(6) Perform an ECG and request a CXR.

MANAGEMENT

(1) Give high-flow oxygen via a face mask.

(2) Replace fluid orally, or via a nasogastric tube in stable asymptomatic patients.

(3) Give hypovolaemic patients volume replacement with i.v. normal saline without causing too rapid a reduction in the serum sodium.
    (i) Aim to reduce serum sodium by 0.5–1.0 mmol/h.

HYPONATRAEMIA

DIAGNOSIS

(1) Hyponatraemia is defined by a serum sodium level less than 130 mmol/L.

(2) Causes include:
    (i) Fictitious 'pseudo' hyponatraemia:
        (a) associated with hyperglycaemia, hyperlipidaemia, hyperproteinaemia
        (b) correct the sodium for hyperglycaemia by adjusting the

serum sodium up by 1 mmol/L for every 3 mmol/L elevation in blood sugar.

(ii) *Hypovolaemic hyponatraemia.*

    (a) urinary sodium over 20 mmol/L: renal causes including diuretics, Addison's disease, salt-losing nephropathy, glycosuria, ketonuria

    (b) urinary sodium less than 20 mmol/L: extrarenal losses such as vomiting, diarrhoea, burns, pancreatitis.

(iii) *Normovolaemic hyponatraemia.*

    (a) urine osmolality > serum osmolality:

      – syndrome of inappropriate antidiuretic hormone secretion (SIADH) due to head injury, meningoencephalitis, CVA, pneumonia, COPD, neoplasia, HIV infection, drugs such as carbamazepine, NSAIDs, antidepressants

      – positive-pressure ventilation, porphyria

    (b) urine osmolality < serum osmolality:

      – hyotonic post-operative fluids such as 5% dextrose only, transurethral resection of the prostate (TURP) irrigation fluid, 'tea and toast' diet, psychogenic polydipsia, beer potomania.

(iv) *Hypervolaemic hyponatraemia.*

    (a) urinary sodium below 20 mmol/L: congestive cardiac failure, cirrhosis, nephrotic syndrome, hypoalbuminaemia, hepatorenal syndrome

    (b) urinary sodium over 20 mmol/L: steroids, hypertonic saline, cerebral salt wasting, chronic renal failure, hypothyroidism.

(3) Clinical features progress as the serum sodium level drops, but depend also on the rate of fall, i.e. the more rapid the fall the greater the symptoms:

    (i) Greater than 125 mmol/L: usually asymptomatic.

    (ii) 115–125 mmol/L: lethargy, weakness, ataxia, and vomiting.

    (iii) Lower than 115 mmol/L: confusion, headache, convulsions, and coma.

(4) Assess the underlying volume status. Look at the skin turgor, JVP, measure lying and sitting BP, listen for basal crackles.

(5) Send blood for FBC, U&Es, LFTs, thyroid function and serum osmolality. Send urine for sodium and osmolality.

(6) Perform an ECG and request a CXR.

MANAGEMENT

(1) Commence high-flow oxygen by face mask.
(2) Asymptomatic patients:
  (i) Discontinue implicated drug therapy and treat the underlying medical condition, e.g. antibiotics for sepsis.
  (ii) Restrict fluid intake to 50% of estimated maintenance fluid requirements in SIADH, i.e. around 750 mL/day.
  (iii) Aim to increase the serum sodium gradually by 0.5 mmol/L per hour, to a maximum rate of 12 mmol/L per 24 hours.
(3) Get senior ED doctor help if the patient has neurological symptoms.
  (i) Administer 3% hypertonic saline to raise serum sodium levels by 1 mmol/h.
  (ii) Consult with the Intensive Care team if the patient develops seizures or coma, and give 20% hypertonic saline 10–20 mL by rapid i.v. infusion.

> **(!)** **Warning:** too rapid correction of hyponatraemia may cause coma associated with osmotic demyelination syndrome or central pontine demyelinosis, or the underlying disease process itself.

CALCIUM DISORDERS

Calcium is the most abundant mineral in the body and essential for bone strength, neuromuscular function and a myriad of intracellular processes. Minor degrees of hypercalcaemia may be the first clue to an underlying diagnosis of malignancy or hyperparathyroidism.

HYPERCALCAEMIA

DIAGNOSIS

(1) Hypercalcaemia is defined by a serum level of more than 2.6 mmol/L after correction for albumin.
(2) Causes include:
  (i) Malignancy, sarcoidosis, thyrotoxicosis and TB.
  (ii) Primary or tertiary hyperparathyroidism.
  (iii) Drugs, e.g. thiazides.
  (iv) Addison's disease.
(3) Patients present with anorexia, thirst, weakness, abdominal pain,

constipation, lethargy and confusion or psychosis. Coma occurs at serum calcium levels of more than 3.5 mmol/L.

(4) Insert a large-bore i.v. cannula and send blood for FBC, U&Es, LFTs, calcium, lipase and thyroid function.

(5) Perform an ECG. Typical changes include:
  (i) Bradycardia.
  (ii) Short QT interval with a widened QRS.
  (iii) Flattened T waves, atrioventricular block and cardiac arrest.

(6) Request a CXR that may show an underlying cause.

MANAGEMENT

(1) Commence rehydration with 0.9% normal saline i.v. at 500 mL/h.

(2) Give frusemide (furosemide) 20–40 mg i.v. after urine output is established to maintain a diuresis.

(3) Refer the patient to the Medical team for longer-term therapy with steroids, biphosphonates or dialysis.

HYPOCALCAEMIA

DIAGNOSIS

(1) Hypocalcaemia is defined by a serum level of less than 2.1 mmol/L after correction for albumin.

(2) Causes include:
  (i) Chronic renal failure, acute pancreatitis.
  (ii) Rhabdomyolysis, tumour lysis syndrome and toxic shock syndrome.
  (iii) Calcium-channel blocker overdose.

(3) Patients present with paraesthesiae of the extremities and face, muscle cramps, carpopedal spasm, stridor, tetany, seizures, and cardiac failure.

(4) Look for hyper-reflexia and positive Chvostek's and Trousseau's signs:
  (i) Chvostek's sign is facial twitching from percussing the facial nerve in front of the ear.
  (ii) Trousseau's sign is carpal spasm after 3 min of inflation of a BP cuff above systolic pressure.

(5) Insert a large-bore i.v. cannula and send blood for FBC, U&Es, LFTs, CK, magnesium and lipase.

(6) Perform an ECG and look for:
  (i) QT interval prolongation, T wave inversion.
  (ii) AV block, torsades de pointes (cardiac arrest can occur).

MANAGEMENT
(1) Commence rehydration with 0.9% normal saline i.v. at 250 mL/h.
(2) Look for and treat the underlying cause.
(3) Administer calcium in asymptomatic patients by oral calcium supplements, or vitamin D-rich milk.
    (i) Symptomatic patients:
       (a) give 10% calcium gluconate 10–40 mL i.v.
       (b) discuss further elemental calcium infusion regimen with the Medical team or ICU admitting team.

MAGNESIUM DISORDERS

Magnesium is the second most abundant intracellular cation and essential for stabilizing excitable cellular membranes and facilitating the movement of calcium, potassium and sodium into and out of cells.

HYPERMAGNESAEMIA

DIAGNOSIS
(1) Hypermagnesaemia occurs at a serum level of more than 1.1 mmol/L.
(2) Causes include:
    (i) Renal failure.
    (ii) Iatrogenic magnesium administration.
    (iii) Rhabdomyolysis and tumour lysis syndrome.
(3) Patients present with muscular weakness, confusion, ataxia and hypotension.
    (i) Extreme magnesium toxicity of more than 5.0 mmol/L may be associated with bradycardia, respiratory depression, altered conscious level, and cardiac arrest.
(4) Insert a large-bore i.v. cannula and send blood for FBC, U&Es, LFTs, magnesium and thyroid function.
(5) ECG changes are similar to hyperkalaemia.

MANAGEMENT
(1) Commence i.v. rehydration with normal saline at 500 mL/h.
(2) Give 10% calcium chloride 10 mL i.v. for life-threatening arrhythmias and severe magnesium toxicity.
(3) Otherwise give a combination of normal saline i.v. and frusemide (furosemide) 1 mg/kg i.v. to increase the renal excretion of magnesium, provided the urine output is normal.

(i) Check regularly calcium levels to prevent hypocalcaemia, which will worsen the symptoms of magnesium toxicity.

(4) Refer the patient to the Medical team or ICU for consideration of dialysis in severe toxicity with levels more than 5.0 mmol/L.

HYPOMAGNESAEMIA

DIAGNOSIS

(1) Hypomagnesaemia occurs at a serum level of less than 0.6 mmol/L.

(2) Causes include:
(i) Increased magnesium losses:
(a) gastrointestinal loss from vomiting, diarrhoea, and pancreatitis
(b) ATN and chronic renal failure
(c) drugs, e.g. alcohol, diuretics, gentamicin, digoxin.
(ii) Reduced magnesium intake in starvation, malnutrition and chronic alcoholism.
(iii) Metabolic with low levels of calcium, phosphate and potassium.
(iv) Endocrine such as DKA, thyrotoxicosis, hyperparathyroidism, hypothermia.

(3) Clinical manifestations are non-specific and may mimic hypocalcaemia and hypokalaemia. Look for paraesthesia, tetany, altered mental state, ataxia, nystagmus and seizures.

(4) Insert a large-bore i.v. cannula and send blood for FBC, U&Es, LFTs, CK, magnesium, lipase and thyroid function.

(5) Perform an ECG and look for:
(i) Prolongation of PR and QT intervals.
(ii) ST segment depression.
(iii) Widened QRS and torsades de pointes.

MANAGEMENT

(1) Commence rehydration with 0.9% normal saline i.v. at 250 mL/h.

(2) Look for and treat the underlying cause.

(3) Administer oral magnesium supplements to asymptomatic patients.

(4) Start parenteral magnesium in more severe cases:
(i) Give patients with seizures, torsades de pointes, or cardiac arrest 50% magnesium sulphate 8 mmol or 2 g i.v. over 5–10 min.
(ii) Give other symptomatic patients 50% magnesium sulphate 8 mmol (2 g) i.v. at a slower rate over 30–60 min.

(5) Refer the patient to the Medical team and discuss further elemental magnesium treatment.

ACUTE RENAL FAILURE

DIAGNOSIS

(1) Acute renal failure leads to an abrupt, sustained increase in serum urea and creatinine secondary to decreased glomerular filtration rate (GFR), usually associated with oliguria or anuria.

(2) Causes include:

(i) *Pre-renal failure* (decreased renal perfusion)

(a) shock, burns, sepsis, dehydration, low-output cardiac failure

(b) renal disease such as renal artery stenosis, renal artery emboli.

(ii) *Intrinsic renal failure*

(a) ATN secondary to ischaemia, sepsis and toxins, e.g. gentamicin, radiographic contrast, myoglobin, ethylene glycol

(b) acute interstitial nephritis, infection, drugs, sarcoidosis, and autoimmune disease, e.g. SLE

(c) acute cortical necrosis secondary to protracted renal hypoperfusion

(d) acute glomerulonephritis

(e) malignant hypertension, vasculitis, e.g. Wegener's, renal vein thrombosis.

(iii) *Post-renal failure*

Obstruction may be extramural, intramural, or intraluminal at any point from the renal tubules to the distal urethra:

(a) causes include retroperitoneal fibrosis, ureteric strictures, calculi or crystal deposition, tumours such as uterine cancer, prostatic disease such as benign prostatic hypertrophy or malignancy

(b) proximal obstructions cause renal failure to single kidneys, or bilaterally to both kidneys.

(3) Take a thorough drug history to elucidate potential nephrotoxic agents, a common aetiology for intrinsic renal disease. Get an accurate weight on arrival as this will help monitor treatment progress.

(4) As acute renal failure is associated with multiple pathologies it may present in a variety of ways.

  (i) Pre-renal failure with symptoms and signs of hypovolaemia such as confusion, dehydration, orthostatic hypotension, oliguria and anuria.

  (ii) Nephritic syndrome with haematuria, hypertension, and generalized oedema from acute glomerular disease.

  (iii) Flank pain and haematuria.

(5) Examine patients systematically looking at:

  (i) Volume status:

    (a) signs of volume depletion include hypotension, tachycardia, decreased skin turgor, dry mucous membranes in patients with decreased renal perfusion associated with pre-renal conditions

    (b) signs of volume overload include a raised JVP, peripheral oedema and respiratory crepitations in intrinsic renal disease.

  (ii) Clinical manifestations of uraemia such as altered mental status, confusion, asterixis (flap) and seizures.

  (iii) Signs of post-renal obstruction such as an enlarged prostate on p.r. and cervical or uterine mass lesions on vaginal examination in females.

(6) Insert an i.v. cannula and send bloods for FBC, U&Es, LFTs, blood sugar, CK, calcium and uric acid. Take an arterial blood gas analysis. Attach a cardiac monitor to the patient.

(7) Organize a bedside bladder scan to determine the presence of urinary retention in post-renal obstructive renal failure.

(8) Insert an indwelling catheter and send an MSU for urinary osmolality and electrolyte screen to help distinguish pre-renal from intrinsic renal causes of renal failure. Request microscopy for signs of glomerulonephritis such as red cell casts or more than 70% dysmorphic red cells, myoglobinuria or infection.

(9) Perform an ECG to look for signs of hyperkalaemia, or an arrhythmia such as atrial fibrillation (AF) that may, for instance, be associated with renal embolic disease.

(10) Request a CXR to look for volume overload, metastatic disease and pulmonary–renal syndromes such as Wegener's granulomatosis.

(11) Arrange a renal tract ultrasound to look at the size of the kidneys, particularly for evidence of obstruction, or of shrunken kidneys suggesting an acute on chronic process.

MANAGEMENT

(1) Determine the need for urgent treatment.
   (i) Treat severe hyperkalaemia with 10% calcium chloride 10 mL i.v. (see p. 115).
   (ii) Arrange urgent dialysis for patients with refractory pulmonary oedema, pericarditis, or cardiac tamponade.
   (iii) Treat accelerated hypertension and any suspected sepsis including urinary.
(2) Otherwise, commence fluid resuscitation with caution.
   (i) Aim to optimize renal perfusion by treating any hypovolaemia, taking care not to precipitate life-threatening fluid overload.
(3) Closely monitor urine output.
(4) Refer the patient to the Medical, Renal or Urology team depending on the suspected underlying pathology, response to resuscitation, and any urgent requirement for dialysis.

FURTHER READING

American Heart Association (2005). Guidelines for cardiopulmonary resuscitation and emergency cardiovascular care. Part 10.1: Life-threatening electrolyte abnormalities. *Circulation* 112:IV-121–5.

American Heart Association. http://www.circulationaha.org/ (guidelines for cardiopulmonary resuscitation and emergency cardiovascular care).

European Resuscitation Council (2005). Guidelines for resuscitation. Section 7: Cardiac arrest in special circumstances. *Resuscitation* 67(Suppl 1):S135–70.

European Resuscitation Council. http://www.erc.edu/ (ERC guidelines and resuscitation practice 2005).

Resuscitation Council UK. http://www.resus.org.uk/ (resuscitation guidelines 2005).

INFECTIOUS DISEASE AND FOREIGN TRAVEL EMERGENCIES

FEBRILE NEUTROPENIC PATIENT

Neutropenia has a significant generalized infection risk with a temperature above 100°F (38°C) in patients with an absolute neutrophil count below 0.5×10^9/L, or below 1.0×10^9/L if the count is rapidly falling.

DIAGNOSIS

(1) Neutropenic patients may already know their diagnosis and/or be receiving treatment, or can present as a new case. Causes of neutropenia include:
  (i) Reduced neutrophil production:
     (a) aplastic anaemia
     (b) leukaemia, lymphoma
     (c) myeloproliferative syndrome
     (d) metastatic bone marrow disease
     (e) drug-induced agranulocytosis, including chemotherapy
     (f) megaloblastic anaemia crisis.
  (ii) Reduced neutrophil survival:
     (a) systemic lupus erythematosus (SLE)
     (b) immune-mediated
     (c) drug-related
     (d) Felty syndrome.
  (iii) Reduced neutrophil circulation:
     (a) septicaemia
     (b) hypersplenism.
(2) Ask about constitutional symptoms including fever and malaise, plus organ-specific features such as cough, frequency and dysuria, diarrhoea or headache and confusion.
  (i) Take a detailed drug history, contact and travel history.
(3) Record the vital signs and note any focal sources of sepsis including the skin, ears, throat and perineum, indwelling catheters, and evidence of anaemia or bruising suggesting a pancytopenia.
(4) Establish venous access with strict asepsis, and send blood for FBC, coagulation profile, ELFTs and two sets of blood cultures.
(5) Request a CXR and send an MSU.

MANAGEMENT

(1) Start initial empiric antibiotic therapy, unless there is a clear focal site of infection, after discussion with an Infectious Disease

physician or Microbiologist.

  (i) Give ticarcillin 3 g with clavulanic acid 100–200 mg i.v. q.d.s. *plus* gentamicin 5 mg/kg i.v. once daily
  (ii) Give ceftazidime 2 g i.v. t.d.s. if penicillin-sensitive, *plus* gentamicin 5 mg/kg i.v. once daily

(2) Admit the patient under the Medical team, even if the patient looks well with only a fever, as rapid deterioration may occur.

  (i) Refer haemodynamically unstable patients to the ICU.

HEPATITIS

DIAGNOSIS

(1) Causes of hepatitis include:

  (i) Viruses such as enterically transmitted hepatitis A or E, or parenterally spread hepatitis B, C, D or G, and infectious mononucleosis, cytomegalovirus (CMV) or herpes simplex virus (HSV).
  (ii) Bacteria such as leptospirosis, or amoebae.
  (iii) Toxins and drugs such as alcohol, *Amanita* mushrooms, methyldopa, statins, chlorpromazine, isoniazid, and paracetamol (remember the possibility of acute poisoning).

(2) Hepatitis presents with anorexia, malaise, nausea, vomiting, abdominal pain and joint pain.

(3) Look for a raised temperature, jaundice, tender hepatomegaly and splenomegaly. Assess for confusion or an altered conscious level.

(4) Send blood for serology for hepatitis A, B or C, plus FBC, coagulation profile, ELFTs and lipase.

(5) Test the urine for bilirubin and urobilinogen.

MANAGEMENT

(1) Refer unwell patients to the Medical team.

  (i) This should include those with persistent vomiting, dehydration, encephalopathy or a bleeding tendency with a prolonged prothrombin time.

(2) Otherwise, discharge the patient with advice to avoid preparing food for others and to use their own knife, fork, spoon, cup and plate (assuming the patient could have hepatitis A or E).

(3) Advise the patient to avoid alcohol and cigarettes.

(4) Give the patient a referral letter to Medical outpatients or to their GP for definitive diagnosis and follow-up.

GASTROINTESTINAL TRACT INFECTION

The commonest manifestation is sudden acute diarrhoea, often with vomiting.

DIAGNOSIS

(1) The causes of infectious diarrhoea include:

(i) *Toxin-related* diarrhoea from staphylococcal food poisoning which has a precipitate onset in hours, as does *Bacillus cereus* enterotoxin from rice, in which vomiting and abdominal cramps predominate.

(ii) *Viral* diarrhoea from the rotavirus in very young children and Norwalk-like viruses in older children and adults, with an incubation period of 1–2 days, sometimes occurring in outbreaks of non-bloody diarrhoea.

(iii) *Salmonella* with an incubation period of 6–72 hours and *Shigella* infections with an incubation period of 1–3 days result in fever, malaise, diarrhoea (which may be blood-stained), vomiting and abdominal pain.

(iv) *Campylobacter* infection has an incubation period of 2–5 days and presents with colicky abdominal pain, which may precede the onset of diarrhoea, that is watery and offensive, and sometimes blood-stained.

(v) *Giardiasis* has an incubation period of 3–25 days and causes explosive watery diarrhoea, which often persists for weeks. Chronic infection may eventually cause malabsorption with steatorrhoea. Ask about travel to Russia or North America.

(vi) *Amoebiasis* may also cause a chronic, recurring diarrhoea, with stools containing blood and mucus. Ask about travel to Africa, Asia or Latin America.

(vii) '*Traveller's diarrhoea*' is most often due to enterotoxigenic *Escherichia coli*, and is usually self-limiting over 2–5 days, causing watery stools and occasionally vomiting. Fever is not a feature.

(2) The most important feature, apart from ascertaining a contact or travel history, is assessing the patient for dehydration in all cases.

   (i) Dehydration causes thirst, lassitude, dry lax skin, tachycardia, and postural hypotension, leading to oliguria, confusion and coma when critical.

(3) Also consider the non-infectious causes of acute diarrhoea including drug-related, *Clostridium difficile* antibiotic-related diarrhoea (CDAD), Crohn's disease, ulcerative colitis, ischaemic colitis, irritable bowel syndrome, and 'spurious' from faecal impaction.

(4) Send blood for FBC and ELFTs, and commence an i.v. infusion of normal saline in all dehydrated, febrile, or toxic patients.

   (i) Send a stool specimen for *Clostridium difficile* toxin assay, if antibiotic-associated diarrhoea is suspected following any antibiotic use in the previous 3 months.

MANAGEMENT

(1) Admit dehydrated, toxic, very young or elderly, and immunosuppressed patients for rehydration.

(2) Allow other patients home and encourage them to drink plenty of fluid.

   (i) Alternatively, give the patient an oral glucose and electrolyte rehydration solution, which may also be purchased over-the-counter.

   (ii) Give an antimotility agent such as loperamide 4 mg initially, followed by 2 mg after each loose stool to a maximum of 16 mg/day (not in children).

(3) Ask the patient to return within 24–48 hours if symptoms persist:

   (i) Send stools for microscopy and culture now.

   (ii) Consider empirical treatment for moderate to severe systemic illness with bloody diarrhoea or for associated rigors.

      (a) give ciprofloxacin 500 mg orally b.d. for 5–7 days (not in children).

   (iii) Give tinidazole 2 g orally once if *Giardia* is suspected.

   (iv) Arrange follow-up in Medical outpatients or by the local GP.

SEXUALLY TRANSMITTED DISEASES

DIAGNOSIS

(1) A sexually transmitted disease (STD) may be caused by non-specific infection, *Chlamydia*, gonococcus, herpes simplex, human papilloma virus, *Trichomonas*, scabies or lice, syphilis, and of course HIV.

(2) Males may present with dysuria, urethral discharge, penile ulceration, warts, epididymo-orchitis and balanitis.

(3) Females may present with vaginal discharge, vaginal pruritus, ulceration, warts, menstrual irregularities and abdominal pain.
   (i) Pelvic inflammatory disease is commonly sexually acquired (see p. 383).

(4) Take swabs for bacterial, viral and chlamydial studies for microscopy, culture and nucleic acid amplification, if you intend to commence treatment.
   (i) Discuss the swabs and transport medium with your microbiology lab if you are unsure.

MANAGEMENT

(1) All STDs deserve expert diagnosis, treatment, follow-up and partner-contact tracing readily available in the Genitourinary Medicine clinic (Special Clinic).

(2) As many patients are reluctant to attend these clinics, explain carefully the local appointment system, what to expect, and how to locate the clinic, and refer the patient on.
   (i) Advise males not to empty the bladder for at least 4 hours before attendance.

(3) Commence empiric antibiotic treatment in the homeless or itinerant patient considered unlikely to attend any clinic.
   (i) Give azithromycin 1 g orally as a single dose *plus* ceftriaxone 250 mg i.m. or ciprofloxacin 500 mg orally one dose for urethritis.

(4) In addition, consider treating the patient with an immediately painful condition such as genital herpes simplex:
   (i) Give aciclovir 200 mg orally five times a day or famciclovir 125 mg orally b.d. for 5 days.

(5) Admit patients under the Medical or Gynaecology team for

treatment of the acute manifestations of HIV infection, secondary syphilis, acute Reiter syndrome, disseminated gonococcal infection, severe primary genital herpes, or acute severe salpingitis.

HUMAN IMMUNODEFICIENCY VIRUS (HIV) INFECTION

DIAGNOSIS

(1) HIV is a cytopathic RNA retrovirus. It is transmitted by sexual contact, by syringe sharing in intravenous drug abusers, transplacentally, and rarely now by blood transfusion.

(2) HIV risk groups include:
- (i) Homosexual and bisexual males.
- (ii) Intravenous drug abusers.
- (iii) Heterosexual partners of HIV patients.
- (iv) Children of affected mothers.
- (v) Haemophiliacs and transfusion recipients in the early 1980s.

(3) The original CDC classification of HIV infection (Centers for Disease Control and Prevention 1986) is:
- (i) Group 1: acute infection.
- (ii) Group 2: asymptomatic infection.
- (iii) Group 3: persistent generalized lymphadenopathy (PGL).
- (iv) Group 4: symptomatic infection:
  - (a) subgroup A – non-specific constitutional disease
  - (b) subgroup B – neurological disease
  - (c) subgroup C – secondary infectious diseases categories C1 and C2
  - (d) subgroup D – secondary cancers
  - (e) subgroup E – other conditions.

(4) The revised Classification System for HIV Infection and Expanded Surveillance Case Definition for AIDS Among Adolescents and Adults was published by the CDC in 1993:
- (i) This emphasized the clinical importance of the absolute CD4+ T-lymphocyte count or its percentage of the total lymphocyte count.
- (ii) Three categories of CD4+ count were recognized for medical management purposes:

      (a) CD4 count ≥ 500/μL

      (b) CD4 count 200–499/μL

      (c) CD4 count below 200/μL.

    (iii) A CD4+ count under 200/μL or 14% may be used to define acquired immune deficiency syndrome (AIDS).

(5) Presentation varies according to the disease group.

    (i) Group 1 – Acute infection:

      (a) 50–70% of patients infected with HIV develop an acute illness with lethargy, fever, pharyngitis, myalgia, rash and lymphadenopathy about 2 weeks after exposure. Acute meningitis or encephalitis are occasionally seen

      (b) although the patient is infectious, serology for HIV antibodies at this early stage will be negative.

    (ii) Group 2 – Asymptomatic infection:

      (a) the acute infection symptoms usually resolve by 3 weeks

      (b) infected patients seroconvert to HIV-positive over the next 4 months, most within 2–12 weeks of exposure

      (c) 50% of these patients will have fully developed AIDS by 10 years, with a near 100% mortality, although disease progression is slowing with modern highly-active antiretroviral therapy.

    (iii) Group 3 – Persistent generalized lymphadenopathy:

      (a) enlarged nodes in two or more non-contiguous extra-inguinal sites for at least 3 months and not due to a disease other than HIV

      (b) the patient is otherwise relatively well and enters a latency period of 2–10 years or more.

    (iv) Group 4 – Symptomatic infection:

      (a) subgroup A: constitutional disease with persistent fever, unexplained weight loss of 10% body mass or diarrhoea for over 1 month

      (b) subgroup B: neurological disease, including encephalopathy, myelopathy and peripheral neuropathy

      (c) subgroup C: secondary infectious diseases due to opportunistic infections occur as the CD4+ count drops usually below 200/μL. These include *Pneumocystis carinii* pneumonia, recurrent pneumonia, *Mycobacterium tuberculosis*, atypical mycobacteria, toxoplasmosis, cryptosporidiosis, isosporiasis, strongyloidosis, cytomegalovirus, systemic candidiasis, cryptococcosis, and many others

(d) subgroup D: secondary cancers including Kaposi's sarcoma, high-grade non-Hodgkin's lymphoma, primary lymphoma of the brain, and invasive cervical cancer

(e) subgroup E: other conditions such as the HIV-wasting syndrome and chronic lymphoid interstitial pneumonitis.

(6) AIDS-defining illnesses in a HIV-positive patient are in subgroups B to E, most commonly *Pneumocystis carinii* pneumonia and *Cryptococcus neoformans* meningitis.

(7) Thus, patients encountered in the Emergency Department infected with HIV will range from the asymptomatic carrier state in the majority, to non-specific illness or acute problems as varied as collapse, respiratory failure, gastrointestinal bleeding, skin disorders, depression, dementia, stroke and coma.

(8) Always maintain a high index of suspicion to identify the HIV-risk patient, if necessary by direct questioning.

(9) Send blood preferably for HIV antigen if the patient is acutely unwell with possible HIV illness, requesting nucleic acid amplification (NAA) techniques such as polymerase chain reaction (PCR) for HIV, viral RNA or the p24 antigen, rather than simple antibody testing.

(10) Otherwise, routine HIV testing in the Emergency Department is inappropriate as skilled counselling and follow-up are not available.

(i) Also relying on a single serum test for HIV antibody to establish or exclude HIV infection is unwise as:

(a) occasional false positives occur

(b) false negatives occur in those infected due to:
   – early infection
   – lack of seroconversion in the first 4 months.

MANAGEMENT

(1) Consider all patients to be potentially infected and adopt Universal Blood and Body Fluids Precautions with *every* patient to prevent any disease transmission:

(i) Always wash hands before and after contact with patients.

(ii) Wear gloves when handling blood specimens and body fluids.

(iii) Wear disposable aprons if there is likely to be contamination of clothing (e.g. from bleeding), and face masks and goggles if splashing is a possibility.

(iv) Take great care handling needles or scalpel blades, particularly

on disposal.
(v) Clean blood spills immediately with a suitable chlorine-based disinfectant.
(2) Refer the patient to the Medical team in the usual way if he or she is acutely ill.
(i) Otherwise refer the patient to the Genitourinary Medicine clinic (Special Clinic), Infectious Disease clinic or to the appropriate Medical outpatient clinic for complete and ongoing care.

NEEDLESTICK AND SHARPS INCIDENTS

INOCULATION INCIDENT WITH HIV RISK

DIAGNOSIS
(1) The risk of seroconversion is 0.1–0.5% following accidental inoculation of blood or infectious material from a suspected HIV-positive person.
(2) This risk depends on the nature and extent of the inoculation, and the viral disease activity of the HIV-positive source.
(3) Take 10 mL clotted blood from the injured person, and if possible 10 mL with consent from the source. Send for HIV, Hep B and Hep C testing, clearly marking the specimen as 'needlestick/sharps injury'.

MANAGEMENT
(1) Use a skin antiseptic such as 0.5% chlorhexidine in 70% alcohol and encourage bleeding by local venous occlusion.
(2) When the source is known to be HIV-positive with a high viral load or late-stage disease, and higher-risk exposure has occurred, e.g. deep needlestick or laceration with blood inoculated, proceed as follows:
(i) Discuss the situation with an Infectious Diseases specialist.
(ii) On their advice, commence immediate (within hours) triple antiretroviral therapy such as zidovudine 300 mg orally b.d., lamivudine 150 mg orally b.d. and nelfinavir 1.25 g orally b.d. or indinavir 800 mg orally t.d.s., all for 4 weeks. Check your local policy for regional variations.

(iii) The side effects of these drugs are complex and significant, including fatigue, headache, anorexia, nausea, vomiting, and blood dyscrasias.

(3) When the source is HIV-positive with a low viral load and lower-risk exposure has occurred, e.g. superficial scratch or mucous membrane contamination, commence zidovudine and lamivudine only, as above, or according to local policy.

(4) Refer the injured person to Occupational Health for follow-up with repeated serology and monitoring blood tests for up to 6 months, advice and counselling with psychological support.

(i) Report the incident to the senior ED doctor and Infection Control officer.

(ii) The exposed person needs follow-up for 6 months, should practise safe sex, should not donate blood, and should avoid pregnancy.

(iii) Assure confidentiality and sensitivity for all concerned.

(5) Consider the additional possibility of transmission of hepatitis B and the need for tetanus prophylaxis (see p. 323).

INOCULATION INCIDENT WITH HEPATITIS B RISK

DIAGNOSIS

(1) The risk of seroconversion in a non-immunized person following a needlestick injury with HBV-positive blood is 5–40%, and following injury with HCV-positive blood is 3–10%.

(2) Take 10 mL clotted blood from the injured person, and if possible 10 mL with consent from the source. Send for Hep B, Hep C and HIV testing, clearly marking the specimen as 'needlestick/sharps injury'.

MANAGEMENT

(1) Wash the area with soap and water, dress the wound, and give tetanus prophylaxis.

(2) Use Table 3.1 to determine the need for hepatitis B prophylaxis following significant percutaneous, ocular or mucous membrane exposure in persons without adequate immunity, i.e. anti-HBs levels unrecordable or less than 10 IU/mL. Check your local policy for regional variations.

(3) Refer the injured person to Occupational Health for follow-up, with repeated serology and monitoring blood tests for up to 6 months.

(i) Inform the senior ED doctor and Infection Control officer.

(ii) The exposed person needs follow-up for 6 months, should practise safe sex, should not donate blood, and should avoid pregnancy.

(iii) Assure confidentiality and sensitivity for all concerned.

Table 3.1 Hepatitis B prophylaxis following significant percutaneous, ocular or mucous membrane exposure for persons without adequate immunity

Exposure source	Exposed person
Test for **HBsAg**	Test for **anti-HBs** (unless recent satisfactory level of ≥ 10 IU/mL is known)
HBsAg +ve, or cannot be identified and tested rapidly	**anti-HBs** –ve or < 10 IU/mL, give: **HBIG**[a] **HB vaccine**[b]
HBsAg –ve	**anti-HBs** –ve, offer: **HB vaccine**[c]

anti-HBs, antibody to HbsAg; HB vaccine, hepatitis B vaccine; HBIG, hepatitis B immunoglobulin; HBsAg, hepatitis B surface antigen.
[a]HBIG: 400 IU i.m. for adults, or 100 IU i.m. for children under 30 kg, within 72 hours.
[b]HB vaccine: 1 mL i.m. within 7 days, then at 1–2 months, and a third dose at 6 months.
[c]Injury indicates evidence that the work area represents a significant exposure risk, so full vaccination is encouraged for the injured (exposed) person.

COMMON IMPORTED DISEASES OF TRAVELLERS

Ask patients who have been travelling abroad specifically about the time, place and type of travel. Also ask how much time they spent in each foreign country and how long they have been back for.

Enquire specifically about malaria prophylaxis and whether it was taken for 4 weeks after leaving the malarial zone, and about immunizations before going abroad.

Advice on tropical diseases is always available from local Infectious Disease physicians, specialist Tropical Disease hospitals and now the Internet. The CDC travellers' health website (open access) has information covering all aspects of foreign travel, including lists of recent disease outbreaks, and details on illnesses in alphabetical order from African sleeping sickness to yellow fever (see http://www.cdc.gov/travel/index.htm).

Remember that the returned traveller is as likely to have a condition that is not considered 'tropical', such as an STD including HIV infection, meningococcal infection, pneumonia, pyelonephritis, and simple gastrointestinal infection.

The tropical diseases discussed below may be endemic but are more frequently contracted abroad.

MALARIA

DIAGNOSIS

(1) Falciparum malaria is the most dangerous form of malaria and may prove rapidly fatal. Most cases are imported from sub-Saharan Africa, South-East Asia, Papua New Guinea, the western Pacific, the Amazon basin and Oceania.

  (i) Large numbers of destroyed red cells affect the capillary circulation, leading to damage to the brain, kidneys, liver, heart, gastrointestinal tract, and lungs.

  (ii) Abrupt onset of encephalopathy with headache, confusion, seizures and coma may occur, known as cerebral malaria.

  (iii) Other presentations include an influenza-like illness, diarrhoea and vomiting, jaundice, acute renal failure, acute respiratory distress, arthralgia, postural hypotension or shock, progressive anaemia and thrombocytopenia.

  (iv) The patient may not appear ill in the first few days, but non-immune or splenectomized patients may then deteriorate rapidly over a few hours and die.

(2) The patient usually presents within 4 weeks of returning from a malarious area with fever, rigors, nausea, vomiting, diarrhoea, and headache. Hepatosplenomegaly is common.

(3) However, symptoms may manifest months or even years later due to release of parasites from the exoerythrocytic phase in the liver. This does *not* occur in falciparum malaria.

(4) Send blood for FBC, coagulation profile, ELFTs and two sets of blood cultures.

  (i) Request a thick and thin film for malarial parasites in *every* patient returning from abroad with fever and with any of the above symptoms or signs.

(5) Request an MSU.

MANAGEMENT

(1) Falciparum malaria is a medical emergency requiring prompt treatment with oral or i.v. quinine therapy.

    (i) Call the senior ED doctor for help.

    (ii) Give immediate i.v. treatment with quinine 20 mg/kg up to 1.4 g infused over 4 hours, if there is altered conscious level, respiratory distress, jaundice, vomiting, oliguria, severe anaemia from haemolysis, over 2% red cells parasitized, hypoglycaemia or acidosis. Admit these severe cases to the ICU.

    (iii) Admit other patients under the Medical team when falciparum malaria is even considered as being possible, and begin treatment immediately – if necessary before the blood results are available.

(2) Refer patients with other types of malaria to the Medical team, although some will be treated as outpatients.

(3) Ask patients with initial negative films, but a suggestive history, to return for repeat blood films if symptoms persist.

    (i) Inform the GP of the possibility of malaria by fax and letter.

> **Warning:** do not diagnose the 'flu in a febrile patient without asking about travel and considering malaria.

TYPHOID

DIAGNOSIS

(1) The incubation period is up to 3 weeks following travel to India, Latin America, the Philippines and South-East Asia. There is an initial insidious onset of fever, malaise, headache, anorexia, dry cough, and constipation in the first week.

(2) The illness then progresses to abdominal distension and pain associated with diarrhoea, splenomegaly, a relative bradycardia, bronchitis, confusion or coma.

    (i) The characteristic crop of fine rose-pink macules on the trunk is rare.

(3) Send blood for FBC that may show a leucopenia with a relative lymphocytosis. Send ELFTs and two sets of blood cultures in all suspected cases.

(4) Request an MSU and a stool culture if diarrhoea is prominent.

    (i) Blood cultures are positive in up to 90% in the first week.

(ii) Stool culture becomes positive in 75% and urine culture in 25% in the second week.

MANAGEMENT

(1) Commence i.v. rehydration with normal saline or Hartmann's.
(2) Refer all suspected cases to the Medical team for ciprofloxacin 500 mg b.d. orally for 7–10 days or ciprofloxacin 400 mg i.v. 12-hourly.

DENGUE

DIAGNOSIS

(1) Dengue occurs after a short 1-week incubation period from infection by one of four serotypes of mosquito-borne flavivirus, particularly in Central or South America and South-East Asia.
(2) There is abrupt fever, chills, retro-orbital or frontal headache, myalgia, back pain, lymphadenopathy and rash.
  (i) The initial rash is transient, blanching and macular.
  (ii) A secondary rash on days 3–6 is maculopapular.
(3) Dengue haemorrhagic fever (DHF) and dengue shock syndrome occur in repeat infections with a different serotype.
(4) Send blood for FBC, coagulation profile, ELFTs, two sets of blood cultures and dengue serology.

MANAGEMENT

(1) Admit the patient under the Medical team for supportive care with i.v. fluids and antipyretic analgesics.
(2) Admit patients with DHF or dengue shock syndrome to the ICU.

HELMINTH INFECTIONS

DIAGNOSIS

(1) *Schistosomiasis* (bilharzia) rarely presents acutely, but should be suspected in cases from endemic areas such as Africa, South America, the Middle East and Asia presenting with fever and diarrhoea associated with eosinophilia (Katayama fever).
  (i) Chronic infection may present up to years later with painless terminal haematuria or obstructive uropathy, portal or pulmonary hypertension and seizures.

(2) *Roundworm infection* is discovered when the adult worm is passed in the stool, although occasionally allergic pneumonitis, abdominal pain or urticaria occur.

(3) *Tapeworm infection* usually presents with lassitude, weight loss and anaemia or with specific disease complications such as seizures in cysticercosis, and mass effects in hydatid disease (*Echinococcus*).

MANAGEMENT

(1) Discuss your suspicions with an Infectious Disease specialist and take advice about which laboratory tests are indicated.

PANDEMIC THREATS

A pandemic is a global outbreak of a new type of infection in susceptible individuals, with rapid person-to-person spread and the potential to affect millions.

Severe acute respiratory syndrome (SARS) affected 8400 humans during 2002–2003 in 29 countries with a 10% case fatality rate. Person-to-person spread occurred.

Avian influenza A (H5N1) has spread from poultry to humans since the end of 2003 in several Asian and eastern European countries, but person-to-person spread has been rare.

SARS AND BIRD 'FLU (AVIAN INFLUENZA)

DIAGNOSIS

(1) SARS has an incubation period of 7–10 days, and causes fever, headache, malaise, myalgia and rigors.
    (i) Dry cough, dyspnoea and confusion occur 3–7 days later, with CXR abnormality by day 7 of the illness.
    (ii) Diarrhoea may also occur as a presenting feature.

(2) Bird 'flu (avian influenza) has an incubation period of up to 7 days, causing sudden fever, headache and myalgia, followed by cough. An altered conscious level may occur.

(3) Ask patients presenting with fever or respiratory symptoms specifically about travel, ideally at triage *before* entering the Emergency Department.
    (i) Check the status of the current 'at risk' countries at

http://www.cdc.gov/travel/index.htm or refer to local policy information concerning these global infectious threats.

MANAGEMENT

(1) Place suspected cases of either SARS or avian influenza in isolation, preferably a negative-pressure room, and give them a high-filtration N95 mask to wear.

(2) All attending staff must wear a correctly fitted, high-filtration mask (N95), long-sleeved gown, gloves, and full eye protection.

(3) Inform the senior ED doctor, the local Infectious Disease physician, and Hospital Infection Control officer.

 (i) Call the duty microbiologist and take FBC, ELFTs, blood cultures and 30 mL for serology including for atypical pneumonia.

 (ii) Send a nasopharyngeal aspirate (NPA), nose/throat swab (NTS) and sputum, and arrange a CXR. Alert the radiographer to the infection risk.

(4) Specialist consultation will determine the further management.

FURTHER READING

Australian Department of Health and Ageing (2003) *The Australian Immunisation Handbook*, 8th edn. http://immunise.health.gov.au/handbook.htm/ (hepatitis B).

Centers for Disease Control and Prevention. http://www.cdc.gov/travel/index.htm/ (travellers' health).

Department of Health UK. http://www.dh.gov.uk/PolicyAndGuidance/HealthAndSocialCareTopics /Immunisation/ImmunisationGeneralInformation/fs/en/ Immunisation against infectious diseases 2006 '*The Green Book*'. (hepatitis B).

Health Protection Agency. http://www.phls.co.uk/ (infectious diseases).

TOXICOLOGY

ACUTE POISONING: GENERAL PRINCIPLES

Most cases of acute poisoning are acts of deliberate self-harm in the adult, but they are usually accidental in children. All cases are initially managed as medical emergencies and require substance identification, risk assessment, resuscitation, specific and non-specific treatment, and a period of observation. Thereafter, cases will require psychiatric assessment. Remember that an apparently trivial act of self-harm may still indicate serious suicidal intent (see p. 444).

DIAGNOSIS

(1) Consider acute poisoning in any unconscious patient or one exhibiting bizarre behaviour, or in unexplained metabolic, respiratory or cardiovascular problems.

(2) Obtain specific information from the patient, witnesses, and ambulance personnel regarding:
   (i) Pharmaceutical agent or toxin ingested:
      (a) remember that two or more drugs are taken in 30% of cases
      (b) alcohol is a common adjunct.
   (ii) Quantity of agent ingested (look for empty blister packets).
   (iii) Time since ingestion.
   (iv) History of any toxic effects experienced from the poisoning.
   (v) Specific events prior to arrival in the Emergency Department (ED), such as:
      (a) rapid deterioration in conscious level
      (b) seizures.
   (vi) Clinical features on presentation.

(3) Corroborate the history in the cooperative patient, but do not be misled, as information supplied may be incomplete or deliberately false.

(4) Focus the examination on immediate life threats, identification of clinical signs specific to certain drugs, and obtaining baseline vital signs.
   (i) Rapidly assess airway patency, respiratory function and conscious level.
   (ii) Record the pulse, blood pressure, respiratory rate, temperature and blood sugar level, and attach a cardiac monitor and pulse oximeter to the patient.

(a) hypoglycaemia and hyperthermia are common findings in the collapsed patient with a drug overdose, and are often overlooked.

(iii) Look for signs of seizure activity, assess upper and lower limbs for signs of hypertonicity and clonus, and examine the pupils.

(iv) Look for clues to the substance taken:
    (a) dilated pupils: tricyclics, amphetamine, antihistamines, anticholinergic agents
    (b) pinpoint pupils: opiates, organophosphates
    (c) nystagmus: alcohol, benzodiazepines, phenytoin
    (d) hyperventilation: salicylates
    (e) nasal bleeding or perioral sores: solvent abuse.

(5) Gain i.v. access and send blood for FBC, U&Es, LFTs, a paracetamol level in *all* poisonings, and a salicylate level only if symptomatic of salicylism or when comatose (see p. 155).

(6) Perform an arterial blood gas to rapidly determine metabolic acidosis, respiratory function and electrolyte imbalance.
    (i) Metabolic acidosis is associated with many poisonings including salicylates, methanol, ethanol, iron, and ethylene glycol.

(7) Request other specific measurable serum drug levels in ingestion of phenytoin, sodium valproate, digoxin, carbamazepine, iron, methotrexate and theophylline.

(8) Perform an ECG looking for tachycardia, bradycardia and potential cardiac conduction abnormalities such as QT prolongation and widening of the QRS complex.

(9) Request a CXR if clinical signs of aspiration are present.

(10) Request an abdominal X-ray (AXR) when potentially radio-opaque tablets such as iron or potassium have been ingested.

MANAGEMENT

(1) Start immediate resuscitation if risk assessment indicates ingestion of a potentially lethal drug, or if the patient is obtunded with signs of cardiorespiratory distress.

(2) Unconscious or collapsed patient:
    (i) Clear the airway by extending the head, remove dentures, vomit or blood by a quick sweep round the mouth with a Yankauer suction catheter, and give oxygen via a face mask.
    (ii) Insert an oropharyngeal Guedel airway if the patient is not breathing or the gag reflex is reduced, and use a bag–valve

mask system to ventilate the patient, aiming for an oxygen saturation above 94%.

(iii) Call an airway-skilled doctor urgently to pass a cuffed endotracheal tube to protect and maintain the airway and to optimize ventilation.

(3) Administer the following without delay:

(i) 50% dextrose 50 mL i.v. if the blood sugar level is low.

(ii) Naloxone 0.4–1.2 mg i.v. if the pupils are pinpoint, the respiratory rate is below 10 and opioid intoxication is suspected (see p. 159).

(iii) Normal saline to treat hypotension and maintain the circulation. If hypotension is secondary to an arrhythmia or myocardial depression, specific drug therapy and inotropic support may be needed.

(4) Treat toxic seizures with:

(i) Intravenous benzodiazepines such as lorazepam 0.07 mg/kg up to 4 mg i.v., diazepam 0.1–0.2 mg/kg, or midazolam 0.05–0.1 mg/kg.

(ii) Second-line treatment such as phenobarbitone (phenobarbital) 10–20 mg/kg i.v. at no faster than 100 mg/min. Phenytoin is contraindicated in the treatment of toxic seizures.

(5) Gastrointestinal decontamination:

This is not routine, and it is only instituted once basic resuscitative and supportive care has been performed and the airway is secure.

(i) *Activated charcoal*

(a) this is used to reduce the absorption of many drugs. Consider in patients presenting within 1 hour of taking a potentially toxic overdose of an agent known to be adsorbed to charcoal

(b) give 50 g for adults (1 g/kg body weight in children) in 100–200 mL water administered orally or via a nasogastric tube. Warn the patient that charcoal is somewhat unpalatable and will turn the stools black

(c) charcoal administration is contraindicated when:

– an oral antidote such as methionine is to be given

– the patient has an altered level of consciousness or an unprotected airway

– the patient has ingested substances not adsorbed to charcoal, such as iron, lithium, alcohols, acid, alkali, petroleum, pesticides, or cyanide.

(ii) *Whole bowel irrigation* (WBI):

   (a) WBI is not used routinely, but may be useful in poisonings with:
      - sustained-release or enteric-coated medications
      - toxic ingestion of agents such as iron, lithium, sodium valproate and calcium-channel blockers, particularly if charcoal is known to be ineffective
      - 'body-packers' who have ingested wrapped illicit drugs.

   (b) WBI is contraindicated in patients with:
      - an unprotected airway
      - haemodynamic instability
      - bowel obstruction, perforation or ileus.

(6) *Enhanced elimination*

   Consider for specific poisonings in consultation with the ICU. Obtain additional advice from a Poisons Information Service.

   (i) Multiple-dose activated charcoal: give repeated 25–50 g charcoal every 4 hours. This may be useful in severe salicylate, theophylline, digoxin, carbamazepine, quinine and phenytoin poisoning.

   (ii) Haemodialysis, charcoal haemoperfusion and urinary pH modification are alternatives in certain severe poisonings.

(7) *Antidotes*

   These drugs counter the effects of the poison, but only exist for a few specific agents.

(8) Admit the patient following ED resuscitation, supportive care, decontamination and antidote administration to the ED observation unit, Medical team or ICU, depending on the clinical severity of poisoning.

(9) All patients require psychiatric evaluation and management following their medical care.

> (!) **Warning:** gastric lavage is rarely if ever used, and induced emesis is positively contraindicated.

151

SPECIFIC POISONS

Obtain advice as necessary from agencies such as the UK National Poisons Information Service (NPIS), comprising six Poisons Centres (Belfast, Birmingham, Cardiff, Edinburgh, London and Newcastle). The NPIS coordinates an Internet and telephone service to assist in the diagnosis, treatment and management of all types of poisonings.

(1) TOXBASE® is an online resource for the routine diagnosis, treatment and management of patients exposed to toxic substances. Use this as the first point of contact for poisons advice. It is available on the Internet at http://www.spib.axl.co.uk/.

(2) Specialist consultants are available for telephone advice in more complex clinical cases. A 24-hour number **0870 600 6266** will direct callers to the relevant local centre.

In Australia, obtain advice regarding toxic ingestions 24 hours a day from the Poisons Information Centre on **13 11 26**, and in New Zealand on **03 479 7248** (or **0800 764 766** within New Zealand only).

PARACETAMOL

DIAGNOSIS

(1) Paracetamol overdose is common and potentially lethal.

(2) Hepatocellular necrosis is the major complication of paracetamol toxicity. Factors that enhance the potential for hepatotoxicity, and therefore morbidity and mortality, include:

    (i) Late presentation with delayed antidote administration, especially if over 24 hours.

    (ii) Staggered overdose: multiple supra-therapeutic ingestions over a number of days.

    (iii) Glutathione deficiency in starvation and debilitating illness such as AIDS.

    (iv) Enzyme-inducing drugs such as phenytoin, carbamazepine, phenobarbitone (phenobarbital) or rifampicin.

    (v) Regular alcohol use.

(3) Determine the time since ingestion, total paracetamol consumed, the patient's weight, and any increased hepatotoxicity risk factors:

    (i) Patients who have taken more than 12 g (24 tablets) or more than 150 mg/kg are considered at risk for severe liver damage.

(ii) Hepatotoxicity may occur in patients at enhanced risk following as little as 7.5 g (15 tablets).

(4) The patient is usually asymptomatic, but can present in fulminant hepatic failure with abdominal pain, vomiting, hypoglycaemia, tender hepatomegaly, jaundice and encephalopathy.

(5) Gain i.v. access and send bloods for FBC, U&Es, LFTs, PTI (INR) and a blood sugar level. Check the paracetamol level when 4 hours or more have elapsed since overdose.

MANAGEMENT

(1) Resuscitation is rarely required unless the patient is in fulminant hepatic failure.

(2) Administer 50% dextrose 50 mL i.v. if the patient is hypoglycaemic.

(3) Review the blood results:
    (i) Plot the serum paracetamol level on the paracetamol nomogram for all patients presenting between 4 and 24 hours after an acute, single ingestion of paracetamol.
    (ii) Treat patients who have enhanced hepatotoxicity risk factors with any level above line C, or other patients with a level above line B (see Fig. 4.1).
    (iii) A raised PTI (INR) or ALT levels greater than 1000 IU/L define hepatotoxicity.

(4) N-acetylcysteine (NAC), the antidote for paracetamol, is most effective when commenced within 8 hours of poisoning. Administer NAC in the following circumstances:
    (i) Patients presenting within 8 hours of ingestion, with a 4–8-hour serum paracetamol level above the relevant nomogram treatment line (see Fig. 4.1).
    (ii) A potentially toxic ingestion of paracetamol (more than 24 tablets or 150 mg/kg) in patients presenting 8–24 hours after overdose, or if the serum paracetamol level will not be available within 8 hours of the original ingestion:
        (a) commence treatment immediately without waiting for the blood results
        (b) cease treatment if the serum paracetamol level turns out to be below the relevant treatment line, and the alanine aminotransferase (ALT) and PTI (INR) are normal.
    (iii) Patients presenting with deranged ALT and PTI (INR) more than 24 h after acute overdose, or following staggered overdose.

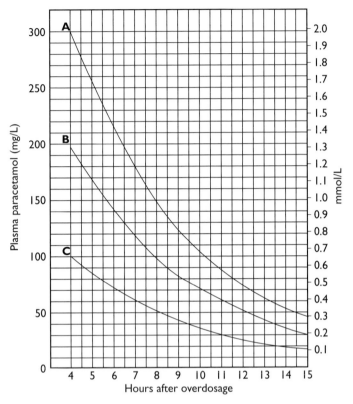

Figure 4.1 Treatment nomogram for paracetamol poisoning
Line (B): specific treatment is indicated above this line. Line (C): specific treatment is indicated above this line in patients who regularly take enzyme-inducing drugs, such as phenytoin, carbamazepine, phenobarbitone (phenobarbital) and rifampicin, or alcohol. Line (A): 90% of untreated patients will develop alanine transaminase (ALT) levels over 1000 units/L, and most fatal cases will be above this line. Reproduced with permission from Proudfoot AT (1993) *Acute Poisoning Diagnosis and Management*, 2nd edn. Oxford, Butterworth Heinemann.

(a) serum paracetamol levels are difficult to interpret in cases of staggered ingestion. Monitor the PTI (INR) and ALT regularly instead and seek specialist toxicologist advice (see below).

(5) Consult a clinical toxicologist for patients presenting with staggered overdoses, with delayed presentation of more than

24 hours, and patients with severe liver dysfunction and an elevated PTI (INR).

(6) Use the adult infusion protocol for NAC below.

   (i) Take care with the dose calculation. Or simply read from the drug-insert infusion dosage guide the volume in mL of NAC 200 mg/mL to be added to the 5% dextrose, according to the patient's weight:

     (a) 150 mg/kg in 5% dextrose 200 mL i.v. over 15 min.

     (b) 50 mg/kg in 5% dextrose 500 mL i.v. over 4 hours.

     (c) 100 mg/kg in 5% dextrose 1000 mL i.v. over 16 hours.

(7) Side effects are mostly from non-allergic anaphylaxis, occurring in the first 30 min of administering high-dose NAC, and include nausea, flushing, itching, urticaria, wheeze and hypotension.

   (i) Stop the infusion.

   (ii) Give promethazine 25 mg i.v. and hydrocortisone 200 mg i.v.

   (iii) Once symptoms have settled, re-commence the infusion at a lower rate of 50 mg/kg over 4 hours.

SALICYLATES

DIAGNOSIS

(1) The clinical features of salicylate toxicity following acute ingestion are dose related:

   (i) Less than 150 mg/kg: usually asymptomatic.

   (ii) 150–300 mg/kg: moderate symptoms such as tachypnoea, nausea, vomiting and tinnitus.

   (iii) 300–500 mg/kg: severe toxicity with hyperthermia, marked dehydration, agitation, confusion and an altered level of consciousness, which may lead to coma.

   (iv) More than 500 mg/kg is associated with pulmonary and cerebral oedema and may be fatal.

(2) Gain i.v. access and send bloods for U&Es, blood sugar, coagulation profile and a salicylate level. ABGs are useful to detect respiratory alkalosis or a metabolic acidosis.

MANAGEMENT

(1) Call an airway-skilled doctor immediately to pass a cuffed endotracheal tube if the patient is obtunded, unconscious, or unable to protect their airway.

(2) Commence a normal saline infusion to replace insensible losses associated with hyperthermia, hyperventilation, and vomiting.

(3) Administer charcoal as soon as possible, even in patients with a delayed presentation. Consider repeat-dose activated charcoal every 4 hours to reduce salicylate absorption in the following situations:

    (i) Overdose of sustained-release aspirin.

    (ii) Evidence of continued absorption with rising serum salicylate levels.

(4) Urinary alkalinization may reduce salicylate elimination from 20 to 5 hours. Consider in patients with signs and symptoms of salicylate toxicity, or a serum salicylate level of more than 300 mg/L (2.2 mmol/L).

    (i) Give a bolus of 8.4% sodium bicarbonate 1 mmol/kg (1 mL/kg) i.v.

    (ii) Follow with an infusion of 8.4% sodium bicarbonate 100 mmol (100 mL) in 5% dextrose solution 1 L, at a rate of 100–250 mL/h.

    (iii) Titrate this bicarbonate infusion to maintain urinary pH above 7.5 and urine output greater than 1 mL/kg per hour.

(5) Monitor serum electrolytes, salicylate level and urinary pH every 2–4 hours.

    (i) Salicylate level:

        (a) symptoms occur at 300 mg/L (2.2 mmol/L)

        (b) significant toxicity occurs at 500 mg/L (3.6 mmol/L)

        (c) repeat the level at least once. Rising levels indicate continued drug absorption.

    (ii) Potassium: significant hypokalaemia hinders salicylate elimination so potassium may need to be replaced.

(6) Patients with no clinical evidence of salicylate toxicity, normal arterial blood gases (ABGs) and falling serum salicylate levels 4 hours apart may be ready for psychiatric review.

(7) Otherwise observe all patients with clinical salicylate toxicity for a minimum of 12 hours until they demonstrate resolution of symptoms and a falling serum salicylate level, before considering medically fit.

(8) Consult a clinical toxicologist for patients with salicylate levels above 500 mg/L (3.6 mmol/L), severe symptoms or obtunded. Consider haemodialysis for severe poisoning with a metabolic acidosis or a salicylate level over 700 mg/L (5.1 mmol/L).

TRICYCLIC ANTIDEPRESSANTS

DIAGNOSIS

(1) Tricyclic antidepressant (TCA) overdose is associated with significant mortality. Ingestion of 15–20 mg/kg or more is potentially fatal.

(2) The onset of symptoms is usually rapid, and in large overdoses deterioration occurs within 1–2 hours. Significant toxicity is heralded by cardiotoxicity, convulsions and coma.

(3) Clinical features include:
  (i) Anticholinergic: warm dry skin with absent sweating, dilated pupils, urinary retention, sinus tachycardia, and delirium.
  (ii) CNS: seizures are usually associated with an altered level of consciousness and rapid development of coma, especially with a large overdose.
  (iii) Cardiovascular: cardiac arrhythmias are common and occur as a result of sodium-channel blockade. They are often associated with hypotension.

(4) Perform an ECG. Look for tachycardia, heart block, torsades de pointes and junctional rhythms.
  (i) A QRS interval of more than 120 ms indicates cardiotoxicity and is predictive of ventricular arrhythmias and seizures.

(5) Gain i.v. access and send blood for FBC, U&Es and a paracetamol level and attach a cardiac monitor and pulse oximeter to the patient.

(6) Perform an arterial blood gas to monitor for hypoxia and acidosis, both of which exacerbate any cardiotoxicity.

MANAGEMENT

(1) Give high-dose oxygen and commence a normal saline infusion.

(2) Call an airway-skilled doctor to pass an endotracheal tube in patients with a reduced conscious level, inadequate respiratory effort or convulsions, with or without cardiac arrhythmias.

(3) Administer oral activated charcoal as soon as possible, provided the airway is secured, to all patients with significant TCA ingestion, even with a delayed presentation.

(4) Give a loading dose of 8.4% sodium bicarbonate 1–2 mmol/kg (1–2 mL/kg), followed by an infusion of 20–100 mmol/h (20–100 mL/h) to maintain an arterial pH of between 7.50 and 7.55.
  (i) Sodium bicarbonate is a specific antidote in TCA poisoning

and provides high concentrations of sodium ions, which help reduce cardiotoxicity.

(ii) Indications for sodium bicarbonate administration include:

(a) cardiac arrhythmia or cardiac arrest

(b) widened QRS interval of greater than 120 ms

(c) persistent hypotension despite saline or colloid fluid administration.

(5) Repeat the ABGs and electrolytes regularly to ensure resolution of acidosis and prevent hypernatraemia.

(6) Perform repeated ECGs to monitor for cardiac arrhythmias and to ensure the resolution of any QRS prolongation.

(7) Refer patients with significant cardiovascular or CNS toxicity to the ICU or CCU, for ECG monitoring and supportive care.

(8) Observe patients with drowsiness and non-progressive or absent ECG changes in the ED observation unit for a minimum of 6 hours.

BENZODIAZEPINES

DIAGNOSIS

(1) These are comparatively safe if taken alone. Reported deaths are associated with mixed overdoses with other CNS depressants such as opioids and alcohol.

(2) Clinical manifestations include drowsiness, respiratory depression, ataxia and dysarthria.

(3) Coma is unusual unless combined with other sedatives or alcohol, or in the elderly.

(4) Gain i.v. access and send blood for U&Es and a paracetamol level. No specific investigations are required unless co-ingestion is suspected. Attach a cardiac monitor and pulse oximeter to the patient.

(5) Perform a baseline ECG.

MANAGEMENT

(1) Give high-dose oxygen and nurse in the left lateral position to prevent aspiration, unless the airway is protected.

(2) Administer normal saline to maintain a normal BP.

(3) Gastrointestinal decontamination is rarely necessary unless there is co-ingestion or the patient is deeply unconscious, in which case protect the airway first by endotracheal intubation.

(4) Admit the patient to the ED observation unit overnight, followed by subsequent psychiatric evaluation.

(5) The use of flumazenil, a specific benzodiazepine receptor antagonist, is controversial. It is rarely if ever indicated, and must be discussed with the senior ED doctor.

    (i) Flumazenil may induce ventricular tachycardia, elevate intracranial pressure, precipitate benzodiazepine withdrawal in chronic abusers, and may invoke seizures, particularly with co-ingestion of tricyclic antidepressants.

    (ii) Potential roles for flumazenil are thus restricted to:

        (a) reversal of excessive benzodiazepine sedative effect following procedural sedation

        (b) reversal of respiratory depression and coma in a pure benzodiazepine overdose, to prevent the need for intubation. The difficultly is knowing when no other drugs were ingested.

OPIOIDS

DIAGNOSIS

(1) Opioid drugs include opium alkaloids such as morphine and codeine; semi-synthetic opioids such as heroin (diamorphine) and oxycodone and fully synthetic opioids such as pethidine and methadone.

(2) Opioids produce euphoria, pinpoint pupils, sedation, respiratory depression and apnoea with increasing doses.

(3) Complications of opioid intoxication include hypotension, convulsions, non-cardiogenic pulmonary oedema and compartment syndrome from prolonged immobility.

(4) Perform a thorough examination to evaluate potential complications, and to exclude alternative causes of an altered mental state with bradypnoea such as sepsis, neurotrauma, stroke and metabolic disease (see p. 54).

(5) Send bloods for U&Es, blood sugar and serum paracetamol level. Perform an ECG.

MANAGEMENT

(1) Commence supportive care with oxygen and assisted ventilation.

(2) Give naloxone 0.4–2 mg i.v. as a bolus or in 0.1 mg increments. Carefully titrate response to achieve improved airway control and

adequate ventilation, without precipitating an acute agitated withdrawal state.

    (i) Naloxone is a short-acting opioid antagonist that may be administered by the intramuscular, intravenous, subcutaneous or endotracheal routes.

    (ii) It is safe and rarely associated with complications.

    (iii) Use it to reverse severe respiratory depression, apnoea and oversedation, or for cases of undifferentiated coma with respiratory depression and pinpoint pupils.

(3) Continue to monitor for respiratory depression and hypoxia. Further doses of naloxone or an infusion may be required due to its short half-life.

(4) Observe all patients for a period, because re-sedation with respiratory depression may occur as the naloxone wears off.

IRON

DIAGNOSIS

(1) Acute iron overdose is a potentially life-threatening condition, particularly in children who mistake iron tablets for sweets.

(2) The clinical course following iron overdose includes:

    (i) Gastrointestinal toxicity: haemorrhagic gastroenteritis with vomiting, abdominal pain and bloody diarrhoea. Failure to develop significant GI symptoms within 6 hours of ingestion effectively rules out significant iron poisoning.

    (ii) Systemic toxicity: hypotension, shock, lethargy, metabolic acidosis, seizures, coma, and acute liver and renal failure.

(3) Toxicity is determined by the quantity of elemental iron ingested:

    (i) Less than 20 mg/kg: usually asymptomatic.

    (ii) 20–60 mg/kg: gastrointestinal symptoms predominate.

    (iii) 60–120 mg/kg: systemic toxicity and high lethality.

(4) Send blood for FBC, U&Es, LFTs, a serum iron level, coagulation profile, blood sugar level, G&S and ABGs.

    (i) Serum iron levels peak at 4–6 hours after ingestion.

    (ii) Levels greater than 90 µmol/L are associated with systemic toxicity.

(5) Most iron preparations are radio-opaque. Request a plain AXR to show residual whole tablets or a concretion, although a negative AXR does not rule out ingestion.

MANAGEMENT

(1) This is dependent on the initial assessment, potential elemental iron ingested, and clinical manifestations.

(2) Start aggressive fluid resuscitation in patients with signs of gastrointestinal or systemic toxicity, and institute decontamination and chelation measures. Discuss these with the senior ED doctor or a clinical toxicologist:

(i) Decontamination:

(a) do not administer charcoal or attempt to induce vomiting

(b) perform gastric lavage provided the airway is protected, or whole bowel irrigation if there are significant numbers of tablets beyond the pylorus.

(ii) Chelation therapy:

Start a desferrioxamine infusion at 2 mg/kg per hour and increase to a maximum of 15 mg/kg per hour in severe cases.

(3) Most patients will remain asymptomatic, or develop mild gastrointestinal symptoms only. Give intravenous fluids to replace vomiting and diarrhoea losses, provide supportive care and observe for a minimum of 6 hours.

(i) Refer all moderate-to-severe cases to the ICU team.

DIGOXIN

DIAGNOSIS

(1) Toxicity occurs from acute overdose or secondary to long-term therapy. Foxglove and oleander ingestion will also cause acute cardiac glycoside poisoning.

(2) Acute digoxin overdose in adults is usually intentional. Clinical manifestations include:

(i) Nausea and vomiting.

(ii) Hyperkalaemia.

(iii) Bradycardia and ventricular arrhythmias.

(3) Chronic digoxin overdose occurs particularly in the elderly and may be precipitated by renal impairment, hypokalaemia, hypercalcaemia and drugs such as amiodarone and quinidine. Clinical manifestations include:

(i) Nausea, vomiting, diarrhoea.

(ii) Sedation, confusion, delirium.

(iii) Visual disturbances, such as yellow haloes (xanthopsia).

(iv) Cardiac automaticity and a wide range of ventricular and supraventricular arrhythmias.

(4) Gain i.v. access and send bloods for U&Es and a serum digoxin level.

   (i) Therapeutic range for digoxin is 0.5–2.0 ng/mL.

   (ii) The serum digoxin level is most accurate at 6 hours post-ingestion.

   (iii) Take serum levels early to confirm poisoning, and repeat in 4 hours if acute ingestion is suspected.

(5) Perform an ECG:

   (i) Any cardiac arrhythmia may be seen in both acute and chronic ingestions.

   (ii) The most common arrhythmias are bradycardia, heart block, paroxysmal atrial tachycardia, ventricular ectopics, and ventricular tachycardia.

MANAGEMENT

(1) Treatment depends on haemodynamic stability, conscious state, and whether it is an acute or chronic intoxication.

(2) Gain i.v. access in all patients and start fluid resuscitation for hypotension, continuous cardiac monitoring, and perform regular ECGs.

(3) Acute digoxin intoxication:

   (i) Administer oral activated charcoal if presentation is within 1 hour of significant overdose. This may be impossible if the patient is vomiting continuously. Repeated administration should not delay other interventions.

   (ii) Treat hyperkalaemia with a dextrose–insulin infusion (see p. 115). Do *not* use intravenous calcium solutions as they may precipitate asystole.

   (iii) Administer digoxin-specific antibody fragments (Digibind™) for:

      (a) cardiac arrest

      (b) haemodynamic instability with cardiac arrhythmia

      (c) serum potassium greater than 5.5 mmol/L

      (d) serum digoxin level greater than 15 nmol/L (11.7 ng/mL)

      (e) ingested digoxin dose greater than 10 mg (4 mg in a child).

   (iv) Calculate the number of vials of Digibind™ required from the estimated ingested dose or the serum digoxin concentration, if obtained at least 6 hours post acute poisoning.

(v) Admit all acute poisonings for cardiac monitoring and close observation for a minimum of 12 hours.

(4) Chronic digoxin intoxication:

(i) Cease the digoxin medication.

(ii) Correct any hypokalaemia with potassium chloride 10 mmol/h i.v., and hypomagnesaemia with magnesium sulphate 10 mmol in 100 mL normal saline i.v. over 30 min.

(iii) Administer two vials of digoxin-specific antibody fragments (Digibind™) i.v. over 30 min to symptomatic patients with an altered mental state, cardiac arrhythmia or gastrointestinal symptoms.

(iv) Patients usually recover quickly. Admit under the Medical team for treatment of any cardiac instability, renal impairment and electrolyte disturbances.

LITHIUM

DIAGNOSIS

(1) Lithium toxicity may be acute or chronic. Chronic toxicity is associated with significant morbidity and mortality, and acute overdose of more than 250 mg/kg.

(2) Acute overdose:

(i) Clinical manifestations of acute overdose include:

(a) gastrointestinal: anorexia, nausea, vomiting

(b) CNS: similar to chronic intoxication, but only manifests in delayed presentations.

(3) Chronic toxicity:

(i) This is commonly associated with renal impairment, dehydration, diuretics and congestive cardiac failure.

(ii) Clinical manifestations of chronic toxicity include:

(a) CNS:

– mild: tremor, hyper-reflexia, ataxia, muscle weakness

– moderate: rigidity, hypotension, stupor

– severe: myoclonus, coma and convulsions.

(b) gastrointestinal symptoms are not present in chronic toxicity.

(4) Gain i.v. access and send bloods for U&Es, blood sugar, and serum lithium level.

(5) Perform an ECG.

MANAGEMENT

(1) Acute overdose:

   (i) Do not administer activated charcoal.

   (ii) Commence normal saline to correct hypotension, salt and water deficits, and to maintain a good urine output. Monitor the fluid and electrolyte status closely.

   (iii) Most patients recover quickly with adequate fluid resuscitation. Observe until they have a normal mental status, the serum lithium level is falling, and is below 2.5 mmol/L.

   (iv) Consider haemodialysis in patients with impaired renal function, late presentation, a serum lithium level of more than 3.5 mmol/L or progressive neurological signs. Contact the ICU.

(2) Chronic toxicity:

   (i) Discontinue lithium medications. Commence normal saline to correct hypotension, salt and water deficits, and to maintain a good urine output.

   (ii) Refer the following to ICU for consideration of haemodialysis:

      (a) patients with neurological abnormalities such as an altered mental state, coma or convulsions

      (b) patients with a serum lithium level of greater than 3.5 mmol/L and significant neurotoxicity.

THEOPHYLLINE

DIAGNOSIS

(1) Theophylline toxicity may result from acute ingestion or chronic use. Both are associated with significant morbidity and mortality.

   (i) Chronic ingestion is exacerbated by intercurrent illness or the concomitant administration of drugs that interfere with hepatic metabolism.

(2) Clinical manifestations include:

   (i) Gastrointestinal tract: nausea, abdominal pain, intractable vomiting.

   (ii) Cardiovascular: sinus tachycardia, hypotension and cardiac arrhythmias.

   (iii) CNS: anxiety, agitation and insomnia.

   (iv) Hyperventilation, gastrointestinal bleeding, convulsions, coma and ventricular tachycardia in severe toxicity.

(3) Clinical signs of significant toxicity may be delayed by up to

12 hours in acute overdose, when sustained-release tablets have been ingested.

(4) Gain i.v. access and send bloods for U&Es, LFTs, blood sugar and a theophylline level. Look for hypokalaemia, hypomagnesaemia, hyperglycaemia and metabolic acidosis, especially in severe acute ingestions.

(5) Determine the serum theophylline level.

   (i) In acute poisoning:

      (a) toxic symptoms occur with theophylline levels over 25 mg/L

      (b) levels of 40–60 mg/L are serious and levels over 80 mg/L are potentially fatal.

   (ii) In chronic toxicity, levels over 20 mg/L cause symptoms and levels over 40 mg/L may be life threatening.

(6) Perform an ECG and cardiac monitoring. Cardiac arrhythmias are common and include sinus tachycardia, supraventricular tachycardia, atrial flutter and ventricular tachycardia.

MANAGEMENT

(1) Ensure the airway is secure and administer high-flow oxygen. Correct fluid depletion and hypokalaemia with normal saline and potassium under ECG control.

(2) Administer oral activated charcoal in acute overdose, even if presentation is delayed. Give repeat doses at 4-hourly intervals.

(3) Give high-dose metoclopramide 10–40 mg i.v. for intractable vomiting. Consider ondansetron 4 mg i.v. if this fails.

(4) Give lorazepam 0.07 mg/kg i.v. up to 4 mg, diazepam 0.1–0.2 mg/kg i.v. or midazolam 0.05–0.1 mg/kg for seizures, although endotracheal intubation may be required.

(5) Administer a beta-blocker such as propranolol 1 mg i.v. over 1 minute, repeated up to a maximum of 10 mg *only* in non-asthmatic patients with supraventricular tachycardia, hypokalaemia and hyperglycaemia.

(6) Admit all patients with signs of toxicity for cardiac monitoring.

   (i) Refer patients with severe toxicity, obtundation and seizures to ICU for haemodialysis or charcoal haemoperfusion.

BETA-BLOCKERS

DIAGNOSIS

(1) Significant beta-blocker toxicity is associated particularly with propranolol ingestion, coexistent cardiac disease, and in polypharmacy overdose with calcium-channel blockers and TCAs.

(2) Clinical evidence of toxicity usually presents within the first 6 hours of overdose. Toxicity is associated with:
  (i) Bradycardia, arrhythmias, hypotension and cardiogenic shock.
  (ii) Sedation, altered mental status, coma and convulsions.

(3) Gain i.v. access and send blood for U&Es and a blood sugar level, as hypoglycaemia may occur, especially with atenolol. Attach a cardiac monitor and pulse oximeter to the patient.

(4) Perform an ECG. Look for toxic conduction defects such as AV block, right bundle branch block, prolongation of the QRS (propranolol) and ventricular arrhythmias (especially with sotalol).

MANAGEMENT

(1) Ensure the airway is secure and administer high-flow oxygen. Commence intravenous fluid administration in cases of hypotension.

(2) Administer oral activated charcoal to all patients as soon as possible.

(3) Give atropine 0.6–1.2 mg i.v. for bradycardia, up to a maximum of 0.04 mg/kg.

(4) Give glucagon 50–150 μg/kg i.v. bolus followed by an infusion at 1–5 mg/h.

(5) Titrate adrenaline (epinephrine) and isoprenaline infusions to maintain organ perfusion in resistant cases. Cardiac pacing may be necessary.

(6) Admit all symptomatic patients to coronary care or ICU.

CALCIUM-CHANNEL BLOCKING DRUGS

DIAGNOSIS

(1) Toxicity is related to underlying cardiac disease, co-ingestants, delay to treatment, increased age, and the specific calcium-channel blocker ingested. Sustained-release verapamil is associated with the majority of significant poisonings.

(2) Clinical signs of toxicity usually present within 2 hours, but may

be delayed up to 8 hours with sustained-release preparations. Features include:

(i)   Gastrointestinal: nausea and vomiting.

(ii) Cardiovascular: hypotension, sinus bradycardia and complex cardiac arrhythmias.

(iii) CNS: lethargy, slurred speech, confusion, coma and convulsions.

(3) Gain i.v. access and send blood for U&Es, LFTs and a blood sugar level. Take an arterial blood gas.

(i)   Hyperglycaemia and metabolic acidosis are common with significant toxicity.

(4) Perform an ECG. Look for toxic conduction defects such as high-grade AV block, complete heart block, and accelerated atrioventricular nodal rhythms.

MANAGEMENT

(1) Ensure the airway is secure and administer high-flow oxygen. Commence intravenous fluid administration.

(2) Administer oral activated charcoal to all patients as soon as possible. More aggressive decontamination, such as whole bowel irrigation, may be required with large ingestions of s.r. tablets.

(3) Give 10% calcium chloride 10 mL i.v. bolus, and repeat up to 30 mL i.v. followed by an infusion. Calcium increases cardiac output and restores perfusion to vital organs.

(4) If hypotension and reduced myocardial contractility persist:

(i)   Commence an adrenaline (epinephrine) infusion at up to 0.5–1.0 µg/kg per minute, titrated to maintain organ perfusion.

(ii) Give glucagon 50–150 µg/kg i.v. bolus followed by an infusion at 1–5 mg/h.

(5) Admit the patient to the Coronary Care unit (CCU) or ICU for continuous cardiac monitoring.

CARBON MONOXIDE

DIAGNOSIS

(1) Carbon monoxide poisoning is usually associated with the combustion of fuel with an inadequate flue, e.g. a blocked domestic heater, or from the fumes of a car exhaust. It is a colourless odourless gas and the most common poison used for successful suicide in the UK and Australia.

(2) Clinical manifestations are related directly to arterial blood gas carboxyhaemoglobin (COHb) concentration levels around the time of exposure. Later COHb levels lack the same prognostic value:

   (i) 0–10%: asymptomatic (may be seen in smokers).

   (ii) 10–25%: throbbing frontal headache, nausea, shortness of breath on exertion.

   (iii) 25–40%: cognitive impairment, auditory and visual disturbances, dizziness, aggression and psychosis.

   (iv) 40–50%: confusion, coma and seizures.

   (v) 50–70%: hypotension, respiratory failure, cardiac arrhythmias and cardiac arrest.

   (vi) Greater than 70%: death.

(3) History and strong clinical suspicion are important in establishing the diagnosis. Suspect carbon monoxide toxicity if several members of one household present in a similar fashion.

(4) Remember a pulse oximeter does not distinguish between carboxyhaemoglobin and oxyhaemoglobin, and will record misleadingly normal oxygen saturations.

   (i) Therefore send an arterial blood gas sample in all cases. Look for evidence of metabolic acidosis and elevated carboxyhaemoglobin levels.

(5) Gain i.v. access and send blood for FBC, U&Es, LFTs, cardiac enzymes, serum lactate and blood sugar level. Perform a beta-HCG pregnancy test in women.

(6) Perform an ECG. Look for evidence of cardiac arrhythmias, myocardial ischaemia and myocardial infarction.

(7) Request a CXR and arrange a CT brain scan in comatose patients.

MANAGEMENT

(1) Secure the airway and give 100% oxygen by tight-fitting mask with reservoir bag.

   (i) Call the senior ED doctor and prepare for endotracheal intubation in comatose patients, to protect and maintain the airway and to optimize ventilation with 100% oxygen.

(2) Commence fluid resuscitation for hypotension and to correct acid–base disturbances. Hypotension usually responds to fluids, but may require inotropic support.

(3) Give 20% mannitol 0.5–1.0 g/kg (2.5–5 mL/kg) for clinical or radiographic evidence of cerebral oedema.

(4) Refer the patient to a Hyperbaric Oxygen (HBO) unit if the patient was found unconscious, has significant neurological symptoms, or is pregnant.
  (i) However, local referral practices will vary as the efficacy of HBO is challenged.

CYANIDE

DIAGNOSIS
(1) Cyanide is a metabolic poison associated with a high mortality.
(2) Features of toxicity include:
  (i) Cardiovascular: initial hypertension followed by profound hypotension, bradycardia, arrhythmias, cardiovascular collapse and cardiorespiratory arrest.
  (ii) CNS: headache, anxiety, sedation, respiratory depression, seizures and coma.
(3) Gain i.v. access and send blood for serum lactate levels and arterial blood gas analysis.
(4) A raised anion gap metabolic acidosis and raised lactate levels relate closely to clinical signs of intoxication and serum cyanide levels (which are not measurable acutely).

MANAGEMENT
(1) Assess and secure the airway immediately. Give oxygen and commence fluid resuscitation.
(2) Call for immediate senior ED doctor help, and/or advice from a clinical toxicologist if time allows. Give the following:
  (i) Hydroxocobalamin 70 mg/kg up to 10 g i.v. over 30 min or as a bolus in severe cases. Although unlicensed, it is preferable to dicobalt edetate.
  (ii) 25% sodium thiosulphate 12.5 g (50 mL) i.v. at a rate of 2–5 mL/min.
(3) Refer patients with significant toxicity to ICU.

CHLOROQUINE

DIAGNOSIS
(1) Overdose with quinine, chloroquine and hydroxychloroquine is potentially fatal with as little as 2.5–5 g ingested, and is associated with significant morbidity.

(2) Clinical manifestations ('*cinchonism*') are dose related and include:
  (i) Mild: flushed and sweaty skin, tinnitus, blurred vision, confusion, reversible high-frequency hearing loss, abdominal pain, vertigo, nausea and vomiting.
  (ii) Severe: hypotension, skin rashes, deafness, blindness, anaphylactic shock, cardiac arrhythmias and cardiac arrest.
(3) Gain i.v. access and send blood for FBC, U&Es, LFTs, blood sugar level and beta-HCG in females. Attach a cardiac monitor and pulse oximeter to the patient.
(4) Perform an ECG. Look for QRS and QT prolongation and ventricular arrhythmias.

MANAGEMENT

(1) Assess and secure the airway and give high-flow oxygen. Commence intravenous fluid resuscitation for hypotension.
(2) Give oral activated charcoal to patients presenting within 1 hour of overdose.
(3) Administer lorazepam 0.07 mg/kg up to 4 mg, diazepam 0.1–0.2 mg/kg i.v. or midazolam 0.05–0.1 mg/kg i.v. to treat seizures and agitation, and to reduce the tachycardia.
(4) Commence an isoprenaline infusion for torsades de pointes, or arrange for overdrive cardiac pacing for the QT prolongation, because magnesium is contraindicated.
(5) There are no specific treatment modalities to reverse blindness and deafness in severe toxicity, other than supportive care.
(6) Admit the patient to CCU or ICU.

COCAINE

DIAGNOSIS

(1) Cocaine hydrochloride is a fine white powder, which may be mixed with baking soda to make 'crack'. It rapidly reaches the cerebral circulation and has a half-life of 90 min.
(2) Complications following cocaine abuse include:
  (i) Respiratory: dyspnoea, pneumothorax, pneumonitis and thermal airway injury.
  (ii) Cardiovascular: palpitations, hypertension, ischaemic chest pain, arrhythmias and cardiac arrest.
  (iii) Nervous system: agitation, altered mental state, syncope, seizures, focal neurological signs, intracranial haemorrhage and coma.

(3) Base the diagnosis on history and clinical suspicion. Monitor the core temperature for hyperthermia.

(4) Gain i.v. access and send blood for FBC, ELFTs, blood sugar level and cardiac enzymes as indicated clinically. Attach a cardiac monitor and pulse oximeter to the patient.

(5) Perform an ECG and look for signs of myocardial ischaemia, infarction and cardiac arrhythmias.

(6) Request a CXR.

MANAGEMENT

(1) Assess and secure the airway and give high-flow oxygen.

(2) Give lorazepam 0.07 mg/kg up to 4 mg, diazepam 0.1–0.2 mg/kg i.v. or midazolam 0.05–0.1 mg/kg i.v. to treat seizures, agitation and to reduce the tachycardia, hypertension and hyperthermia.

(3) Treat persistent myocardial ischaemia with sublingual or intravenous nitrates and benzodiazepine sedation.

   (i) Ideally arrange for percutaneous coronary intervention (angioplasty) if myocardial infarction occurs.

   (ii) Further intravenous nitrates or sodium nitroprusside may be required to treat hypertension.

(4) Admit all patients requiring high-dose benzodiazepine therapy and patients with evidence of cardiovascular instability for cardiac monitoring and observation.

ORGANOPHOSPHATES

DIAGNOSIS

(1) Organophosphates are extremely toxic pesticides, which produce acetylcholine excess with muscarinic, nicotinic and CNS effects.

(2) They are rapidly absorbed through the skin, bronchi and small intestine when ingested orally.

(3) Patients present with degrees of cholinergic crisis, usually within 4 hours of ingestion or exposure. Specific manifestations include:

   (i) Muscarinic:

      (a) bronchospasm, bradycardia, vomiting, profuse diarrhoea, pinpoint pupils

      (b) excessive sweating, lacrimation, salivation and urination.

   (ii) CNS: initial agitation followed by sedation and altered mental status leading to convulsions and coma.

   (iii) Nicotinic: weakness, muscle paralysis and tachycardia.

(4) Gain i.v. access and send blood for FBC, ELFTs, and a plasma cholinesterase level, which is a good marker of exposure, but a poor indicator of severity.

(5) Perform an ECG to evaluate cardiac arrhythmias.

(6) Request a CXR as aspiration pneumonitis is common.

MANAGEMENT

(1) Instruct all staff to wear a gown and gloves to remove soiled clothing and when washing the skin.

(2) Give oxygen, and call an airway-skilled doctor to pass an endotracheal tube for respiratory failure and severe bronchorrhoea.

(3) Commence a normal saline infusion to manage hypotension and replace losses.

(4) Treat seizures with lorazepam 0.07 mg/kg up to 4 mg, diazepam 0.1–0.2 mg/kg i.v. or midazolam 0.05–0.1 mg/kg i.v.

(5) Give atropine 2 mg i.v. repeated until the skin becomes dry, and bronchial secretions are minimal.

    (i) Massive doses may be necessary, but do not rely on pupillary dilatation and tachycardia as indicative end points, as they may not reflect adequate atropinization.

(6) Give pralidoxime 2 g (30 mg/kg) i.v. over 15 min and then 1 g every 8 hours for the next 48 hours, in all moderate-to-severe cases (except for carbamate poisoning).

    (i) Monitor serial plasma or red cell cholinesterase levels and look for signs of clinical improvement before ceasing treatment.

(7) Admit the patient to ICU.

> **(!)** **Warning:** staff treating patients exposed to organophosphates may develop mild headache, eye irritation and pulmonary symptoms secondary to the hydrocarbon solvent and *not* the organophosphate itself. These resolve with simple analgesia and by removing the staff from the exposure source.

PARAQUAT

DIAGNOSIS

(1) Paraquat is an extremely toxic herbicide. Significant oral ingestion is associated with fulminant multi-organ failure. If patients survive

this, they develop progressive pulmonary fibrosis, and may die 4–6 weeks later from hypoxaemia.

(2) Clinical effects depend on the route of exposure:
  (i) Skin: localized irritation, erythema, blistering, ulceration.
  (ii) Eyes: corneal inflammation, oedema, ulceration.
  (iii) Systemic from oral ingestion:
    (a) Less than 15 mL of 20% solution: nausea, vomiting and diarrhoea and reversible pulmonary irritation
    (b) More than 15 mL of 20% solution: pharyngeal ulceration, hypersalivation, intractable vomiting, haematemesis, severe abdominal pain and bowel perforation.

(3) Gain i.v. access and send blood for FBC, U&Es, LFT, coagulation profile and blood sugar level. Request a serum paraquat level.
  (i) A serum level of greater than 5 mg/L is invariably fatal.

(4) A qualitative urine test may be performed by adding 1 mL of 1% sodium dithionite solution to 10 mL of urine. Paraquat ingestion is confirmed if the urine turns blue.

(5) Perform an ECG.

(6) Request a CXR to look for evidence of mediastinitis, aspiration, pulmonary opacities and abdominal viscus perforation.

MANAGEMENT

(1) Early gastrointestinal decontamination is paramount. Give activated charcoal 50–100 g immediately with 20% mannitol 200 mL orally or via an NGT.
  (i) The traditional alternative adsorbing agent 15% aqueous suspension Fuller's earth (bentonite) 1000 mL is rarely available now.

(2) Administer oxygen only if the SaO_2 is less than 90%. Oxygen enhances the pulmonary toxicity.

(3) Refer the patient immediately for admission to ICU.

CHEMICAL BURNS

DIAGNOSIS

(1) These occur at home, in schools, in laboratories and in industrial accidents.

(2) Most agents are strong acids or alkalis, although occasionally

phosphorus and phenol are responsible.

(3) Alkali burns are generally more serious than acid as they penetrate deeper.

MANAGEMENT

(1) Wear gloves to remove any contaminated clothing. Treat by copious irrigation with running water. Continue irrigating for at least 30 min.

(2) Do *not* attempt to neutralize the chemical, as most resultant reactions produce heat and will exacerbate the injury, except in the case of hydrofluoric acid.

(3) *Hydrofluoric acid burns*
   (i) Neutralize these as follows:
      (a) convert hydrofluoric acid to the calcium salt by covering the affected area with dressings soaked in 10% calcium gluconate solution, or by rubbing in 2.5% calcium gluconate gel
      (b) inject subcutaneous 10% calcium gluconate if the pain and burning persist.
   (ii) Dermal absorption of fluoride ions may result in systemic fluorosis with hypocalcaemia, hypomagnesaemia, hyperkalaemia and cardiac arrest.
      (a) *systemic fluorosis* may follow burns affecting as little as 2% of body surface area from concentrated 70% hydrofluoric acid
      (b) seek immediate senior ED doctor help, and give large amounts of i.v. calcium chloride and magnesium sulphate as indicated clinically, and from blood testing.

(4) Refer all patients to the Surgical team unless the area burnt is minimal and the patient is pain free.

(5) Refer patients with systemic fluorosis to ICU. The hyperkalaemia may require haemodialysis.

FURTHER READING

American Heart Association (2005) Guidelines for cardiopulmonary resuscitation and emergency cardiovascular care. Part 10.2: Toxicology in ECC. *Circulation* **112**:IV-126–32.

American Heart Association. http://www.circulationaha.org/ (CPR and ECC guidelines).

European Resuscitation Council (2005) Guidelines for resuscitation. Section 7: Cardiac arrest in special circumstances. *Resuscitation* 67(**Suppl 1**):S135–70.

European Resuscitation Council. http://www.erc.edu/ (CPR and ECC guidelines).

MediTox/HyperTox© Poisons Information. http://www.hypertox.com/ (information on common and serious poisonings) (subscription necessary).

National Poisons Information Service TOXBASE®. http://www.spib.axl.co.uk/ (poisons information).

Resuscitation Council (UK). http://www.resus.org.uk/ (Resuscitation Guidelines 2005).

TOXINOLOGY EMERGENCIES

SNAKE BITES

These are exceedingly rare in the UK, but may present in zookeepers and herpetologists, or following a mishap with an exotic pet. Advice on management is always available from the UK National Poisons Information Service (24 hours) on **0870 600 6266**.

Snakebite is much more common in warmer countries, including Australia, where management advice is again available from the Poisons Information Centre (24 hours) on **13 11 26**. There are no endemic venomous snakes in New Zealand, although toxinology advice is still available from the National Poisons Centre on **03 479 7248** (or **0800 764 766** within New Zealand only).

VIPER (ADDER) SNAKE BITES

DIAGNOSIS

(1) Snakes of the viper species include the North American rattlesnake, the African rhinoceros viper and the adder, which is the only naturally occurring venomous snake in the UK.

(2) Local effects of an adder bite include pain, bruising, swelling and local lymphadenopathy within hours of the bite. However, fewer than 50% of bites are associated with envenomation, and occasionally systemic poisoning may occur with no local reaction.

(3) Systemic envenomation causes:
  (i) Early features including non-allergic anaphylaxis with transient syncope and hypotension, angioedema, urticaria, abdominal pain, vomiting and diarrhoea.
  (ii) Late features including recurrent or persistent hypotension, ECG changes, spontaneous bleeding, coagulopathy, adult respiratory distress syndrome and acute renal failure.

(4) Gain i.v. access, and send blood for FBC, clotting screen, U&Es and LFTs.

(5) Perform an ECG and a CXR in severe cases.

MANAGEMENT

(1) Reassure the patient, apply a firm bandage proximal to the bite, immobilize the dependent limb, and transport the patient rapidly to hospital.

(2) Treat non-allergic anaphylaxis reactions with oxygen, adrenaline

(epinephrine) and fluids (see p. 89).

(3) Give European viper venom antiserum for significant adder envenomation:

    (i) Indications for viper venom antiserum include:

        (a) hypotension

        (b) ECG changes

        (c) vomiting

        (d) bleeding

        (e) extending limb swelling within 4 hours of the bite.

    (ii) Add one 10-mL vial to normal saline 5 mL/kg diluent and infuse over 30 min, repeated as indicated.

    (iii) Have adrenaline (epinephrine) immediately available for anaphylactic reactions to the antivenom.

(4) Give tetanus prophylaxis, and refer all patients to the Medical team for admission, even in the absence of initial symptoms or signs.

ELAPID SNAKE BITES

DIAGNOSIS

(1) The top ten venomous snakes in the world are all elapid snakes found in Australia!

    (i) Elapids have permanently erect front fangs and produce venom containing neurotoxins, myotoxins and haemotoxins.

        (a) they include the brown, black, taipan, tiger, death adder, copperhead and rough-scaled snakes.

(2) Local signs following a snakebite are usually minimal, with fine scratches or small puncture marks only. Some bites such as from the tiger snake and black snake may cause immediate local pain, bruising or swelling within hours.

(3) The majority of venomous snake bites are actually 'dry' as systemic envenomation occurs in only 10–20% of cases.

(4) Look for the following signs that do indicate systemic envenomation, although these may fluctuate:

    (i) General findings such as headache, nausea, vomiting, abdominal pain and transient hypotension.

    (ii) Sudden collapse, convulsions and cardiac arrest in severe envenomation (especially brown snakes).

    (iii) Tissue-specific findings:

        (a) neurotoxic effects including ptosis, diplopia, dysphagia and paralysis progressing to respiratory arrest

       (b) haematoxic effects including asymptomatic coagulopathy, bite- or venepuncture-site oozing, haematemesis, melena and haematuria

       (c) myotoxic effects including rhabdomyolysis, myoglobinuria and renal failure.

(5) Gain i.v. access and send blood for FBC, U&Es, LFT, creatinine kinase (CK) and coagulation profile including fibrinogen. Attach a cardiac monitor and pulse oximeter to the patient.

(6) Send urine for protein, haemoglobin and myoglobin estimation.

(7) Attempt to identify the snake species with a venom detection kit (VDK) analysis on urine or from a bite-site swab, carefully taken from under the pressure–immobilization bandage.

       (i) Visual inspection and an amateur 'guess' at the species is unreliable, is misleading, and is a waste of time – unless you are a trained herpetologist.

(8) Perform an ECG, CXR and spirometry in significant envenoming.

MANAGEMENT

(1) Make sure that first aid using the pressure–immobilization technique has been applied to impede the spread of venom through local lymphatics.

       (i) Apply a broad firm bandage around the bite site and extend proximally up the limb to cover it completely, as tight as one would bandage a sprained ankle.

       (ii) Splint the dependent limb and organize for transport to be brought to the patient.

       (iii) Keep the immobilization bandage in place until definitive treatment has been instituted and the patient is systemically improved.

(2) Give high-flow oxygen via face mask and watch for any signs of airway compromise.

(3) Give antivenom for definite systemic envenomation. Do *not* use antivenom for a positive VDK result alone, if no other abnormal clinical or laboratory features are present:

       (i) Indications for antivenom include the presence of any clinical signs, especially refractory hypotension, cardiac arrhythmias, renal failure and impending respiratory or cardiac arrest *or* abnormal laboratory findings, particularly coagulopathy.

       (ii) Give the appropriate species-specific monovalent antivenom if the snake species has been positively identified by an expert herpetologist or on VDK.

(a) start with five vials (5000 units) in brown snake envenoming, up to ten vials (10 000 units) for critical cases

(b) give up to four vials (12 000 units) for tiger snake envenoming; one or two vials (12 000 to 24 000 units) for taipan; and start with one vial for envenoming of black snake (18 000 units) and death adder (6000 units).

(iii) Give tiger and brown snake monovalent antivenoms only at the above starting doses in Victoria, when the species has not been identified, or give tiger snake antivenom alone in Tasmania.

(a) get expert advice urgently in the other Australian states if the species is still unknown. Giving polyvalent antivenom two to four vials i.v. is expensive and may not be effective.

(iv) Give antivenom slowly by i.v. infusion over 30 min after 1 in 10 dilution with normal saline.

(a) give an undiluted neat bolus of antivenom as a life-saving measure if the patient is in cardiac arrest or has circulatory collapse.

(v) Pre-treat the patient with 1 in 1000 adrenaline (epinephrine) 0.1–0.3 mg (0.1–0.3 mL) s.c. especially if there has been a previous reaction to antivenom, as anaphylaxis occurs in 1–5% cases.

(4) Give tetanus prophylaxis according to the patient's immune status.

(5) Refer all patients with signs of systemic envenomation to the local Toxicology unit or ICU.

(6) Remove the pressure–immobilization bandage and observe carefully in all other patients who remain systemically well, with no clinical signs of envenomation and normal initial laboratory blood tests.

(i) Repeat all the laboratory tests again 2 hours after bandage removal.

(ii) Observe the patient for a further 6–12 hours prior to discharge if all blood tests and clinical examination still remain normal, looking particularly for delayed neurotoxicity.

SPIDER ENVENOMATION

The majority of spider bites are associated with local symptoms of pain and erythema. Certain species are associated with significant envenomation, and may be fatal.

DIAGNOSIS

(1) The *Lactrodectus* species includes the red-back (Australia), the black widow (America), and the katipo (New Zealand) spiders. Envenomation is by the female. Clinical features of lactrodectism include:
  (i) Local pain, erythema, sweating, lymphadenopathy and piloerection.
  (ii) Systemic features including headache, nausea, vomiting, abdominal pain, generalized sweating and hypotension.

(2) Over 40 species of funnel-web spider occur in Australia, with the most significant envenomation from the male Sydney funnel-web spider. Clinical features of funnel-web spider envenomation include:
  (i) Severe localized pain, with erythema.
  (ii) Generalized muscle fasciculations, nausea, vomiting, abdominal pain, sweating, lacrimation and salivation.
  (iii) Initial tachycardia and hypertension progressing to hypotension and pulmonary oedema and finally convulsions and coma.

(3) Base the diagnosis on history and clinical examination, because no laboratory tests are helpful.

(4) Perform an ECG and request a CXR if funnel-web spider bite is suspected.

MANAGEMENT

(1) Apply a pressure–immobilization bandage immediately after a funnel-web spider bite to retard the spread of the venom. *Never* use this in red-back spider envenomation.

(2) Otherwise, give first-aid treatment with the application of ice or heat and the administration of oral analgesia to provide symptomatic relief.

(3) Observe all patients in a monitored resuscitation area, assess and secure the airway, and administer oxygen. Gain i.v. access only if antivenom is indicated.

(4) Antivenom administration:
  (i) *Red-back spider antivenom*
    (a) administer red-back spider antivenom to patients with clinical manifestations of systemic toxicity or severe uncontrolled local symptoms
    (b) give one to two vials (500–1000 units) red-back spider antivenom i.m.
      – i.v. administration diluted in 100 mL normal saline over 30 min may be used, particularly if the initial response to i.m. antivenom by 90 min was poor
      – discuss additional management with a clinical toxicologist if symptoms continue
    (c) observe all patients given antivenom until symptoms have gone
    (d) discharge all the other patients with mild or absent symptoms. Advise them to return if symptoms worsen, as antivenom may work even many days after envenoming.
  (ii) *Funnel-web spider antivenom*
    (a) administer funnel-web spider antivenom to patients with clinical manifestations of systemic toxicity or severe uncontrolled local symptoms
    (b) give two vials (250 units) i.v. slowly (four if severe) and repeat every 15 min until symptoms have resolved
    (c) refer all patients with persistent local symptoms or significant systemic envenomation to the Medical team or to the ICU
    (d) discharge other patients who remain systemically well, with absence of signs of envenoming by 4 hours after removal of any first-aid bandage applied.

MARINE ENVENOMATION

Several hazardous marine animals are found in coastal waters in the UK and around the world. Clinical manifestations of various envenomations are outlined on the following pages.

DIAGNOSIS

(1) Jellyfish:
  (i) *Irukandji syndrome* (Australia). This causes mild local pain followed 30–40 min later by severe generalized muscle cramps, back and abdominal pain, hypertension and pulmonary oedema. It is potentially fatal.
  (ii) *Box jellyfish* (Australia). This causes severe local pain and cross-hatched erythematous dermal lesions, associated with cardiovascular and respiratory collapse. It is also potentially fatal.
  (iii) *Bluebottle* or *Portuguese man-of-war* (worldwide). These cause severe local stinging pain, erythema, and elliptical blanched wheals, rarely associated with a muscle-pain syndrome and hypotension.
(2) Poisonous fish such as the stonefish, lionfish, bullrout (Australia) or lesser weever (UK):
  (i) These fish have venomous spines that can cause extreme local pain and oedema.
  (ii) Systemic effects include diarrhoea, respiratory depression and hypotension.
(3) Sea urchins, fire coral (worldwide):
  (i) Sea urchins cause local erythema and pain from the many tiny spines which may break off and enter a joint cavity or the deep palmar or plantar spaces.
  (ii) Fire coral causes local burning similar to a jellyfish sting.

MANAGEMENT

(1) Assess and secure the airway first and provide basic life support to patients with cardiovascular collapse and systemic toxicity.
(2) Jellyfish first aid:
  (i) Box jellyfish and Irukandji: rinse jellyfish wounds with seawater, remove adherent tentacles, and prevent further nematocyst discharge with 5% acetic acid (vinegar).
  (ii) Bluebottle: rinse with seawater (*not* vinegar), remove adherent tentacles, and immerse the affected area in warm water at 40–45°C without scalding.
(3) Jellyfish systemic envenomation:
  (i) Irukandji:
    (a) administer oxygen and give opiate analgesia, e.g. with fentanyl 5 µg/kg i.v. every 10 min until pain is controlled

(b) commence a GTN infusion if severe hypertension is not controlled with pain management (see p. 46).

(ii) Box jellyfish:
(a) administer oxygen and commence intravenous fluid resuscitation for hypotension. Give morphine 5–10 mg i.v. for severe local pain
(b) administer box jellyfish antivenom if the pain is refractory to opiates, the patient is shocked, or in cardiac arrest:
– give three vials (60 000 units) diluted 1 in 10 with normal saline i.v. over 30 min or six vials as a bolus in cardiac arrest.

(4) Poisonous fish:
(i) Immerse the affected area in warm water at 40–45°C without scalding. If pain persists, perform a regional block with 2% lignocaine (lidocaine) and give morphine 5–10 mg i.v.
(ii) Debride the wound, remove spines and give tetanus prophylaxis according to the patient's immune status.
(iii) Systemic stonefish envenomation: give one vial (2000 units) of stonefish antivenom i.m. for every 2 puncture marks visible.

(5) Sea urchins and fire coral:
(i) Relieve pain by immersion in hot water at 40–45°C without scalding or by using a local anaesthetic block, followed by exploration, irrigation and debridement as necessary, and give tetanus prophylaxis.
(ii) Give an antibiotic such as doxycycline 100 mg orally once daily for 5 days (not in children or pregnant patients), for deep or necrotic wounds.

BEE AND WASP STINGS

DIAGNOSIS

(1) There are more deaths in Britain and the USA from anaphylaxis following bee or wasp stings than from all the other venomous bites and stings put together.

(2) Local pain predominates and may be followed by a severe anaphylactic reaction causing laryngeal oedema, bronchospasm, hypotension and collapse (see p. 89).

MANAGEMENT

(1) Remove a bee sting by scraping the sting out with a knife, without squeezing.

(2) Anaphylaxis:

   (i) Assess and secure the airway, give oxygen, gain i.v. access and commence fluid resuscitation in all cases.

   (ii) Give 1 in 1000 adrenaline (epinephrine) 0.3–0.5 mg (0.3–0.5 mL) i.m. early. Give 1 in 10 000 adrenaline (epinephrine) or 1 in 100 000 adrenaline (epinephrine) 0.75–1.5 µg/kg, i.e. 50–100 µg slowly i.v. if circulatory collapse occurs.

(3) Arrange for patients prone to anaphylaxis from bee or wasp stings to carry a pre-filled adrenaline (epinephrine) syringe (EpiPen®) at all times.

FURTHER READING

DEY® (affiliate of Merck KGaA). http://www.anaphylaxis.com/ (anaphylaxis information).

University of Adelaide Clinical Toxinology Resources. http://www.toxinology.com/.

ENVIRONMENTAL EMERGENCIES

HEAT ILLNESS

This is predisposed to by hot weather, exercise, obesity, fever, lack of physical fitness or acclimatization, alcohol intake, and drugs such as anticholinergic agents.

DIAGNOSIS
(1) Mild to moderate heat illness:
  (i) Thermoregulatory mechanisms remain intact.
  (ii) *Heat cramps*
    (a) pain develops in heavily exercising muscles in hot weather secondary to sodium depletion.
  (iii) *Heat exhaustion*
    (a) thirst, cramps, headache, vertigo, anorexia, nausea and vomiting occur
    (b) the patient is flushed and sweating, with rectal temperature of 38–39°C
    (c) tachycardia and orthostatic hypotension occur secondary to dehydration.
(2) Severe heat illness:
  (i) *Heat stroke*
    (a) thermoregulatory mechanisms fail
    (b) *classic (non-exertion) heat stroke* (CHS) usually occurs in the elderly during a heat wave secondary to high environmental temperatures
    (c) *exertion heat stroke* (EHS) is associated with young adults exercising in high temperatures
    (d) symptoms include headache, vomiting and diarrhoea, progressing to aggressive or bizarre behaviour, collapse, seizures and coma. The rectal temperature is over 40°C
    (e) hot dry skin is usual, but profuse sweating occurs in up to 40% of patients with exertion heat stroke
    (f) the patient is flushed, tachypnoeic, tachycardic and hypotensive. Muscle rigidity, transient hemiplegia, dilated pupils and disseminated intravascular coagulation (DIC) may all occur

(g) gain i.v. access and send blood for FBC, coagulation profile, U&Es, blood sugar, LFTs and creatinine kinase (CK), and check ABGs. Attach an ECG monitor and pulse oximeter to the patient.

MANAGEMENT

(1) *Heat cramps*
   (i) Rest in a cool environment, and replace fluid orally with added salt or give 1 L normal saline i.v.
   (ii) The patient is usually able to go home.

(2) *Heat exhaustion*
   (i) Rest in a cool environment and give up to 3 L cooled normal saline i.v.
   (ii) Cool the patient with tepid sponging and fanning.
   (iii) Admit for observation, particularly when elderly or if orthostatic hypotension persists.

(3) *Heat stroke*
   (i) Give oxygen and aim for an oxygen saturation above 94%. Call the senior ED doctor for help and arrange for endotracheal intubation for airway protection.
   (ii) Commence urgent cooling with tepid sponging, fans and cold packs to the groin and axillae until the temperature is less than 38.5°C.
   (iii) Give 1 L cooled 4% dextrose 0.18% normal saline over 20 min, then according to the blood pressure, serum sodium level and urine output.
   (iv) Give lorazepam 0.07 mg/kg up to 4 mg i.v., diazepam 0.1–0.2 mg/kg up to 20 mg i.v. or midazolam 0.05–0.1 mg/kg up to 10 mg i.v. for seizures.
      (a) give chlorpromazine 25 mg i.v. to suppress shivering, if the rate of cooling is inadequate.
   (v) Admit the patient to the ICU.

HYPOTHERMIA

This is present when the core temperature drops to less than 35°C (95°F). Mild hypothermia is classified as 32–35°C (89.6–95°F), moderate hypothermia as 30–32°C (86–89.6°F), and severe hypothermia as less than 30°C (86°F).

DIAGNOSIS

(1) Hypothermia is predisposed to in the following situations:
  (i) Exposure to low air temperatures, particularly with wind and rain.
  (ii) Exposure in cold water.
  (iii) Unconscious patients, or patients who have taken sedative drugs, especially alcohol.
  (iv) Babies or the elderly with intercurrent illness, e.g. stroke, pneumonia, diabetic ketoacidosis (DKA).
  (v) Endocrine disorders, such as myxoedema or hypopituitary coma (rare).

(2) Clinical manifestations include:
  (i) Mild hypothermia: lethargy, ataxia, shivering and tachypnoea.
  (ii) Moderate hypothermia: bradycardia, hypotension, bradypnoea, and confusion. Shivering is absent.
  (iii) Severe hypothermia: the patient is comatose and may appear dead with an undetectable pulse, absent reflexes, unrecordable BP and fixed pupils.

(3) Record the core temperature rectally with a low-reading thermometer; this is more accurate than a tympanic membrane device.

(4) Send blood for FBC, U&Es, CK, coagulation profile and blood sugar level. Check serum lipase/amylase, as pancreatitis may be associated. Send ABGs.

(5) Perform an ECG.
  (i) Look for evidence of bradycardia, low-voltage complexes, atrial fibrillation and prolongation of the QT interval.
  (ii) Osborne 'J' waves (a slurred notching of the terminal portion of the QRS complex) may be present at core temperatures of less than 32°C.
    (a) the size of the wave is proportional to the degree of hypothermia and may be used to monitor the response to re-warming.

(6) Request a CXR.

MANAGEMENT

(1) Give high-flow, warmed 42–46°C (108–115°F), humidified oxygen, if the core temperature is 32°C or less.

(2) Take extreme care with endotracheal intubation, as this may precipitate cardiac arrhythmias including ventricular fibrillation in

severe hypothermia. Call the senior ED doctor for help.

(3) Remove wet clothing and cover the patient in warm blankets and layers of polythene.

    (i) Use a forced-air re-warming blanket, e.g. Bair Hugger®, minimize handling, and aim for a core temperature rise of 1°C/h in younger patients and 0.5°C per hour in the elderly.

(4) Give i.v. fluids cautiously through a warming device at 43°C (109°F). Pulmonary oedema may be precipitated by excessive fluid administration.

(5) Cardiac arrest in hypothermic patients:

    (i) *Severe hypothermia* (core temperature less than 30°C).

        (a) attempt defibrillation once, delivering 150–200 J biphasic or 360 J monophasic

        (b) standard resuscitation drugs are usually ineffectual as the efficacy of adrenaline (epinephrine) and amiodarone are reduced, with an increased circulation time

        (c) provide aggressive active internal re-warming with warmed pleural, gastric or peritoneal lavage, even extracorporeal blood re-warming, when available, aiming for a core temperature rise to at least 33°C.

    (ii) *Moderate hypothermia* (core temperature 30–32°C).

        (a) attempt defibrillation with one DC shock

        (b) administer standard resuscitation medications, but double the time between doses.

    (iii) Apply usual resuscitation protocols with core temperatures of 33°C and above.

    (iv) Continue resuscitation attempts until the core temperature rises to at least 33°C or until a senior doctor advises to the contrary:

        (a) this may involve a prolonged period of resuscitation and aggressive measures as outlined.

DROWNING

DIAGNOSIS

(1) Drowning is a common cause of accidental death in Europe and Australasia. It is defined as a process that results in primary respiratory impairment following immersion (face and upper airway) or submersion (whole body) in a liquid medium.

(2) The duration of hypoxia is the most important factor in

determining outcome and full neurological recovery. Victims with spontaneous circulation and breathing on arrival at hospital usually have a good outcome.

(3) The presence of lung crackles indicates likely inhalation of water. The initial difference between sea-water (hypertonic) and fresh-water (hypotonic) drowning is of little clinical significance, as only small amounts of fluid may have been aspirated.

(4) Consider other more relevant factors:

   (i) Preceding injury, especially to the cervical spine in diving accidents.

   (ii) Sudden preceding illness, such as a myocardial infarction, CVA or epileptic seizure that may have led to the drowning.

   (iii) Alcohol or drug use (a contributing factor in up to 70% of drownings).

   (iv) Hypothermia.

(5) Check FBC, U&Es, blood sugar, and ABGs. Attach a cardiac monitor and pulse oximeter to the patient.

(6) Perform an ECG and request a CXR.

MANAGEMENT

(1) Aim to restore oxygenation, ventilation and cerebral and coronary artery perfusion as rapidly as possible.

(2) Commence cardiopulmonary resuscitation if the patient has no detectable cardiac output or is not breathing.

   (i) Take due precautions to control the cervical spine if a neck injury is possible.

   (ii) Be prepared for gastric regurgitation, which is common and occurs in up to 85% of patients requiring basic life support with external cardiac compression and expired air, or bag, valve–mask ventilation.

   (iii) Continue prolonged resuscitation efforts, which may be successful particularly with hypothermia in cold water.

(3) Otherwise, give high-flow oxygen and aim for an oxygen saturation above 94%.

(4) Call an airway-skilled doctor to intubate the patient if they are unconscious or develop respiratory failure with a PaO_2 of less than 10 kPa (75 mmHg) on 50% oxygen, or a rising $PaCO_2$ above 7.5 kPa (56 mmHg).

(5) Record the rectal temperature and re-warm the patient if the core temperature is low.

(6) Refer all patients to the Medical team or ICU for admission.
  (i) Delayed adult respiratory distress syndrome (ARDS) may develop 6–72 hours after submersion 'secondary drowning'.

SPORTS-DIVING ACCIDENTS

Dysbarism is the medical complication of exposure to gases at higher than normal atmospheric pressure. It manifests clinically as decompression illness (DCI), which may be further classified by the acuity, evolution, presence or absence of barotrauma and the organs involved. It is most commonly associated with sports-diving accidents with scuba (self-contained underwater breathing apparatus) diving.

DECOMPRESSION ILLNESS (DCI)

Decompression illness (DCI) occurs when inert nitrogen gas forms bubbles within the venous and lymphatic systems, or body tissues, rather than being eliminated by the lungs.

DIAGNOSIS

(1) Symptoms may occur within minutes of surfacing or up to 48 hours after diving. It is important to look for and treat any patient who presents within hours of a dive as DCI until proven otherwise.
(2) Clinical manifestations include:
  (i) *Mild*
    (a) joint pain, ranging from a dull ache to the crippling 'bends'. Pain usually commences in large joints such as the elbow or shoulder and may migrate
    (b) unusual fatigue and malaise are common
    (c) skin itching, marbling, scarlatiniform rashes, painful lymphadenopathy and local oedema also occur.
  (ii) *Serious*
    (a) cardiopulmonary:
      – *'the chokes'*: retrosternal or pleuritic chest pain, dyspnoea, cough and haemoptysis
      – may be associated with myocardial infarction, hypotension and cardiac arrhythmia, and progress to respiratory failure.

(b) central nervous system:
- *'the staggers'*: labyrinthine damage with deafness, tinnitus, nystagmus, vertigo and nausea
- motor and sensory loss with hemiplegia and paraplegia
- personality disorder, seizures and urinary retention.

(3) Gain i.v. access and take blood for FBC, U&Es, LFTs and blood sugar level.

(4) Perform an ECG and request a CXR in patients with cardiopulmonary symptoms.

MANAGEMENT

(1) Give the patient 100% oxygen by tight-fitting face mask with reservoir bag.

(2) Commence normal saline rehydration, avoiding glucose-containing solutions as they may exacerbate CNS injury.

(3) Give lorazepam 0.07 mg/kg up to 4 mg i.v., diazepam 0.1–0.2 mg/kg i.v. or midazolam 0.05–0.1 mg/kg i.v. for seizures.
   (i) These drugs may also be used for severe labyrinthine disturbance after discussion with a Hyperbaric Medicine unit.

(4) Minimize strong analgesics, particularly opiates, as they mask symptoms.

(5) Fill the endotracheal tube cuff with saline to avoid changes in volume on recompression if endotracheal intubation is required.

(6) Refer every patient, however strange their symptoms, to a Hyperbaric Medicine unit:
   (i) Provide information about any dive in the preceding 48 hours, including the depth and duration, gas mix, time and duration of symptoms.
   (ii) Advice on diagnosis and arrangements for treatment are available by telephoning local or national Hyperbaric Medicine units; or in a dire emergency ring the police or coastguard, who will have the relevant contact details.

DECOMPRESSION ILLNESS WITH BAROTRAUMA

DIAGNOSIS

(1) *Middle ear barotrauma*
   (i) This is the most common medical disorder associated with diving, almost always occurring on descent.

(ii) Symptoms include local pain, bleeding from the ear, and conductive hearing loss.

(iii) The tympanic membrane appears reddened or may rupture.

(2) *Inner ear barotrauma*

(i) This is associated with too rapid descent.

(ii) Vertigo, tinnitus and sensorineural deafness occur secondary to rupture of the round or oval windows and an associated perilymph fistula.

(iii) It mimics labyrinthine CNS decompression illness.

(3) *Sinus barotrauma*

Local pain occurs over the maxillary and frontal sinus, sometimes associated with bleeding.

(4) *Dental barotrauma*

Pain occurs in or around fillings or carious teeth and percussion of the involved tooth is painful.

(5) *Pulmonary barotraumas*

This is the most serious form of barotrauma, and it causes:

(i) Surgical emphysema, pneumothorax or pneumomediastinum associated with chest pain and dyspnoea.

(ii) Arterial gas embolus affecting:

(a) the coronary circulation, with cardiac pain, arrhythmia and cardiac arrest

(b) the cerebral circulation, with sudden onset of neurological symptoms just before or within 5 min of surfacing (without the delay seen in CNS decompression illness)

(c) any neurological symptom or sign from confusion to seizures or coma may occur, and may fluctuate.

(6) Gain i.v. access and take blood for FBC, U&Es, LFTs, blood sugar level and cardiac biomarkers.

(7) Perform an ECG in patients with cardiopulmonary symptoms, and request a CXR to exclude pneumothorax or pneumomediastinum.

MANAGEMENT

(1) *Middle ear barotrauma*

(i) Give an analgesic such as paracetamol 500 mg and codeine phosphate 8 mg.

(ii) Give amoxicillin 500 mg orally t.d.s. for 5 days if tympanic membrane rupture is present, and refer the patient to the next ENT clinic.

(iii) The patient should not dive again until the drum is fully healed.

(2) *Inner ear barotrauma*

Discuss immediately with a Hyperbaric Medicine unit, as labyrinthine CNS decompression illness is possible.

(3) *Sinus and dental barotrauma*

Give an analgesic such as paracetamol 500 mg and codeine phosphate 8 mg.

(4) *Pulmonary barotrauma*

(i) Give oxygen and insert an intercostal drain if a significant pneumothorax is present (see p. 45). Manage a pneumomediastinum and surgical emphysema conservatively.

(ii) If arterial gas embolus is suspected:

(a) keep the patient horizontal on their left side (not head-down, as this raises intracranial pressure)

(b) give 100% oxygen by tight-fitting face mask with reservoir bag

(c) commence normal saline rehydration

(d) give lorazepam 0.07 mg/kg up to 4 mg i.v., diazepam 0.1–0.2 mg/kg or midazolam 0.05–0.1 mg/kg i.v. for seizures

(e) refer the patient to a Hyperbaric Medicine unit, even after apparent recovery, as delayed deterioration can occur and recompression may still be required.

ELECTRICAL BURNS, ELECTROCUTION AND LIGHTNING STRIKE

Factors influencing the severity of electrical injury include whether the current is alternating or direct, resistance to current flow, voltage, the pathway of current through the patient and the area and duration of skin contact. Skin resistance is decreased by moisture which increases the likelihood of injury.

Electrical injury may be considered in four groups:

- Electrical flash burns
- Low-voltage electrocution
- High-voltage electrocution
- Lightning strike

ELECTRICAL FLASH BURNS

DIAGNOSIS

(1) The external passage of current from the point of contact to the ground is associated with arcing. Electrical energy is converted to heat as electricity traverses the skin associated with brief high temperatures that may ignite clothing.

(2) Burns are usually superficial partial-thickness, but they may be deep dermal or even full-thickness. Secondary flame burns may occur if clothing ignites.

MANAGEMENT

(1) Assess the depth and extent of the burn (see p. 246).

(2) Check the eyes for evidence of corneal injury using fluorescein.

(3) Dress the areas as for a thermal burn and treat accordingly.

LOW-VOLTAGE ELECTROCUTION

DIAGNOSIS

(1) Injury primarily occurs in the home through carelessness or faulty electrical equipment, or to inquisitive children.

(2) Household voltage supply is usually 240 volts AC. AC is more dangerous than direct current (DC) and may induce tetanic muscle spasm. The longer the duration of contact, the greater the potential for injury.

  (i) Gripping the electrical source by hand will prevent release and worsens the injury.

(3) Low-voltage electrical injury causes local tissue necrosis manifesting as a contact surface burn that is often full-thickness. The underlying thermal tissue damage may be extensive and include blood vessels and muscle. There may be a similar exit (earthing) burn.

(4) Arrhythmias including VF and unconsciousness may occur if the charge crosses the heart or brain.

(5) Attach a cardiac monitor and pulse oximeter to the patient. Perform a 12-lead ECG.

(6) Request a CT head scan if there is coma, confusion or focal neurological signs.

MANAGEMENT

(1) Manage cardiac or respiratory arrest as for cardiopulmonary resuscitation (see p. 2).

(2) Otherwise, give oxygen and aim for an oxygen saturation over 94%.

(3) Give i.v. normal saline for any hypotension, aiming for a urine output of 100 mL/h if there is evidence of myoglobinuria (tea-coloured urine with a false-positive urine dipstick test for blood).

(4) Treat muscle pain with simple analgesia such as paracetamol 500 mg and codeine phosphate 8 mg.

(5) Admit patients with an abnormal ECG or history of arrhythmias for cardiac monitoring.

(6) Discharge the patient if there is no history of altered consciousness or cardiac arrhythmia, and the neurological state and ECG are normal, provided there is no significant thermal soft-tissue burn.

   (i) Lethal delayed cardiac arrhythmias have not been reported in patients with no initial history of arrhythmias.

> **Warning:** electrical burns may look deceptively innocent. A white blister or small area of broken skin can cover extensive deep-tissue damage requiring admission to hospital.

HIGH-VOLTAGE ELECTROCUTION

DIAGNOSIS

(1) These injuries occur from electric shocks sustained from sources greater than 1000 volts such as electrical cables and power stations. These are serious injuries, and often fatal.

(2) Injuries are associated with:

   (i) Electrical flash burns with full-thickness injury at points of electricity entry and exit, or flame burns secondary to clothing ignition.

   (ii) Extensive tissue damage, deep muscle necrosis, and compartment syndrome requiring fasciotomy and potentially limb amputation.

   (iii) Tetanic muscle spasm causing long-bone fracture, vertebral crush fracture, muscle tears and joint dislocations.

   (iv) Indirect injury from a resultant fall.

(3) According to the pathway the charge follows, other effects include:

   (i) Lungs: asphyxia from respiratory paralysis and lung parenchyma burns.

   (ii) Heart: cardiac arrest or arrhythmia. The most common cardiac arrest rhythm is VF.

(iii) Brain and CNS: confusion, coma, cerebral haemorrhage, spinal cord damage and peripheral nerve damage.

(iv) Gastrointestinal tract: bowel perforation and intestinal ileus.

(v) Kidneys: acute renal failure secondary to tubular deposition of myoglobin and haemoglobin.

(vii) Visceral and connective tissue: immediate damage to nerves, muscle and bone from heat, vascular thrombosis or delayed secondary haemorrhage.

(viii) Eyes and ears: dilated pupils, uveitis, vitreous haemorrhage, ruptured eardrum, deafness and the late development of cataracts.

(4) Gain i.v. access and send blood for FBC, U&Es, blood sugar, CK, G&S and arterial blood gases. Attach a cardiac monitor and pulse oximeter to the patient.

(5) Perform an ECG.

(6) Request a cervical spine X-ray, CXR and pelvic or limb X-rays, according to the suspected additional injuries.

MANAGEMENT

(1) Assess the airway, give oxygen, and commence cardiopulmonary resuscitation if there is no pulse or absent respirations.

(2) Commence an i.v. infusion ensuring adequate volume replacement guided by the BP and urine output.

(i) Fluid requirements are higher than they appear from assessment of the burnt areas alone. Aim for a urine output of 100 mL/h if there is myoglobinuria.

(3) Examine for major injuries secondary to falls and treat accordingly.

(4) Refer patients to the Surgical team or specialist Burns unit for admission. Escharotomy, fasciotomy, surgical debridement and limb amputation may all become necessary.

LIGHTNING STRIKE

DIAGNOSIS

(1) Lightning strike can deliver up to 300 million volts DC in a few milliseconds.

(2) Death is secondary to cardiac or respiratory arrest (as in industrial and domestic electrical injuries).

(i) The commonest rhythm in cardiac arrest is asystole, as opposed to VF with a high-voltage injury.

    (ii) Overall mortality is up to 30%, with 70% of survivors sustaining significant morbidity.

(3) Lightning strike can produce a wide range of clinical effects:

    (i) Full-thickness contact burns usually to the head, neck and shoulders.

    (ii) Cardiac arrest secondary to depolarization of the entire myocardium.

    (iii) Respiratory arrest secondary to thoracic muscle spasm and depressed respiratory drive.

        (a) this may persist even after return of spontaneous circulation, and may lead to secondary hypoxic arrest.

    (iv) Massive autonomic stimulation with hypertension, tachycardia and myocardial necrosis.

    (v) Non-specific ECG changes including QT prolongation and T wave inversion.

    (vi) Neurological deficits ranging from initial loss of consciousness, peripheral nerve damage, intracerebral haemorrhage, cerebral oedema and transient total body paralysis.

    (vii) Arborescent, feathery cutaneous burns presenting within the first 6 hours post injury, known as Lichtenberg flowers.

    (viii) Miscellaneous injuries including tympanic membrane rupture, corneal defects, retinal detachment and optic nerve damage.

(4) Send bloods for FBC, U&Es, LFTs, CK, blood sugar and G&S.

(5) Perform an ECG and request a trauma X-ray series including chest, pelvis and cervical spine as clinically indicated.

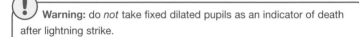

Warning: do *not* take fixed dilated pupils as an indicator of death after lightning strike.

MANAGEMENT

(1) Use standard protocols for VF and asystolic cardiac arrest if there is no pulse or absent respirations (see p. 2).

(2) Assess the airway and give high-flow oxygen. Remove smouldering clothing to prevent secondary thermal injury to skin.

(3) Perform early endotracheal intubation to prevent airway obstruction secondary to soft tissue oedema associated with head and neck burns. Call for urgent senior ED doctor help.

(i) Ventilatory support is also essential to prevent hypoxic cardiac arrest secondary to thoracic muscle paralysis.

(4) Maintain spinal precautions and inline cervical immobilization during endotracheal intubation and physical examination, because of the associated risk of spinal trauma with lightning strike.

(5) Commence an i.v. infusion with normal saline.

(i) Ensure adequate volume replacement guided by BP, urine output and the degree of metabolic and respiratory acidosis.

(ii) Give vigorous fluid resuscitation to enhance excretion of tissue necrosis byproducts such as myoglobin and potassium from extensive rhabdomyolysis.

(6) Examine for major injuries secondary to falls and treat accordingly.

(7) Admit all patients. Survivors of the initial lightning strike have an excellent prognosis provided secondary trauma has not occurred.

> ✓ **Tip:** resuscitate those patients at the scene in cardiac arrest first, the opposite to a mass casualty disaster, where they would be left for dead while other survivable injuries are treated as the priority (see p. 466).

FURTHER READING

American Heart Association (2005) Guidelines for cardiopulmonary resuscitation and emergency cardiovascular care. Part 10.3: Drowning. *Circulation* **112**:IV-133–35.

American Heart Association (2005) Guidelines for cardiopulmonary resuscitation and emergency cardiovascular care. Part 10.4: Hypothermia. *Circulation* **112**:IV-136–38.

American Heart Association (2005) Guidelines for cardiopulmonary resuscitation and emergency cardiovascular care. Part 10.9: Electric shock and lightning strikes. *Circulation* **112**:IV-154–55.

American Heart Association. http://www.circulationaha.org/ (CPR and ECC guidelines 2005).

Emerson GM (2004) Dysbarism. In: Cameron P, Jelinek G, Kelly A-M, *et al. Textbook of Adult Emergency Medicine*, 2nd edn. Churchill Livingstone, Edinburgh: pp. 756–63.

European Resuscitation Council (2005) Guidelines for Resuscitation. Section 7: Cardiac arrest in special circumstances. *Resuscitation* **67(Suppl 1)**:S135–70.

European Resuscitation Council. http://www.erc.edu/ (CPR and ECC guidelines 2005).

Resuscitation Council (UK). http://www.resus.org.uk/ (resuscitation guidelines 2005).

SURGICAL EMERGENCIES

MULTIPLE INJURIES

OVERVIEW

The management of *every* severely injured patient requires a coordinated approach, such as that taught in advanced trauma life support (ATLS) and the equivalent early management of severe trauma (EMST) courses. This involves a rapid primary survey, resuscitation of vital functions, a detailed secondary survey, and the initiation of definitive care.

(1) The primary survey is a rapid patient assessment to identify life-threatening conditions and establish immediate priorities.

   (i) The resuscitation phase optimizes the patient's respiratory and circulatory status. The response to resuscitation is recorded with comprehensive non-invasive monitoring.

   (ii) Once resuscitation is under way, a trauma series of X-rays is taken, bloods are sent, and additional procedures such as a rapid bedside ultrasound, nasogastric tube insertion and urinary catheterization are performed.

(2) The secondary survey commences after the primary survey is complete and the resuscitation phase well under way.

   (i) A detailed head-to-toe examination is made.

   (ii) Special X-rays, repeat ultrasound, CT scan and angiographic studies are performed as indicated.

(3) Definitive care is the management of all the injuries identified, including surgery, fracture stabilization, hospital admission or preparation of the patient for transfer, if required.

(4) Expect serious injuries in patients presenting after the following high-risk mechanisms or with altered physiology:

   (i) Abnormal vital signs: systolic blood pressure under 90 mmHg, GCS score 12 or less, respiratory rate less than 10/min or more than 30/min.

   (ii) Motorcyclist or pedestrian struck.

   (iii) Fall greater than 5 metres (15 feet).

   (iv) Entrapment.

   (v) High-speed impact, ejection or death of another vehicle occupant.

(5) Call senior Emergency Department staff immediately for any multiple-injury patient, to organize an integrated team response incorporating anaesthetic, intensive care, surgical and orthopaedic colleagues.

(6) The time-honoured mnemonic for the initial sequence of care is **ABCDE** (see Table 7.1).

Table 7.1 Mnemonic for initial sequence of care of the multiply-injured patient during the primary survey and resuscitation phases

A	**A**irway maintenance with cervical spine control
B	**B**reathing and ventilation
C	**C**irculation with haemorrhage control
D	**D**isability: brief neurological evaluation
E	**E**xposure/environmental control: completely undress the patient, but prevent hypothermia

IMMEDIATE MANAGEMENT

(1) *Airway*

　(i) Assess the airway to ascertain patency and identify potential obstruction:

　　(a) clear the airway of loose or broken dentures and suck out any debris

　　(b) insert an oropharyngeal airway if the patient is unconscious

　　(c) give 100% oxygen by tight-fitting mask with reservoir bag

　　(d) aim for an oxygen saturation above 94%.

　(ii) Intubation:

　　(a) a definitive procedure to protect and maintain the airway is indicated if the patient is unconscious, or has a reduced or absent gag reflex

　　(b) take great care to minimize neck movements in the unconscious head injury or suspected neck injury by maintaining in-line manual immobilization during airway assessment and endotracheal intubation

　　(c) *rapid sequence induction (RSI) intubation*

　　　– this is the airway technique of choice, provided the operator is skilled in the technique

　　　– use an i.v. induction agent such as thiopentone (thiopental) 0.5–5 mg/kg; etomidate 0.3 mg/kg; or midazolam 0.1 mg/kg plus fentanyl 2.5–5 μg/kg *after* pre-oxygenation ideally for 3 min

– follow with a muscle relaxant, usually suxamethonium
1.5 mg/kg, applying cricoid pressure as muscle tone is
lost

– insert the endotracheal tube under direct vision,
visualizing its passage between the vocal cords, and
inflate the cuff

– confirm correct tube placement using capnography to
measure end-tidal carbon dioxide ($ETCO_2$). Only
release cricoid pressure when happy with tube position

– tie the tube in place and carefully monitor the patient as
a CXR is arranged.

> **⚠ Warning:** *never* attempt RSI unless you have been trained. Use a
> bag–valve mask technique instead while awaiting help.

(iii) Surgical airway: proceed directly to cricothyrotomy if
endotracheal intubation is impossible due to laryngeal injury
or severe maxillofacial injury (see p. 47).

(2) *Maintain the integrity of the cervical spine*

(i) Place the unconscious head injury and the patient with
suspected neck injury in a semi-rigid collar.

(ii) Minimize head movement. When the patient requires turning,
the body should be 'log-rolled', holding the head in the
neutral position at all times.

(3) *Breathing and ventilation*

Look for and treat the following critical conditions:

(i) Tension pneumothorax:

(a) suspect a tension pneumothorax if examination reveals
tachycardia, hypotension, unequal chest expansion, absent
or decreased breath sounds and distended neck veins

(b) insert a wide-bore cannula into the second intercostal space
in the mid-clavicular line on the affected side. Following
initial decompression, proceed to formal intercostal tube
drainage (see p. 45).

(ii) Sucking chest wound with open pneumothorax:

(a) cover with an occlusive dressing such as paraffin gauze
under an adhesive film dressing, secured along three sides
only. Leave the fourth side open for air to escape

(b) proceed to formal intercostal tube drainage (see p. 45).

(iii) Flail chest:
- (a) this causes paradoxical movement of part of the chest wall and may necessitate positive-pressure ventilation
- (b) an associated haemothorax or pneumothorax will require an intercostal tube drain to prevent the development of a tension pneumothorax, if positive-pressure ventilation is used.

(4) *Circulation with haemorrhage control*
- (i) Apply a bulky sterile dressing to compress any external bleeding point (not a tourniquet, as this increases bleeding by venous congestion).
- (ii) Monitor the pulse, blood pressure, pulse oximetry and ECG.
- (iii) Establish an i.v. infusion:
  - (a) insert two large-bore (14- or 16-gauge) cannulae into the antecubital veins
  - (b) one cannula should be below the diaphragm in mediastinal or neck injuries, e.g. in the femoral vein
  - (c) although a central venous (CVP) line is useful both to administer fluids and to monitor the response to resuscitation, only senior ED staff should perform this to minimize the potential complications of arterial puncture and pneumothorax.
- (iv) Infusion fluid:
  - (a) infuse normal saline or Hartmann's (compound sodium lactate) to correct hypovolaemia
  - (b) remember that in healthy adults the only sign associated with the loss of up to 30% of the circulatory blood volume (1500 mL) may be tachycardia with a narrowed pulse pressure. Therefore, a consistent fall in systolic blood pressure indicates that at least 30% of the blood volume has already been lost
  - (c) change infusion fluid to blood if 3000 mL of normal saline or Hartmann's (compound sodium lactate) fail to reverse hypotension. A full cross-match takes 45 min, a type-specific cross-match takes 10 min, and O rhesus-negative blood is available immediately
  - (d) use a blood warmer and macropore blood filter for multiple transfusions. Fresh frozen plasma 5 units and platelets may be required after transfusing 10 units of blood or more, i.e. a 'massive blood transfusion'.
- (v) Send blood for haemoglobin, U&Es, LFTs and blood sugar,

and cross-match at least 4 units of blood according to the suspected injuries. Save serum for a drug screen in case alcohol or drug intoxication is subsequently suspected.

(vi) Cardiac tamponade:

(a) consider cardiac tamponade if there is persistent hypotension with distended neck veins that fill on inspiration (Kussmaul's sign), particularly following penetrating chest trauma

(b) arrange an immediate focussed ultrasound to look for pericardial fluid (blood)

(c) call the Surgical and/or Cardiothoracic team for an urgent thoracotomy if there is persistent haemodynamic compromise.

(5) *Disability: brief neurological evaluation*

(i) Assess the level of consciousness using the Glasgow Coma Scale (see p. 237).

(ii) Examine the eye movements, pupil size, shape and reactivity.

(iii) Assess for abnormal tone, weakness and gross sensory loss, or an asymmetric response to pain if the patient is unconscious. Check the limb reflexes, including the plantar responses.

(iv) Examine the face and scalp for injuries.

(6) *Exposure: completely undress the patient*

(i) Request a lateral cervical spine X-ray, CXR and pelvic X-ray, known as the 'trauma series'. Perform these in the resuscitation bay without interrupting patient care.

(ii) Examine the front of the abdomen, including the perineum, for evidence of penetrating trauma or blunt trauma, e.g. seat-belt bruising or a tyre mark on the skin. Cover any exposed abdominal viscera with saline-soaked packs.

(iii) Log-roll the patient and examine the back for evidence of penetrating or blunt trauma. Palpate the spine for deformity and widened interspinous gaps.

(iv) Perform a rectal examination to assess the position of the prostate, integrity of the rectal wall, anal sphincter tone, and to check for evidence of internal bleeding.

(v) Assess the pelvis by springing to detect instability from major pelvic ring fracture, although this is an unreliable sign.

(vi) Look for associated urethral injury. Suspect urethral transection if there is any bleeding from the urethral meatus, a scrotal haematoma or a high-riding prostate.

> (a) Do not attempt urethral catheterization at this stage.
>
> (vii) Otherwise, insert a urethral catheter and measure the urine output, which should be over 50 mL/h in the adult, and 1 mL/kg per hour in a child.

(7) Pass a large-bore nasogastric or orogastric tube if a basal skull or mid-face fracture is present. This is particularly important in children, who commonly develop acute gastric dilatation following trauma.

(8) Splint major limb fractures, cover compound injuries with sterile dressings, and check the peripheral pulses.

(9) Administer increments of morphine 2.5–5 mg i.v. titrated to analgesic response.

The above procedures will save life during the resuscitation phase, and allow a decision on priorities in proceeding to definitive care. Make sure an ongoing record is kept of all vital signs and clinical findings, and keep re-examining the patient regularly.

Obtain as full a history as possible from ambulance crew, witnesses or relatives, as well as the patient. A useful mnemonic for remembering the components in the history is **AMPLE** (see Table 7.2).

Table 7.2 Mnemonic for components of the history in multiple trauma

A	**A**llergies
M	**M**edications
P	**P**ast history, including alcohol and cigarette use
L	**L**ast meal
E	**E**vents/environment relating to the injury, including time, speed of impact, initial vital signs, and any change in condition

FURTHER DIAGNOSIS AND MANAGEMENT OF MULTIPLE INJURIES: DEFINITIVE CARE

This is considered under the following headings:

- Head and facial injuries
- Neck injuries
- Chest injuries
- Abdominal and pelvic trauma
- Additional orthopaedic injuries

HEAD AND FACIAL INJURIES

DIAGNOSIS AND MANAGEMENT

(1) Scalp.
  (i) Look for lacerations, haematomas, penetrating wounds and foreign bodies.
  (ii) Palpate for evidence of deformity and fracture.
  (iii) Assess the level of consciousness if a major head injury is suspected, and manage as described on p. 236.

(2) Face.
  (i) Check the integrity of the airway again, and remember the possibility of an unsuspected neck injury.
  (ii) Look for bruising, swelling or deformity suggesting orbital, nasal, malar or mandibular fractures (see p. 436).
  (iii) Look for parotid and facial nerve damage in injuries to the face in the area in front of the ear.
  (iv) Clean and evaluate all facial lacerations. They will require meticulous debridement and formal closure when the patient's condition is stable, and all serious injuries have been dealt with.

(3) Eyes.
  (i) Inspect the eyes for evidence of penetrating or blunt injury. Look for specific conditions such as iris prolapse, hyphaema, lens dislocation and traumatic mydriasis (see p. 421).
  (ii) Assess the pupil size and reactions, and examine the fundi for evidence of vitreous or retinal haemorrhage and retinal detachment.
  (iii) Check the visual acuity and eye movements.

(4) Nose.
  (i) Examine for evidence of blood or CSF leakage suggesting a basal skull fracture (see p. 238).
  (ii) Palpate for deformity and nasal bone fracture (see p. 408).
  (iii) Look specifically for a septal haematoma, which, if large, will require incision and drainage to reduce the risk of subsequent cartilage necrosis (see p. 408).

(5) Mouth.
  (i) Examine for broken or missing teeth. They may have been inhaled (see p. 435).
  (ii) Check for dental malocclusion, suggesting maxillary or

mandibular fracture (see p. 436).

   (iii) Assess for nasopharyngeal bleeding, which may be profuse and associated with a basal skull fracture. Look for any tongue lacerations, although they rarely need repairing (see p. 434).

(6) Ears.

   (i) Examine for skin and cartilage damage, which will require drainage and suture later.

   (ii) Consider perforation of the eardrum, although if frank bleeding is seen, do not examine with a speculum to avoid introducing infection. This bleeding may be associated with a basal skull fracture or damage to the external ear canal (see p. 238).

NECK INJURIES

CERVICAL SPINE INJURY

This should be considered in all patients with localized neck pain or pain on palpation following trauma. It should also be *assumed* in any unconscious head injury, multiply injured patient or a patient with a locally distracting injury above the clavicles.

DIAGNOSIS

(1) Ask about local pain or tenderness on palpation if the patient is conscious, and about any associated limb weakness or sensory deficit noticed.

(2) Check the vital signs. A cervical or high thoracic cord lesion will cause respiratory difficulty, tachypnoea and abdominal breathing. Loss of sympathetic tone will cause bradycardia, hypotension and hypothermia from vasodilation if the ambient temperature is low.

(3) Palpate for areas of tenderness, swelling or deformity in the neck. Assess for limb tone, weakness, reflex loss and sensory deficit, including loss of perineal sensation and anal tone.

(4) Describe any motor weakness found by the myotome and reflex abnormalities:

   (i) Myotomes in the upper limb. Nerve roots C5 to T1 supply the muscles of the upper limb (see Table 7.3).

(ii) Use the Medical Research Council scale to grade muscle weakness, so that the same terminology is used by each doctor examining the patient (see Table 7.4).

(iii) Reflexes in the upper limb: assess for the biceps, triceps and supinator upper limb reflexes, which indicate normal or other functioning of certain motor roots (see Table 7.5 for motor roots of the reflexes).

   (a) use reinforcement (Jendrassik manoeuvre) before concluding that a reflex is absent, e.g. ask the patient to clench the teeth hard or hold the knees together when testing a reflex.

Table 7.3 Myotomes in the upper limb and their associated actions

Root	Action
C5	Shoulder abduction
C6, C7	Shoulder adduction
C5, C6	Elbow flexion
C7	Elbow extension
C6	Pronation and supination
(C6), C7	Wrist flexion
C6, (C7)	Wrist extension
C8	Finger flexion
C7	Finger extension
T1	Intrinsic hand muscles

Table 7.4 Medical Research Council (MRC) scale used to grade muscle weakness

Recorded grade	Physical finding
Grade 0	Complete paralysis
Grade 1	A flicker of contraction only
Grade 2	Movement possible only if gravity is eliminated
Grade 3	Movement against gravity
Grade 4	Movement against gravity and resistance
Grade 5	Normal power

(5) Describe sensory deficit by dermatomes:
  (i) Assess sensation by testing pain fibres using pinprick (spinothalamic tracts), and examine fine touch or joint position sense (posterior columns).
  (ii) Dermatomes C5–T1 supply the upper limb (see Table 7.6).
  (iii) Dermatomes C4 and T2 are adjacent on the front of the chest at the level of the first and second ribs.
(6) The myotomes, reflexes and dermatomes in the leg are described on p. 335.
(7) Cervical spine imaging:
  (i) Lateral cervical spine X-ray:
    (a) make sure an adequate view is obtained and that all seven cervical vertebrae and the C7/T1 junction are visualized. A swimmer's view may be required
    (b) look for appropriate alignment of the cervical spine longitudinal lines. Anterior displacement of greater than 3 mm implies ligament disruption and cervical spine instability (see Fig. 7.1)
    (c) observe the bony vertebrae for signs of fractures such as wedge and teardrop. Examine the soft-tissue shadows in front of the vertebral bodies (see Fig. 7.1):

Table 7.5 Reflexes in the upper limb

Reflex	Root
Biceps	C5, (C6)
Supinator	(C5), C6
Triceps	(C6), C7, C8

Table 7.6 Dermatomes supplying the upper limb

Root	Dermatomal distribution
C5	Outer upper arm
C6	Outer forearm
C7	Middle finger
C8	Inner forearm
T1	Inner upper arm

– the retropharyngeal space should be less than 5 mm between C1 and C4/C5

– the retrotracheal space should be less than the width of one vertebral body in adults between C4/C5 and T1.

(ii) Open-mouth odontoid view: examine the odontoid peg and dens of C2, and the lateral masses of C1 for evidence of fractures.

(iii) Anteroposterior cervical spine X-ray: look for rotation of the vertebrae, loss of joint space and transverse process fracture.

(iv) Cervical spine CT scan: perform this in addition to the 3-view plain cervical spine X-rays to help identify bony injury, and to confirm cervical fractures and vertebral subluxations. It is particularly useful to evaluate trauma patients with:

(a) an altered level of consciousness

(b) distracting injuries

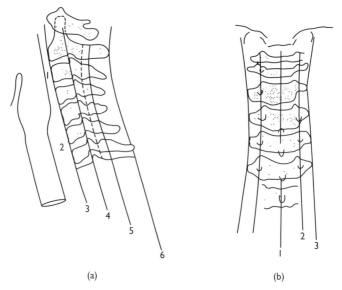

(a)   (b)

Figure 7.1 Cervical spine x-ray in the adult

(a) Lateral view: (1) retropharyngeal space (< 5 mm), (2) retrotracheal space (less than the width of one vertebral body), (3) anterior longitudinal ligament line, (4) posterior longitudinal ligament line, (5) spinolaminar line, (6) posterior spinal line. Lines 3, 4, 5 and 6 should all be parallel, following the normal gentle lordotic curve of the cervical spine. The spinal cord runs between lines 4 and 5. (b) Anteroposterior view: (1) interspinous line, (2) foramen transversarium line, (3) transverse processes line. Lines 1, 2 and 3 should be straight in the normal neck

> (c) neurological deficit
>
> (d) drug/alcohol intoxication.

(v) MRI is more sensitive than CT and plain X-ray for identifying soft-tissue damage such as ligamentous injuries, disc herniation or a haemorrhage causing compression of the spinal cord or cervical nerve roots.

> (a) it is rarely available in the acute situation, but may be arranged subsequently.

MANAGEMENT

(1) Always apply a semi-rigid collar, minimize head movements in any suspected neck injury, and use laterally placed sandbags taped to the forehead to prevent head rotation.

(2) Arrange urgent airway control with orotracheal (or rarely nasotracheal) intubation for the unconscious patient or for profound hypoventilation.

(i) Only an airway-skilled doctor should perform this, usually by a rapid sequence induction (RSI) intubation technique (see p. 205) with in-line manual immobilization to protect the neck from any movement.

(3) Restore the circulatory volume if the patient is hypotensive.

(i) First look for sources of blood loss before deciding that hypotension in a patient with a cervical cord injury is due to loss of sympathetic tone with vasodilation and bradycardia (i.e. neurogenic shock).

(ii) Place a urinary catheter to monitor urinary output.

(4) Severe ligamentous damage with cervical spine instability may occur, with an apparently normal X-ray.

(i) This is more likely in children, in whom up to 50% of serious spinal injuries have normal X-rays (SCIWORA – spinal cord injury without radiological abnormality).

(ii) Neck hyperextension may cause predominant weakness of the arms in elderly patients with cervical spondylosis, without any associated fracture or dislocation, known as the central cord syndrome.

(5) Refer all suspected cervical spine injuries to the Orthopaedic or Surgical team and begin pressure-area nursing.

(6) The value of high-dose methylprednisolone to improve neurological outcome in patients with complete or incomplete spinal cord damage is unconvincing and controversial.

(i) Start treatment within 8 hours of injury, guided by the advice of the regional Spinal Injuries unit.

(ii) Infuse methylprednisolone 30 mg/kg over 15 min, followed 45 min later by 5.4 mg/kg per hour for 23 hours.

AIRWAY INJURY

DIAGNOSIS

(1) Airway injuries may be penetrating or blunt, isolated, or associated with multiple injuries.

(2) Patients may present with pain, stridor, cough, haemoptysis and/or a hoarse voice.

(3) Examine for local swelling, subcutaneous emphysema, pneumothorax or haemothorax.

(4) Perform anteroposterior and lateral cervical spine X-rays and a CXR.

MANAGEMENT

(1) The patient must not be left unattended at any stage. Call for urgent senior ED staff to help.

(2) Perform endotracheal intubation or cricothyrotomy, or insert an endotracheal tube directly into a gaping wound in the trachea to maintain patency of the airway.

(3) Refer the patient immediately to the Surgical team for admission.

VASCULAR INJURY IN THE NECK

DIAGNOSIS AND MANAGEMENT

(1) Vascular injury causes obvious external haemorrhage, or internal bleeding with rapid haematoma formation, which may compromise the airway.

(2) Do *not* attempt to probe or explore any penetrating wounds in the Emergency Department. Leave all penetrating objects *in situ*.

(3) The patient will require angiography and panendoscopy with urgent surgical referral to arrange formal wound exploration in theatre.

NERVE INJURY IN THE NECK

DIAGNOSIS AND MANAGEMENT

(1) Damage to the following nerves causes specific signs and symptoms:
   (i) Recurrent laryngeal branch of the vagus: hoarseness and vocal cord paralysis.
   (ii) Accessory nerve: loss of function of trapezius and sternomastoid.
   (iii) Phrenic nerve: loss of diaphragmatic movement.
   (iv) Hypoglossal nerve: deviation of the tongue to the affected side.
   (v) Cervical sympathetic cord: Horner syndrome, with partial ptosis, a constricted pupil, and decreased sweating on the same side of the face.
(2) Refer any of these injuries to the Surgical team.

OESOPHAGEAL INJURY

DIAGNOSIS AND MANAGEMENT

(1) Oesophageal injury in the neck causes dysphagia, drooling and localized pain, with the development of surgical emphysema.
(2) Refer this rare condition to the Surgical team for immediate admission.

NECK SPRAIN

DIAGNOSIS

(1) Neck sprain is most commonly associated with hyperextension injuries resulting from sudden deceleration in a motor vehicle collision. The lay term for this mechanism of injury is 'whiplash'. In practice, neck sprain occurs with other directions of impact, including hyperflexion.
(2) The resultant neck pain and stiffness often go unnoticed at the time of injury. Patients typically present 12–24 hours after the injury, often with symptoms of headache.
(3) The pain may radiate to the shoulders and arms, causing paraesthesiae, but neurological examination does not show any objective deficit. Neck movements are restricted by pain.
(4) Cervical spine X-ray may show loss of the normal anterior curvature due to muscle spasm.

MANAGEMENT
(1) Treat the patient with a non-steroidal anti-inflammatory analgesic drug (NSAID), such as ibuprofen 200–400 mg orally t.d.s. or naproxen 250 mg orally t.d.s., and encourage early mobilization.
(2) Refer the patient to the Physiotherapy team if the pain fails to settle, for heat treatment and motion exercises.
(3) Unfortunately, symptoms may continue for months, and may be exacerbated by further minor injuries.

CHEST INJURIES

PNEUMOTHORAX

DIAGNOSIS
(1) Tension pneumothorax.
   (i) This causes severe respiratory distress, tachypnoea and hypotension. There is tracheal deviation away from the affected side, distended neck veins, loss of chest expansion on the affected side, a hyper-resonant percussion note, and diminished or absent breath sounds.
   (ii) Perform immediate decompression. Use a large-bore i.v. cannula inserted into the second intercostal space in the mid-clavicular line, followed by placement of an intercostal drain (see p. 45).
(2) Simple pneumothorax.
   (i) This is caused by blunt or penetrating chest trauma, and penetrating abdominal trauma breaching the diaphragm.
   (ii) It is surprisingly easy to miss. Examine for subcutaneous emphysema, decreased chest expansion, and quiet breath sounds.
   (iii) Confirm the diagnosis with an erect CXR to highlight a small apical pneumothorax, provided there is no possibility of spinal injury.
      (a) the supine CXR may, however, appear normal and miss a small pneumothorax lying anteriorly.

MANAGEMENT
(1) Virtually all cases of traumatic pneumothorax require chest-drain insertion to avoid the subsequent development of tension,

particularly if positive-pressure ventilation is necessary.

(2) Insert an intercostal drain into the fifth or sixth intercostal space in the mid-axillary line (see p. 45).

HAEMOTHORAX

DIAGNOSIS

(1) This results from chest wall damage, penetrating or blunt lung injury and great vessel damage.

(2) It causes hypotension, respiratory difficulty with reduced chest expansion, quiet breath sounds, and a dull percussion note at the base of the affected lung.

(3) Request an erect or semi-erect CXR to identify a fluid level, provided there is no possibility of spinal injury.

(4) Look for diffuse ground-glass haziness over one hemithorax if only a supine CXR is possible, which is easy to miss. Alternatively, take a lateral decubitus CXR.

MANAGEMENT

(1) Give high-dose oxygen and commence i.v. fluid, including blood.

(2) Insert a large-bore 32- or 36-French gauge intercostal drain in the fifth or sixth intercostal space in the mid-axillary line, using blunt dissection down to and through the pleura (see p. 45).

(3) Autotransfusion devices are available to collect and return the intrathoracic blood to the circulation, provided contamination from gastrointestinal injury is excluded.

(4) A thoracotomy may be required if bleeding is severe and persists (see p. 225).

RIB AND STERNUM FRACTURES

DIAGNOSIS

(1) These injuries are associated with direct trauma. They cause localized pain and tenderness, worse on breathing or springing the chest wall.

(2) Associated injury may occur with fractures in the following areas:
   (i) Clavicle, first and second ribs: damage to the subclavian vessels, aorta, trachea, main bronchus, and spinal cord or brachial plexus.
   (ii) Sternum: damage to the myocardium, great vessels and upper thoracic spine.

(iii) Right lower ribs: damage to the liver and right kidney.

(iv) Left lower ribs: damage to the spleen and left kidney.

(3) A flail segment with paradoxical chest wall movement from multiple rib fractures in two sites causes hypoxia, mainly from the underlying pulmonary contusion.

(4) Perform an ECG to exclude myocardial contusion (see below).

(5) Request a CXR to look for the complications of pneumothorax, haemothorax and a widened mediastinum, not simply to visualize the fractures. A lateral sternal X-ray is indicated for a suspected sternal fracture.

MANAGEMENT

(1) Give the patient high-flow oxygen by face mask and aim for an oxygen saturation of 94%.

(2) Commence i.v. resuscitation as required, insert an intercostal drain if indicated, and administer adequate analgesia such as increments of morphine 2.5–5 mg i.v.

(3) Refer the following patients to the Surgical team for admission:

(i) Pneumothorax, haemothorax.

(ii) Fractured sternum with severe pain or ECG abnormalities.

(iii) Complications listed in diagnosis point (2) above.

(iv) Pre-existing lung disease with poor respiratory reserve.

(v) Rib fractures with significant pain. These patients may require a thoracic epidural.

(4) Discharge remaining patients with uncomplicated rib fractures or an isolated sternal fracture with a normal ECG and CXR.

(5) Provide an analgesic such as paracetamol 500 mg and codeine phosphate 8 mg two tablets orally q.d.s.

(i) Recommend regular deep-breathing exercises to prevent atelectasis.

(ii) Contact the GP by fax or letter.

(6) Positive-pressure ventilation may be required for deteriorating respiratory function, although an intercostal drain must be inserted first for any pneumothorax, however small.

MYOCARDIAL CONTUSION

DIAGNOSIS

(1) This is due to blunt deceleration injury and is associated with rib fractures, sternal fracture and chest wall contusion. It is difficult to

diagnose as there is no agreed gold standard.

(2) It may be asymptomatic, but can cause chest pain or rarely cause transient right ventricular dysfunction with distended neck veins and hypotension.

(3) Gain i.v. access and send blood for FBC, U&Es, cardiac enzymes and G&S.

    (i) Cardiac enzyme changes including CK and CK-MB isoenzymes are unreliable, non-specific, and do not predict the presence of contusion or its complications.

    (ii) Troponins are a more reliable indicator of cardiac myocyte damage, but again do not stratify the potential risk. They may, however, incidentally diagnose antecedent myocardial infarction.

(4) Perform an ECG.

    (i) Myocardial contusion may result in ventricular conduction abnormalities and malignant arrhythmias.

    (ii) ECG abnormalities range from sinus tachycardia, atrial fibrillation, bundle branch block and ventricular extrasystoles to non-specific ST and T wave abnormalities or ST elevation.

(5) Echocardiography may show wall motion abnormalities, but is most useful to exclude cardiac tamponade or acute valvular rupture.

(6) Request a CXR.

MANAGEMENT

(1) Give the patient high-dose oxygen and administer a cautious fluid challenge if hypotensive.

(2) Give morphine 2.5–5 mg i.v. with an antiemetic such as metoclopramide 10 mg i.v. for pain.

(3) Admit all patients with unstable arrhythmias and haemodynamic instability to the ICU. Obtain an urgent echocardiogram if hypotension persists or cardiac tamponade cannot be excluded.

(4) Refer patients with stable ECG abnormalities, age greater than 50 years or pre-existing cardiac disease to CCU for cardiac monitoring following evidence of significant blunt chest trauma.

(5) Discharge home patients less than 50 years old with normal ECG findings, and without a history of cardiac disease with oral analgesia.

AORTIC RUPTURE

DIAGNOSIS

(1) This occurs following high-speed deceleration injury, when the aorta is torn just distal to the left subclavian artery.

(2) Always consider this diagnosis in any deceleration injury over 45 m.p.h. (60 k.p.h.) or following a fall from over 5 metres (15 feet).

(3) Only 10–15% of patients with rupture of the thoracic aorta survive to reach hospital.

(4) Clinical signs of aortic rupture are subtle or absent and so diagnosis is suspected based on the mechanism of injury, a history of chest or interscapular pain, unequal blood pressures in each arm, or different femoral and brachial pulse volume.

(5) Insert two large-bore i.v. cannulae and cross-match 10 units of blood.

(6) Perform a CXR and look for the following signs of aortic rupture:
  (i) Widened mediastinum (8 cm or more on a 1-metre supine anteroposterior X-ray):
    (a) 10% of these patients will have a contained aortic rupture confirmed
    (b) other causes of a widened mediastinum include a mediastinal haematoma from sternal fracture, lower cervical or thoracic spine fracture, oesophageal injury, local venous oozing and projection artefact.
  (ii) Blurred aortic outline with obliteration of the aortic knuckle.
  (iii) Left apical cap of fluid in the pleural space and a left haemothorax.
  (iv) Depressed left main stem bronchus.
  (v) Displacement of the trachea to the right.
  (vi) Displacement of a nasogastric tube in the oesophagus to the right.

(7) Look for a cervical, thoracic or sternal fracture clinically and on X-ray, although exclusion of aortic rupture is still necessary irrespective of clinical findings if the CXR is suggestive.

(8) Perform a high-speed helical CT scan of the chest to look for blood contiguous with the aorta, or an abnormal aortic wall indicative of rupture.

MANAGEMENT

(1) Administer fluid cautiously.
  (i) Initial hypotension responds to modest fluid replacement in contained aortic rupture.
  (ii) Take care to avoid over-transfusion or hypertension from poorly controlled pain, etc.
(2) Refer the patient to the Surgical team for further evaluation with aortography or transoesophageal echo, if the patient has a high-risk mechanism of injury and positive radiographic findings.
  (i) Urgent thoracotomy and repair are indicated when either of these show a rupture, or endovascular stenting if the expertise is available locally.

DIAPHRAGM RUPTURE

DIAGNOSIS

(1) This may occur from blunt or penetrating chest or abdominal trauma, including crush fracture of the pelvis. Left-sided lesions are more common and allow eventration of the stomach or intestine into the chest.
(2) 75% of patients with ruptured diaphragm have associated intra-abdominal injuries.
(3) It causes difficulty in breathing, and occasionally bowel sounds are audible in the chest.
(4) Perform a CXR and look for any signs of diaphragm rupture:
  (i) Look for evidence of haemothorax, pneumothorax, elevated hemidiaphragm and coils of bowel or a nasogastric tube curled up in the left lower chest.
  (ii) The diagnosis is often missed, as the CXR appears normal in up to 25% of cases.

MANAGEMENT

(1) Decompress the stomach with a nasogastric tube.
(2) Carefully insert an intercostal drain for an associated haemothorax or pneumothorax, using blunt dissection down to and through the parietal pleura (see p. 45). *Never* use the trocar introducer to insert the drain.
(3) Refer the patient to the Surgical team following basic resuscitation.

OESOPHAGEAL RUPTURE

DIAGNOSIS

(1) This rare injury is most commonly associated with penetrating trauma or following blunt trauma to the upper abdomen. Other causes include instrumentation, swallowing a sharp object, and spontaneous rupture from vomiting (Boerhaave syndrome).

(2) The patient complains of retrosternal pain, difficulty in swallowing, and occasionally haematemesis. Look for cervical subcutaneous emphysema.

(3) Establish venous access with a large-bore i.v. cannula.

(4) Request a CXR to look for a widened mediastinum with mediastinal air, a left pneumothorax, pleural effusion or haemothorax. These findings in the absence of rib fracture should suggest the possibility of rupture.

(5) Request a CT scan to look for air in the mediastinum.

MANAGEMENT

(1) Administer oxygen and replace fluids. Give morphine 2.5–5 mg i.v. for pain with an antiemetic.

(2) Commence broad-spectrum antibiotics if rupture is considered likely, such as gentamicin 5 mg/kg i.v., ampicillin 1 g i.v., and metronidazole 500 mg i.v.

(3) Carefully insert an intercostal drain. Particulate matter in the intercostal tube drainage confirms the diagnosis.

(4) Refer the patient to the Surgical team for a gastrografin swallow and/or oesophagoscopy, followed by surgical repair if feasible.

PENETRATING CHEST INJURIES

DIAGNOSIS

(1) Potential injuries arising from penetrating chest injury may be predicted:

   (i) Medial to the nipple line anteriorly or tips of the scapulae posteriorly are at high risk of heart or great vessel injury.

   (ii) Below the fourth intercostal space may also injure the abdominal contents.

   (iii) Above the umbilicus may injure the lungs, heart or great vessels.

(2) Patients usually present with pain and dyspnoea. However, some patients are surprisingly undistressed.

(3) The patient may be hypotensive with signs of a haemothorax or pneumothorax. Hypotension may be secondary to blood loss, cardiac tamponade or the development of tension pneumothorax.

(4) Gain i.v. access and send bloods.

(5) Request a CXR to look for any of the above complications.

MANAGEMENT

(1) Assess and secure the airway, give high-flow oxygen, and perform needle thoracocentesis if required. Commence fluid resuscitation.

(2) 80% of penetrating chest injuries are managed conservatively with the insertion of an intercostal drain (see p. 45).

(3) Injuries involving the heart and great vessels require thoracotomy, either in the Emergency Department or urgently in theatre.

(4) Patients in cardiac arrest secondary to trauma require an immediate *emergency department thoracotomy*:
   (i) Optimum survival rates are found in patients with:
      (a) palpable pulse and spontaneous respirations at the scene of the incident
      (b) elapsed time since cardiac arrest of less than 10 min
      (c) penetrating trauma secondary to stab wound or low-velocity bullet.
   (ii) Traumatic cardiac arrest is nearly always fatal in patients with:
      (a) blunt chest trauma or a high-velocity bullet wound
      (b) absence of palpable pulse or respiratory effort at the scene of the incident
      (c) elapsed time without signs of life greater than 15 min.

(6) Transfer patients with the following injuries immediately to the operating theatre for urgent *operating room thoracotomy*:
   (i) Penetrating cardiac injuries.
   (ii) Massive haemothorax with greater than 1500 mL initial drainage or over 200 mL/h for 2–4 hours.
   (iii) Persistent large air leak suggesting tracheobronchial injury.
   (iv) Cardiac tamponade following trauma that recurs after pericardiocentesis.

ABDOMINAL AND PELVIC TRAUMA

BLUNT ABDOMINAL TRAUMA

DIAGNOSIS

(1) This should be suspected in the following:
   (i) Road traffic crash or a fall from a height, particularly if there is evidence of chest, pelvic or long bone injury (e.g. injuries on either side of the abdomen).
   (ii) Trauma victims with unexplained hypotension in the absence of obvious external bleeding or a thoracic injury.

(2) Ask about referred shoulder-tip pain or localized pain suggesting lower rib, pelvic or thoracolumbar spine injury.

(3) Look for the imprint of clothing or tyre marks as indicators of potential intra-abdominal injury. Bruising from a lap seat belt may be associated with duodenal, pancreatic or small bowel injury, and fracture–dislocation of the lumbar spine.

(4) Examine the chest, pelvis and back as well as the abdomen.

(5) Log-roll the patient to examine the thoracolumbar spine. Inspect the perineum, perform a rectal examination and consider a vaginal examination as well in females, when there are signs of local injury.

(6) Insert two large-bore i.v. cannulae and send blood for FBC, U&Es, LFTs, blood sugar, amylase/lipase, and cross-match at least 4 units of blood.

(7) Request initial radiology including chest, pelvis and thoracolumbar spine X-rays. The plain abdominal film is rarely indicated.
   (i) Erect CXR: this may demonstrate a thoracic injury or free gas under the diaphragm. Look particularly for lower rib fractures associated with liver, splenic and renal injury.
   (ii) Pelvis X-ray: a fractured pelvis may be associated with major intra-abdominal or retroperitoneal injuries, which must be looked for.
   (iii) Plain abdominal film: look for loss of the psoas shadow, transverse process fracture, abnormal renal outlines and free gas within the peritoneal cavity on a lateral decubitus view. It is usually of little value, and rarely performed.

MANAGEMENT

(1) Give high-flow oxygen. Transfuse initially with crystalloid such as normal saline or Hartmann's (compound sodium lactate), then blood when available.

(2) Insert a urethral catheter to measure the urine output and to look for haematuria.

   (i) Omit this if a urethral injury is suspected from blood at the meatus, a scrotal haematoma or a high-riding prostate on rectal examination.

   (ii) Pass a nasogastric tube to drain the stomach.

(3) Consider the need for an immediate laparotomy and alert theatre. Indications include:

   (i) Persistent shock.

   (ii) Rigid, silent abdomen.

   (iii) Radiological evidence of free gas or ruptured diaphragm.

(4) Commonly there are no immediate indications for laparotomy and further investigation is warranted:

   (i) *Ultrasound*

      (a) focussed assessment by sonography for trauma (FAST) ultrasound is ideal for unstable patients unable to be transferred for CT evaluation

      (b) this bedside test is rapid, repeatable, non-invasive and highly sensitive for free intraperitoneal fluid, i.e. blood from a haemoperitoneum

      (c) however, it is operator dependent, and may miss hollow viscus, diaphragmatic and retroperitoneal injuries.

   (ii) *CT scan of abdomen*

      (a) patients must be stable. This investigation takes time and the patient must be transported out of the resuscitation room

      (b) CT provides additional anatomical information of the intra-abdominal organs injured allowing non-operative management

      (c) CT also provides visualization of the retroperitoneum, pelvis and lower chest, but may still miss hollow viscus and diaphragmatic injuries.

   (iii) *Diagnostic peritoneal lavage (DPL)*

      (a) has largely been entirely superseded by FAST and CT scans

      (b) may be used when the above are not available, to diagnose a haemoperitoneum with unexplained hypotension, or

other suspected abdominal injury or when abdominal examination is:
  – unreliable, due to coma, intoxication or spinal injury
  – equivocal, due to fractured lower ribs, pelvis or lumbar spine
  – impractical in planned extra-abdominal radiographic or surgical procedures.

(d) infiltrate local anaesthetic with adrenaline (epinephrine), and then perform open dissection via a mini-laparotomy incision through all the layers of the abdominal wall

(e) the procedure is positive if:
  – 5–10 mL of frank blood or enteric contents are aspirated
  – peritoneal lavage fluid effluent exits via a chest tube or bladder catheter
  – laboratory analysis of lavage fluid shows over 100 000 red blood cells/mm^3.

(f) it is highly sensitive for intraperitoneal bleeding although it provides no indication about its source or volume, and misses retroperitoneal injury to the duodenum, pancreas, kidney and pelvis, or a diaphragm rupture.

(5) Involve the admitting Surgical team at all stages of investigation, as the decision on emergency laparotomy is theirs.

PENETRATING ABDOMINAL TRAUMA

DIAGNOSIS

(1) Penetrating abdominal injury may occur in stabbing injuries, industrial incidents, road traffic crashes, explosions and gunshot wounds.

(2) Gunshot wounds may be divided into three types:
  (i) *High-velocity wound*
    (a) the muzzle velocity of a bullet from a high-velocity rifle exceeds 1000 m/s
    (b) a small entry wound is associated with gross internal tissue damage from cavitation and a large exit wound.
  (ii) *Low-velocity wound*
    (a) the muzzle velocity from a hand gun reaches 250 m/s
    (b) the bullet causes local internal damage by perforation and laceration, often passing through several structures.
  (iii) *Shotgun wound*

    (a) this causes massive superficial internal damage from close range (less than 7 metres) and is usually fatal from a range of less than 3 metres (10 feet)

    (b) there is scattering of shot if the shotgun is fired from more than 7 metres, perforating structures within the abdomen

    (c) a shot from over 40 metres may not even penetrate the peritoneal cavity.

(3) An entry wound may be obvious, with evisceration of bowel, or may be difficult to find especially if hidden by a gluteal fold or in the perineum.

(4) The most important signs to look for are hypotension and shock.

(5) Abdominal examination is often unreliable and abdominal tenderness on examination is absent in up to 50% of patients with acute haemoperitoneum. Positive examination findings include local rigidity and guarding with reduced bowel sounds.

(6) Remember that associated chest injuries can occur with any wound above the umbilicus.

(7) Insert a large-bore i.v. cannula and send blood for FBC, U&Es, amylase/lipase and cross-match.

(8) Request a CXR to look for associated thoracic injury, and an AXR to assess for metallic foreign bodies.

(9) Test gastric aspirate and urine for blood, although haematuria indicating a urological injury is an unreliable sign.

(10) Arrange a CT scan if non-operative management is even considered.

MANAGEMENT

(1) Cover any exposed bowel with saline-soaked pads.

(2) Give oxygen, and replace fluid initially with normal saline. Titrate analgesic requirements by administering 2.5–5.0 mg morphine i.v.

(3) Commence broad-spectrum antibiotics, e.g. gentamicin 5 mg/kg i.v., ampicillin 1 g i.v. and metronidazole 500 mg i.v. Give tetanus prophylaxis.

(4) Refer all patients to the Surgical team for urgent admission and laparotomy for all gunshot wounds and the majority of stab wounds.

PELVIC INJURY

The major complication of a pelvic fracture is massive blood loss, with up to 3 litres or more of concealed haemorrhage, which may continue despite resuscitation.

DIAGNOSIS

(1) Pelvic injuries usually result from high-energy blunt trauma in road traffic crashes, crush injuries, and from falls.

(2) Associated bladder, urethral, vaginal and rectal injuries occur, which account for further morbidity. A ruptured diaphragm must also be excluded.

(3) There is local pain, tenderness and bruising. Bony instability demonstrated by distracting the iliac crests is an unreliable sign that may increase bleeding.

(4) Rectal examination is mandatory to identify rectal or urethral injury.

(5) Insert two large-bore i.v. cannulae and send blood for FBC, U&Es, amylase/lipase, coagulation profile, blood sugar and cross-match at least 6 units of blood.

(6) Request a pelvic X-ray in *all* multi-trauma patients, especially if there is unexplained hypotension.

(7) Pelvic fractures associated with the greatest risk of haemorrhage include:
   (i) Quadripartite 'butterfly' fracture of all four pubic rami.
   (ii) Open-book fracture with diastasis of the symphysis pubis over 2.5 cm.
   (iii) Vertical shear fracture with hemipelvic disruption.

MANAGEMENT

(1) Give high-flow oxygen. Commence i.v. fluid resuscitation.

(2) Do not attempt to catheterize the bladder if urethral rupture is suspected, but await assistance from an experienced ED doctor, or surgical assistance.

(3) Call the Surgical, Orthopaedic and interventional Radiology team immediately.
   (i) Control of haemorrhage secondary to pelvic trauma may require external fixation of pelvic fractures, arterial embolization and laparotomy.

(4) Exclude intraperitoneal bleeding first with a bedside ultrasound (FAST) or failing this a supra-umbilical, open diagnostic peritoneal lavage (DPL).

(5) Fashion a pelvic sling from a sheet secured tightly around the front of the pelvis, or preferably use one of the radiolucent, commercially available pelvic slings.

(6) Alternatively, consider the temporary use of a pneumatic antishock

garment such as MAST (military antishock trousers) in the presence of pelvic ring disruption while definitive care is being organized, if hypotension persists despite fluid resuscitation:

(i) These have three independent compartments, reducing the circulation through the pelvis and legs, thus supporting the blood pressure and splinting any fractures.

(ii) Never deflate the garment until rapid fluid replacement therapy and immediate laparotomy are available.

BLUNT RENAL INJURIES

DIAGNOSIS

(1) These may be associated with injury to the vertebral column, lower ribs, ureters, aorta, inferior vena cava, and the abdominal contents.

(2) Blunt renal trauma causes haematuria, loin pain and tenderness, and rarely a flank mass may be felt.

(3) Hypotension is due to retroperitoneal bleeding or an associated paralytic ileus.

(4) Insert a large-bore i.v. cannula and send blood for FBC, U&Es and cross-match 2–6 units of blood.

(5) Request a thoracolumbar spine X-ray if bony trauma is possible.

(i) A plain abdominal film looking for 11th and 12th rib fracture, loss of the psoas shadow, or an abnormal soft-tissue outline indicating retroperitoneal bleeding is usually unhelpful.

(6) Proceed to special radiological imaging of the kidney and ureters. Indications include:

(i) Significant deceleration injury with the risk of renal pedicle injury.

(ii) Local physical signs.

(iii) Macroscopic haematuria.

(iv) Microscopic haematuria with shock (systolic blood pressure 90 mmHg or less) at any time.

(v) Penetrating proximity trauma (see below p. 232).

(7) Request a CT scan with i.v. contrast to evaluate suspected renal injury in the presence of any of the above. It has virtually replaced the intravenous pyelogram (IVP).

MANAGEMENT

(1) Resuscitate the patient with i.v. fluids and exclude associated intra-abdominal injuries with ultrasound (FAST), CT, or DPL.

(2) Refer the patient to the Surgical team for admission and observation. Over 85% of blunt renal injuries settle on conservative management with bed rest and analgesia.

PENETRATING RENAL INJURIES

DIAGNOSIS

(1) These are rare and usually involve injury to the abdominal contents, ureter or vertebral column. They may be multiple or associated with penetrating anterior truncal injury.

(2) There is usually haematuria, localized pain, and tenderness, although significant renal or ureteric injury may present without haematuria.

(3) Ureteric colic may occur with the passage of blood clots.

(4) Insert a large-bore i.v. cannula and send blood for FBC, U&Es, and cross-match 2–4 units.

(5) Perform special imaging with a CT scan with i.v. contrast or occasionally an IVP if that is all that is available.

(6) Both demonstrate the nature of the renal injury and also confirm the presence and normal function of the other kidney.

(7) CT scan gives essential additional information on intra- or retroperitoneal injury.

MANAGEMENT

(1) Resuscitate the patient with i.v. fluids, commence antibiotics such as gentamicin 5 mg/kg i.v. and ampicillin 1 g i.v. and give tetanus prophylaxis as indicated.

(2) Refer the patient to the Surgical team for admission.

BLADDER AND URETHRAL INJURIES

DIAGNOSIS

(1) These injuries are more commonly associated with direct blunt trauma to the lower abdomen and with major pelvic fractures.

(2) *Bladder rupture* may be intraperitoneal or extraperitoneal.
    (i) Intraperitoneal: associated with shock and peritonism.
    (ii) Extraperitoneal:
        (a) with signs of urine extravasation and local bruising
        (b) more than 95% have macroscopic haematuria.

(3) *Urethral rupture* may occur to the membranous or bulbous urethra.

(i) Membranous urethra:
   (a) associated with difficulty voiding urine and urethral bleeding, which mimics extraperitoneal rupture of the bladder
   (b) rectal examination reveals a high-riding prostate, often with an underlying boggy haematoma.

(ii) Bulbous urethra:
   (a) caused by a straddle injury (falling astride an object)
   (b) results in local perineal bruising, pain and meatal bleeding.

MANAGEMENT

(1) Call for a senior ED doctor and attempt to gently catheterize the bladder, but stop if any resistance at all is encountered.

(2) Treat the patient for pain and shock, and give antibiotics such as gentamicin 5 mg/kg i.v. and ampicillin 1 g i.v.

(3) Refer to the Surgical team for an ascending urethrogram or cystogram, *before* a CT scan of the abdomen with i.v. contrast is performed.

ADDITIONAL ORTHOPAEDIC INJURIES IN MULTIPLE TRAUMA

Pelvic trauma with bony injury particularly associated with haemorrhage requires urgent Orthopaedic team involvement. Other orthopaedic injuries that occur in multiple trauma include thoracic and lumbosacral spine injury and limb injury.

LOWER SPINE INJURIES

DIAGNOSIS AND MANAGEMENT

(1) Always examine the back in multi-trauma patients. Maintain spinal precautions and carefully log-roll all patients with a suspected spinal injury.

THORACIC AND LUMBOSACRAL SPINE INJURY

DIAGNOSIS

(1) This type of injury is caused by blunt trauma from a fall, a direct blow or following a traffic crash. A fractured sternum may

accompany a hyperflexion wedge fracture of the upper thoracic spine.

(2) Look for bruising, deformity and evidence of penetrating injury.

(3) Palpate for localized tenderness and swelling around the vertebral column or for an abnormal gap between the spinous processes suggesting a fracture, or overlying the renal areas suggesting a kidney injury (see p. 231).

(4) Perform a careful neurological examination, assessing for sensory deficit and a sensory level, loss of peri-anal sensation, and for motor and reflex loss in the legs (see p. 335 for the dermatomes, myotomes and reflex roots in the legs).

(5) The spinal cord ends at the level of the first lumbar vertebra, so any injury distal to this involves the cauda equina only.

(6) Send blood for FBC, U&Es, blood sugar and G&S.

(7) Request thoracolumbar spine X-rays in all the following high-risk patients:
    (i)   Fall from 3 metres (10 feet).
    (ii) High-speed motor vehicle crash over 50 mph (80 kph).
    (iii) Ejection from motor vehicle or motor cycle.
    (iv) GCS score of 8 or less.
    (v)   Neurological deficit.
    (vi) Back pain or tenderness (may be absent).

(8) X-rays may show vertebral body fractures, e.g. a distraction 'Chance' fracture or a wedge fracture, transverse process fracture, or a dislocation (particularly between T12/L1, and L4/L5).

(9) Request a CT scan for all significant or potentially unstable fractures.

MANAGEMENT

(1) Treat associated thoracic and abdominal injuries as a priority. Maintain spinal precautions, log-roll the patient and minimize unnecessary movements, as thoracolumbar fractures are commonly unstable.

(2) Commence i.v. fluids if there is hypotension from local or retroperitoneal bleeding, or from loss of sympathetic tone in a high thoracic cord injury.

(3) Consider i.v. methylprednisolone for spinal cord damage within 8 hours of injury, only after consultation with the regional Spinal Injuries unit (see p. 215).

(4) Refer the patient to the Orthopaedic team.

LIMB INJURY

The management of limb injuries does not take precedence over head, thoracic, abdominal or pelvic injuries in the multiply injured patient, even though they may appear more dramatic and attract instant attention. Limb injuries are covered in detail in *Section VIII Orthopaedic Emergencies*.

DIAGNOSIS

(1) Look for obvious deformity, swelling, tenderness, abnormal movement or crepitus (if the patient is unconscious).
(2) Check the distal pulses, particularly in a supracondylar humeral fracture or a dislocated knee.
(3) Remember that closed fractures bleed extensively with little external evidence, and open fractures bleed even more. See Table 7.7 for the amounts of concealed blood loss expected with pelvic and limb injuries in multiple trauma.
(4) Note any neurological deficit, e.g. radial nerve damage in humeral shaft fracture or sciatic nerve damage in posterior hip dislocation.

MANAGEMENT

(1) Restore any deformity to a normal anatomical alignment. This will reduce the risk of neurovascular compromise and maintain skin integrity, reducing long-term complications. Examples include:
  (i) Posteriorly dislocated hip, to prevent sciatic nerve damage.
  (ii) Dislocated knee, to maintain vascular circulation to the distal extremity.
  (iii) Dislocated ankle, to prevent ischaemic pressure necrosis of the skin overlying the malleolus (see p. 314).
(2) Give increments of morphine 2.5–5 mg i.v. for pain with an antiemetic such as metoclopramide 10 mg i.v.

Table 7.7 Expected concealed blood loss from orthopaedic injuries in multiple trauma

Site of closed fracture	Predicted blood loss
Pelvic ring	Up to 6 units or more
Femoral shaft	2–4 units
Tibial shaft	1–3 units

(3) Cover compound fractures with a saline-soaked sterile dressing. Give flucloxacillin 2 g i.v. or cefuroxime 1.5 g i.v. and tetanus prophylaxis.

(4) Immobilize the fracture using a plaster of Paris backslab, or a specially designed splint such as the Donway traction splint for femoral shaft fractures. Splinting reduces pain, making handling easier; it also reduces blood loss and the risk of neurovascular injury.

(5) Obtain urgent vascular and orthopaedic consults if distal ischaemia is present. Otherwise refer the patient when the other major injuries have been stabilized.

(6) *Traumatic amputation of a limb or digit:*
  (i) Control haemorrhage by direct pressure and elevation of the stump.
  (ii) Consider the possibility of replantation, especially in a clean, sliced wound without crushing.
    (a) preserve the amputated part by wrapping in a saline-soaked sterile dressing
    (b) seal the wrapped part in a sterile dry plastic bag, and immerse in a container of crushed ice and water
    (c) give i.v. antibiotics and tetanus prophylaxis as for a compound fracture
    (d) X-ray the limb and severed part
    (e) refer the patient to the Orthopaedic or Plastic Surgery team for consideration of microvascular surgery ideally performed within 6 hours of injury.

HEAD INJURY

The diagnosis and management of head injuries will be considered in two groups:
- Serious head injury
- Conscious head injury

SERIOUS HEAD INJURY

DIAGNOSIS

(1) The head injury may be obvious from the history or on immediate examination.

(2) The possibility of a head injury must also be considered in every instance of coma or abnormal behaviour, in at-risk groups such as drunks and epileptics, non-accidental injury in children, and in falls in the elderly.

(3) Confirm the history from the ambulance crew, police or any witnesses as to the circumstances and nature of the injury, observed loss of consciousness or subsequent seizures.

(4) Obtain any other medical details, if a relative or friend is available, of current medical or surgical conditions, drug therapy, allergies and previous head injury or epilepsy.

(5) Record the temperature, pulse, blood pressure, respiratory rate and level of consciousness using the GCS score (see Table 7.8).

(i) A patient in coma has a score of 8 or less.

(ii) A decrease in score of 2 or more points indicates significant deterioration.

Table 7.8 The Glasgow Coma Scale (GCS) score

		Score
Eye opening	Spontaneously	4
	To speech	3
	To pain	2
	None	1
Verbal response	Oriented	5
	Confused	4
	Inappropriate	3
	Incomprehensible	2
	None	1
Motor response	Obeys commands	6
	Localizes pain	5
	Withdraws (pain)	4
	Flexion (pain)	3
	Extension (pain)	2
	None	1

The maximum score is 15. Any reduction in score indicates deterioration in the level of consciousness.

(iii) Repeated neurological examination, including the GCS, is essential for detecting and managing secondary brain damage.

(6) Perform a neurological examination, including:

  (i) Conscious level: regularly record the GCS and look for any deterioration (decrease in score).

  (ii) Pupil size and reactions: look in particular for an unequal or dilating pupil, indicating a rising intracranial pressure.

  (iii) Eye movements and fundoscopy:

    (a) intact eye movements are one indicator of brainstem function

    (b) fundoscopy may reveal papilloedema, subhyaloid haemorrhage or retinal detachment.

  (iv) Other cranial nerves: include examination of the corneal reflex, facial movements and the cough and gag reflexes.

  (v) Limb movements:

    (a) assess for abnormal tone, weakness or loss of movement, or an asymmetric response to pain if the patient is unconscious

    (b) check the limb reflexes, including the plantar responses.

(7) Examine the scalp for bruising, lacerations and haematomas, and palpate for a deformity indicating a depressed fracture.

(8) Examine the face and mouth for signs of facial fracture or basal skull fracture. A basal skull fracture is indicated by:

  (i) Periorbital and subconjunctival haemorrhage.

  (ii) Haemotympanum, external bleeding, or CSF leak from the ear.

  (iii) Mastoid bruising (Battle's sign), which may not appear for many hours.

  (iv) Haemorrhage or CSF leakage from the nose.

  (v) Nasopharyngeal haemorrhage, which may be profuse.

(9) Perform a head-to-toe assessment for other injuries of the neck, chest, back, limbs, abdomen and perineum, including a rectal examination (loss of anal tone may indicate spinal cord damage).

(10) Insert a large-bore i.v. cannula and send blood for FBC, U&Es, coagulation profile, blood sugar, and G&S, and save serum for a drug screen in case alcohol or drug intoxication is subsequently suspected.

(11) Send ABGs, recording the percentage of inspired oxygen administered at the time the sample was drawn. Attach an ECG monitor and pulse oximeter to the patient.

(12) Request radiological examinations:
  (i) 3-view cervical spine X-rays.
      (a) lateral cervical spine view with an anteroposterior and open-mouth odontoid view should be performed in any unconscious head injury or suspected neck injury
      (b) make sure C1–C7/T1 are visualized, if necessary by traction on the shoulders.
  (ii) CXR and pelvic X-ray in all multiply-injured patients.
  (iii) CT head scan.
      The airway *must* be protected first, before a head CT is performed. Indications for CT include:
      (a) GCS less than 13 at any point since injury
      (b) GCS 14 or less 2 hours post injury
      (c) focal neurological signs
      (d) neurological deterioration, i.e. 2 points or more on the GCS, hemiparesis, diplopia
      (e) fracture known or suspected, including base of skull
      (f) post-traumatic seizure
      (g) coagulopathy (history of bleeding, clotting disorder, or patient on warfarin)
      (h) persistent headache, vomiting
      (i) penetrating injury, known or suspected
      (j) age over 65 years.
  (iv) Skull X-rays are of no additional value in the early management of a major head injury, when there is ready access to CT scanning.
      (a) only ever consider if CT scanning is not available. They may demonstrate a radio-opaque foreign body or depressed skull fracture, but cannot exclude serious injury if normal.

MANAGEMENT

(1) Clear the airway by sucking out any secretions, remove loose or broken dentures, and insert an oropharyngeal airway. Give 100% oxygen by tight-fitting mask with reservoir bag. Aim for an oxygen saturation above 94%.

(2) Immobilize the cervical spine by applying a semi-rigid collar, because up to 10% of patients with blunt head trauma have a concomitant neck injury. Use sandbags in addition on either side of the head taped to the forehead, unless the patient is excessively restless.

(3) The patient must be intubated to protect and maintain the airway, prevent aspiration and guarantee oxygenation and ventilation, if the gag reflex is reduced or absent. Take great care to minimize neck movements by an assistant providing in-line manual immobilization of the neck throughout.

(i) Call the senior ED doctor immediately.

(ii) Prepare for an RSI intubation (see p. 205).

(4) Regularly repeat the temperature, pulse, blood pressure and respirations.

(5) Consider whether a tension pneumothorax (see p. 206), open pneumothorax (see p. 206), massive haemothorax (see p. 219) or flail chest (see p. 220) is responsible if the respirations are rapid or ineffectual.

(6) Shock is rarely due to isolated head injury. Search for associated injuries, including chest, abdominal or pelvic bleeding, long-bone fracture and cardiac tamponade if the patient is hypotensive:

(i) Occasionally, brisk scalp bleeding alone is found to be responsible, usually in children.

(ii) Alternatively, a cervical or high thoracic spinal cord injury with loss of sympathetic vascular tone may be the cause.

(iii) Commence i.v. fluid to restore normotension. Use a crystalloid such as normal saline or Hartmann's.

(a) aim for a mean arterial pressure of greater than 90 mmHg, to ensure adequate cerebral perfusion pressure

(b) avoid excessive fluid administration if the patient is normotensive, as this may contribute to cerebral oedema.

(7) Treat the following complications immediately, as they worsen the existing primary cerebral injury and lead to secondary brain damage:

(i) *Hypoglycaemia*

(a) perform a bedside glucose test; if it is low, send a formal blood glucose to the laboratory and give 50% dextrose 50 mL i.v.

(b) remember this especially if the patient has been drinking alcohol.

(ii) *Hypoxia*

(a) PaO_2 of less than 9 kPa (70 mmHg) breathing air or 13 kPa (100 mmHg) on supplemental oxygen and hypercarbia with $PaCO_2$ over 6 kPa (45 mmHg) in the spontaneously breathing patient requires active intervention

   (b) call for urgent senior ED doctor help and prepare for
       endotracheal intubation using an RSI technique (see
       p. 205), if not already performed to protect the airway.
(iii) *Seizures*
   (a) give lorazepam 0.07 mg/kg i.v. up to 4 mg, diazepam
       0.1–0.2 mg/kg i.v. or midazolam 0.05–0.1 mg/kg i.v.
   (b) follow with phenytoin 15 mg/kg i.v. (see p. 70).
(iv) *Pinpoint pupils*
   (a) give naloxone 0.8–2 mg i.v.
   (b) no response may indicate pontine or cerebellar damage.
(v) *Restless or aggressive behaviour*
    Consider if any of the following are present:
   (a) hypoxia: check that the airway is still patent and high-flow
       oxygen is being delivered
   (b) hypotension: repeat the blood pressure
   (c) pain: catheterize the bladder, and exclude a constricting
       bandage or tight cast.
(vi) *Gastric distension*
   (a) pass a large-bore nasogastric tube
   (b) use an orogastric tube if a basal skull or mid-face fracture is
       present.
(8) Look out for signs of increasing intracranial pressure and uncal
    transtentorial herniation ('coning') such as a deteriorating level of
    consciousness, bradycardia, hypertension and focal neurological
    signs, e.g. a dilated pupil:
    (i) Arrange for a skilled doctor to perform an RSI intubation, if
        an endotracheal tube is not already positioned.
    (ii) Mildly hyperventilate the patient to maintain $PaCO_2$ at
         4.0–4.7 kPa (30–35 mmHg).
    (iii) Give 20% mannitol 0.5–1 g/kg (2.5–5 mL/kg) as an osmotic
          diuretic, provided adequate circulatory volume resuscitation
          has occurred.
    (iv) Arrange immediate neurosurgical intervention.
(9) Give flucloxacillin 1 g i.v. or cefuroxime 1.5 g i.v. if a penetrating
    or compound skull fracture or intracranial air is found, and tetanus
    prophylaxis.
(10) Refer all the following patients to the Neurosurgery team.
     Criteria for neurosurgical consultation:
     (i) Coma continues after resuscitation (GCS less than 9).
     (ii) Deterioration in neurological status, e.g. worsening in

conscious state (2 points or more decrease in GCS), seizures, increasing headache, focal neurological signs.

(iii) Skull fracture:

    (a) compound depressed fracture

    (b) basal skull fracture (see p. 238)

    (c) any skull fracture with confusion, decreased level of consciousness or focal neurological signs.

(iv) Penetrating head injury.

(v) Confusion or other neurological disturbance (GCS 9–13) for more than 2 hours with no defined skull fracture.

(vi) Radiological abnormality on CT head scan.

(11) Stabilize the patient's condition *first* and make sure any associated injuries have been dealt with before transferring the patient, if transfer is necessary.

    (i) The transport team must be trained and suitably experienced and carry appropriate monitoring equipment (see p. 465).

(12) Refer all other patients for admission under the care of the Surgical team.

CONSCIOUS HEAD INJURY

The aim is to differentiate patients requiring admission from those who could be allowed home.

DIAGNOSIS

(1) *History*

Enquire about:

    (i) The nature and speed of impact.

    (ii) Subsequent loss of consciousness, drowsiness, vomiting or seizures.

    (iii) The length of post-traumatic amnesia (PTA) from the time of injury to the time of the return of memory for consecutive events. This is often underestimated. Over 10 min PTA is significant.

    (iv) Associated alcohol or drug intoxication.

    (v) Relevant medical conditions and drug therapy, including warfarin.

(2) *Examination*

    (i) Record the temperature, pulse, blood pressure and respirations.

    (ii) Assess higher mental functions, including the level of

consciousness, using the GCS score (see p. 237).

(iii) Check the pupil size and reactions, eye movements, cranial nerves and the limbs for lateralizing neurological signs.

(iv) Examine the scalp for bruising, lacerations or palpable fractures and haematomas.

(v) Exclude associated neck or other injuries.

(3) *Radiological imaging*

(i) Request a CT scan of the head as the investigation of choice for the detection of acute, clinically important brain injuries.

(ii) Indications for CT head scan in the conscious head injury include:

(a) any loss of consciousness or significant PTA; history unknown or unreliable (e.g. under the influence of alcohol or drugs); on warfarin

(b) high-speed injury, injury from a sharp or heavy object, or a suspected penetrating injury

(c) deep scalp laceration, large haematoma, or fracture suspected on palpation

(d) focal neurological signs

(e) repeated vomiting or headache

(f) cerebrospinal fluid or blood loss from the nose or ear

(g) difficulty assessing the patient, e.g. children, elderly, epileptic patients.

(iii) Skull X-rays.

These really now only have a limited role if any:

(a) in detection of non-accidental injury in children

(b) when CT scanning services are unavailable, in conjunction with inpatient observation

(c) look for a linear fracture, the double shadow of a depressed fracture, suture diastasis, an air-fluid level in a sinus, a traumatic aerocoele, shift of the pineal or a foreign body.

MANAGEMENT

(1) Clean scalp lacerations thoroughly, trim the edges and remove any foreign bodies. Then suture in layers using a monofilament synthetic non-absorbable material such as nylon or polypropylene.

(2) Give tetanus prophylaxis according to the patient's immune status.

(3) Try to avoid giving patients with suspected head injury excessive parenteral analgesia until fully assessed, to allow an accurate measure of consciousness and to look for other neurological signs.

(4) *Admission*
  (i) Refer patients with a minor head injury and any of the following features to the Surgical team and admit for neurological observation:
    (a) confusion or any other decreased level of consciousness
    (b) neurological symptoms or signs, including persistent headache or vomiting
    (c) difficulty assessing, e.g. alcohol, drugs, epilepsy
    (d) other medical conditions, e.g. warfarin, coagulation defects
    (e) skull fracture
    (f) abnormal CT head scan
    (g) age under 5 or over 50 years
    (h) no responsible observation available outside hospital
    (i) significant associated injuries.
  (ii) Make certain all of the above have radiological imaging with a CT head scan. Some will have been discussed with the Neurosurgery team.
(5) *Discharge*
  (i) Send the following patients with a minor head injury home, provided there is someone with them and home circumstances are suitable:
    (a) fully conscious and oriented
    (b) normal CT head scan
    (c) normal skull X-ray (when CT unavailable)
    (d) no other significant injuries
    (e) no seizures or focal neurological signs
    (f) no persistent headache or vomiting.
  (ii) Give each patient a standard head injury advice card.
    (a) these cards advise patients to return if complications such as confusion, drowsiness, seizure, visual disturbance, vomiting or persistent headache occur in the subsequent 24 hours after discharge.
  (iii) This still leaves some patients with a minor head injury to be dealt with. Admit these patients to the Emergency Department short-stay ward for regular neurological observations:
    (a) no one to accompany them
    (b) poor home circumstances
    (c) other significant injuries to the face or nose, etc.
    (d) an unreliable history, particularly if they were under the influence of alcohol or drugs.

(6) *Always remember*
  (i) To look for the cause of any preceding fall in the elderly, such as a TIA, Stokes–Adams attack or other syncopal episode. These require diagnosis and management in their own right, in addition to the resultant head injury.
  (ii) A head injury may be due to non-accidental injury in a child (see p. 375).
  (iii) Cervical spine injuries are commonly associated with head injuries and appropriate examination and investigation should be performed based on clinical grounds.

BURNS

These are considered in the following categories:
- Major burns
- Minor burns and scalds
- Minor burns of the hand
- Minor burns of the face
- Bitumen burns

MAJOR BURNS

DIAGNOSIS
(1) Determine the nature of the fire, how it started, whether there was any explosion, the time of the incident and delay in reaching hospital.
(2) Ask if the patient was in an enclosed place and, if so, for how long. Ascertain whether smoke or fumes, which predispose to carbon monoxide and cyanide poisoning, were present and the duration of exposure.
(3) Examine for signs of a respiratory burn.
  (i) Look for burns around the face and neck, burnt nasal hairs, and soot particles in the nose and mouth.
  (ii) Look for signs of tachypnoea, hoarseness, stridor or wheezing.
  (iii) Assess for headache and confusion suggesting carbon monoxide poisoning.
(4) Consider the possibility of cyanide poisoning from burning plastics and fabrics, especially in patients with:

     (i) Tachypnoea, respiratory failure, cardiac arrhythmias, hypotension, convulsions, and coma.

     (ii) Severe, persistent, raised anion gap metabolic acidosis with a venous lactate level of more than 10 mmol/L despite fluid resuscitation.

(5) Check for associated injuries, particularly if burns occurred from an explosion or blast injury.

(6) Determine the extent of the burn.

     (i) Use Wallace's *Rule of Nines* in adults, ignoring areas of mere erythema (see Fig. 7.2).

     (ii) Use comparison with the size of the child's palm, equal to 1%

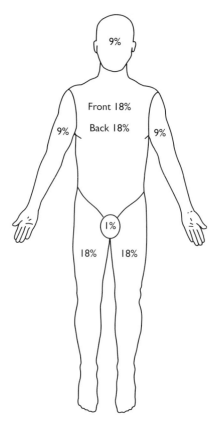

Figure 7.2 Wallace's *Rule of Nines* in adults, for estimating the percentage of body surface area burned

of body surface area (BSA), when estimating the extent of a burn in children. A child's head is relatively larger than an adult's (12–14%) and the legs are relatively smaller (14%).

(iii) Or use a body map such as a Lund and Browder chart.

(7) Determine the depth of the burn.

(i) *Full-thickness*: the skin is white or brown, dry, leathery, and anaesthetic with no capillary refill. This will require skin grafting.

(ii) *Partial-thickness*

(a) deep dermal – the skin is pink or white, feels thickened, does not blanch, and has reduced sensation. This should heal over in about 3 weeks, but some areas may require grafting to avoid leaving a scar

(b) superficial – the skin is red and blistered, blanches and is painful. This should heal spontaneously in 10–14 days.

(iii) *Superficial*: erythema, blanching and pain occur, followed by peeling as in sunburn. This should heal rapidly in 5–7 days.

(8) Insert one or two large-bore i.v. cannulae and send blood for FBC, U&Es, CK, blood sugar, G&S and a drug screen if there is suspected alcohol or drug abuse.

(i) The cannula may be placed through burned skin if absolutely necessary, or use a cut-down technique if no vein is found.

(ii) Avoid central line insertion because there is a high risk of sepsis from this procedure.

(9) Check ABGs. An elevated carboxyhaemoglobin level will confirm exposure to carbon monoxide (see p. 167).

(10) Monitor the ECG and attach a pulse oximeter to the patient.

(11) Request a CXR.

MANAGEMENT

(1) Confirm the adequacy of the airway and give 100% oxygen by tight-fitting mask with reservoir bag.

(2) Give salbutamol 5 mg nebulized for wheeze.

(3) Organize for an airway-skilled person to perform urgent endotracheal intubation using a RSI technique with an uncut endotracheal tube in patients with:

(i) Significant burns involving the face, tongue and pharynx.

(ii) Stridor, hoarseness, respiratory distress, or a deteriorating level of consciousness.

(iii) Evidence of cyanide toxicity from smoke and fume inhalation.

(4) Commence i.v. fluids in any burn over 10% BSA in a child or 15% BSA in an adult, or for associated injuries causing hypovolaemia.

(5) Determine the rate of fluid administration using the Parkland formula:

    (i) Give fluid at 4 mL/kg per percentage of body surface area burned.

    (ii) Administer the first 50% in the initial 8 hours and the remaining 50% in the subsequent 16 hours.

    (iii) More rapid fluid replacement may be required to catch up if there has been a delay in reaching hospital.

    (iv) Give additional maintenance fluid at 1.0–1.5 mL/kg per hour of 4% dextrose 1/5 normal saline.

    (v) The Parkland formula and other fluid resuscitation formulae such as the Muir and Barclay are a guide only. Aim for at least 1 mL/kg per hour urine output.

(6) The quantity of fluid is more important than the type.

    (i) Consider albumin initially in extensive, deep (e.g. electrical) burns, or when resuscitation is delayed.

    (ii) Otherwise, use a crystalloid solution alone, such as Hartmann's (compound sodium lactate).

(7) Insert a urinary catheter to assess the adequacy of resuscitation, aiming for a urine output of 50 mL per hour in adults, or 1 mL/kg per hour in children less than 30 kg.

(8) Pass a nasogastric tube in patients with burns over 20%, who may develop gastric stasis.

(9) Give morphine 0.1 mg/kg i.v. with an antiemetic such as metoclopramide 10 mg i.v. Remember that under-transfusion or hypoxia are more common causes of restlessness than pain.

(10) Give tetanus prophylaxis to all burn patients (see p. 323).

(11) Consider the need for escharotomy in the following:

    (i) Circumferential, leathery, full-thickness burns that may cause respiratory compromise by constricting chest wall movements, and distal ischaemia in limbs or digits by restricting blood flow.

    (ii) Ask the Surgical team to perform relieving incisions through the burn area.

(12) Leave any adherent clothing alone and do not break blisters in the burnt area. Remove constricting articles such as rings, bracelets and watches.

    (i) Cover the burn with a non-adherent, paraffin-impregnated gauze dressing or plastic cling wrap. Beware of hypothermia in children if wet soaks were left on.

(ii) Avoid silver sulfadiazine cream at this stage until the patient has been assessed by the Surgical or Burns unit team.

(13) All full-thickness burns of over 1–2% body surface area require hospital admission by the Surgical team. Refer patients on to a specialist Burns unit with:

(i) Burns over 10% in children and 15% in adults.

(ii) Burns of important functional areas, such as the face, hands, feet, perineum and genitalia.

(iii) Respiratory burns.

(iv) Chemical burns and electrical burns, including lightning injury.

(14) Assess all serious burns with care and resuscitate fully before departure, similar to the precautions taken when transferring serious head injuries to a Neurosurgical unit.

(i) Avoid any risk of sudden respiratory obstruction during transit.

(ii) Make sure a senior doctor has assessed the need for endotracheal intubation in any significant respiratory burn, prior to departure.

> **Tip:** burn injuries are always frightening and unexpected, and relatives (particularly the parents of children) may feel guilty and angry. Special counselling and reassurance are helpful from the start to aid coming to terms with the injuries and to allay anxiety, so they are useful as a support to the victim.

MINOR BURNS AND SCALDS

These include full-thickness burns under 1% or partial-thickness burns under 15% body surface area in adults and under 10% in children. The aim is to manage them as outpatients, as distinct from patients with major burns, who require admission (see above).

INITIAL MANAGEMENT

(1) Irrigate the wound immediately with copious running cold water until the pain is relieved.

(2) Assess the extent and depth of the burn (see p. 246). In general,

superficial partial-thickness burns heal spontaneously, deep dermal partial-thickness burns heal slowly with scar formation, and full-thickness burns do not heal at all, unless under 1–2 cm in diameter, when epithelium will cover the area from the edges. Otherwise grafting is required.

(3) Clean with sterile saline or an antiseptic such as chlorhexidine.

(4) Give adequate analgesia. Give adults paracetamol 500 mg with codeine 8 mg two tablets orally q.d.s. and/or ibuprofen 200–400 mg orally t.d.s. Give children 15 mg/kg of paracetamol elixir.

(5) De-roof large blisters that have broken, or aspirate the fluid if the blister is tense. Otherwise leave blisters intact to protect the healing epithelium.

(6) Apply silver sulfadiazine cream and cover the burn with a non-adherent paraffin-impregnated gauze dressing.

(7) Then apply gauze and an absorbent layer consisting of a cotton-wool and gauze combine pad, overlapping the paraffin-impregnated gauze dressing by 3 cm at either end.

(8) Finally, keep the absorbent layer in place with a firm crêpe bandage, again overlapping each end by 3 cm, and seal with adhesive tape.

(9) Always elevate the limb using a high-arm sling for arm and hand burns.

(10) Give tetanus prophylaxis and oral analgesics such as paracetamol 500 mg and codeine phosphate 8 mg two tablets q.d.s. to take home.

(11) Remember that burns of the perineum, feet or hands in children may be due to non-accidental injury.

   (i) Suspect this when there has been a delay in seeking treatment and the explanation is tenuous, or there is absence of any evidence of splashing.

   (ii) Refer the child to the Paediatric team for admission if non-accidental injury is possible, however trivial the burn (see p. 375).

FOLLOW-UP MANAGEMENT

(1) Review the patient after 24–48 hours to clean the affected site, to reassess the condition of the burn, and to ensure that no evidence of secondary infection is present. Re-dress the site, but omit the silver sulfadiazine.

(2) Thereafter, change the dressing every 5 days, unless the wound becomes painful, or smells, or the bandage becomes soaked ('strike through'), when the dressing should be renewed immediately.

   (i) Leave the paraffin-impregnated gauze in place when changing the dressing, if it has become adherent to the skin, to avoid destroying the delicate new epithelium forming underneath.

   (ii) Otherwise, replace the paraffin-impregnated gauze, the gauze and cotton-wool absorbent layer, and the crêpe bandage.

(3) When the wound is healing and has become epithelialized, leave it exposed or cover it with a dry, non-adherent dressing.

(4) Refer burns that have not healed in 10–12 days to a Plastic Surgery unit for review and consideration for skin grafting.

(5) Warn the patient that healed burns will initially be both hypersensitive and photosensitive, will have dry scaly skin, and that there may be depigmentation in dark-skinned races.

MINOR BURNS OF THE HAND

DIAGNOSIS AND MANAGEMENT

These are difficult to dress.

(1) Cover the hand with silver sulfadiazine cream and place the hand inside a sterile polythene bag, bandaged over a gauze ring as a seal at the wrist.

(2) Elevate the hand and encourage the patient to move the fingers regularly.

(3) Give tetanus prophylaxis and analgesia.

(4) Replace the silver sulfadiazine cream and bag daily, as turbid fluid collects in the bag.

MINOR BURNS OF THE FACE

DIAGNOSIS AND MANAGEMENT

(1) Leave these alone and exposed to heal in 10 days. A proprietary moisturizing lotion may be used.

(2) Exclude corneal damage by staining with fluorescein.

(3) Warn the patient that facial swelling may develop the following day.

BITUMEN BURNS

DIAGNOSIS AND MANAGEMENT

(1) Road-laying and roofing accidents are usually responsible.
(2) Irrigate the area immediately with cold water.
(3) Leave the black bitumen alone and cover it with paraffin-impregnated gauze.
(4) Await blister formation or re-epithelialization, which will allow the bitumen to drop off.
(5) Assess subsequently for the depth of the burn, which is usually partial-thickness.

THE ACUTE ABDOMEN

The aim is to resuscitate critically ill patients and to differentiate those patients requiring surgical, gynaecological, or medical referral from those patients who can be allowed home.

SERIOUSLY ILL PATIENTS

(1) Clear the airway, give oxygen, and attach a cardiac monitor and pulse oximeter to the patient. Check the temperature, pulse, blood pressure, respiratory rate and blood sugar level.
(2) Obtain a brief history of the onset, duration, nature and character of the pain, prior episodes of pain, relevant previous operations and illnesses, present medication and known drug allergies.
(3) Examine the chest and heart, and then lay the patient flat to examine the abdomen, including the femoral pulses.
(4) Consider ruptured abdominal aortic aneurysm, pancreatitis, inferior myocardial infarction, mesenteric infarction or ruptured ectopic pregnancy in a shocked patient with acute abdominal pain.
(5) Perform a rectal examination.
(6) Catheterize the bladder. Test the urine for sugar, blood, protein, bile and urobilinogen, and send for microscopy and culture. Perform a urinary beta-HCG pregnancy test in females of reproductive age.
(7) Insert one or two large-bore i.v. cannulae and send blood for FBC, U&Es, LFTs, blood sugar and lipase/amylase. Cross-match blood if

haemorrhage is suspected. Send blood cultures if pyrexial. Check arterial blood gases.

(8) Commence an i.v. infusion with normal saline.
   (i) Arrange insertion of a CVP line by an experienced doctor in older patients with pre-existing cardiac disease, to avoid precipitating heart failure from fluid overload.

(9) Perform an ECG.

(10) Request an erect CXR or lateral decubitus abdominal film if the patient is unable to sit upright, to look for free gas.
   (i) Or consider an AXR in suspected bowel obstruction, volvulus or for abnormal air such as the 'double-wall sign' in a perforation.

(11) Insert a nasogastric tube if there is evidence of intestinal obstruction, ileus or peritonitis.

(12) Commence broad-spectrum antibiotics such as gentamicin 5 mg/kg, ampicillin 1 g i.v. and metronidazole 500 mg i.v. for generalized peritonitis.

(13) Refer the patient immediately to the Surgical team.

THE STABLE PATIENT WITH AN ACUTE ABDOMEN

(1) Determine the onset and nature of pain:
   (i) Explosive and excruciating pain: consider myocardial infarction, ruptured aortic aneurysm, perforated viscus, and biliary or renal colic.
   (ii) Rapid, severe and constant pain: consider pancreatitis, strangulated bowel, mesenteric infarction and ectopic pregnancy.
   (iii) Gradual, steady pain: consider cholecystitis, appendicitis, diverticulitis, hepatitis and pelvic inflammatory disease (salpingitis).
   (iv) Intermittent pain with crescendos: consider mechanical obstruction.

(2) Ask about the location and radiation of pain:
   (i) Central abdominal pain radiating to the back suggests an aortic aneurysm or pancreatitis.
   (ii) Flank pain radiating to the genitalia suggests ureteric colic, or rarely ruptured aortic aneurysm.
   (iii) Otherwise pain tends to localize over the organ affected, provided there is peritoneal involvement, with radiation to a

shoulder tip if the diaphragm is irritated, e.g. by cholecystitis or a ruptured spleen.

(3) Look for associated features such as:
   (i) Nausea and vomiting:
      (a) pain tends to precede the nausea and vomiting in the surgical acute abdomen
      (b) a medical condition such as gastroenteritis or gastritis is more likely if the nausea and vomiting precede the pain.
   (ii) Fever and rigors:
      (a) a low-grade pyrexia is usual in appendicitis or diverticulitis
      (b) a high fever and rigors suggest cholecystitis, cholangitis, diffuse peritonitis, pyelonephritis or acute pelvic inflammatory disease (salpingitis).

(4) Check the temperature, pulse, blood pressure and respiratory rate.

(5) Inspect for visible peristalsis and distension, palpate for local tenderness, guarding and masses, percuss for free gas, and listen for increased or absent bowel sounds. Examine the hernial orifices, particularly in cases of intestinal obstruction.

(6) Perform a rectal examination, external genitalia examination in male patients, and consider a vaginal examination in female patients.

(7) Insert an i.v. cannula and send blood for FBC, U&Es, LFTs, blood sugar and lipase/amylase.
   (i) Their true discriminatory value in differentiating between the various conditions is limited apart from the amylase/lipase.

(8) Test the urine for sugar, blood, protein, bile and urobilinogen, and send for microscopy and culture in suspected UTI. Perform a pregnancy test in females with abdominal pain.

(9) Record an ECG.

(10) Radiology.
   Only request the following for the specific indications outlined:
   (i) An erect CXR – to show evidence of pulmonary disease, a secondary pleural reaction from intra-abdominal disease and free gas under the diaphragm indicating a perforation.
   (ii) Erect and supine abdomen films – to look specifically at the gas pattern for obstruction or volvulus, splenic shadow, renal outlines and psoas shadows, and for calcification and opacities.
   (iii) Upper abdominal ultrasound to confirm biliary colic or cholecystitis.
   (iv) Pelvic ultrasound – to look for a gynaecological cause in

females with acute abdominal pain (remember to do the beta-HCG first).

(v) CT scan – without contrast to confirm ureteric colic; or with i.v. contrast particularly for suspected aortic aneurysm, provided the patient is haemodynamically stable; and with or without oral contrast for the difficult diagnoses such as suspected bowel cancer or for other complex masses.

(11) Give all patients i.v. analgesia as required, such as morphine 2.5–5 mg i.v. with metoclopramide 10 mg i.v. This does not interfere with the surgical diagnosis, which may even be facilitated.

(12) Refer all cases to the Surgical team if an acute surgical condition is suspected or cannot be excluded.

CAUSES OF ACUTE ABDOMINAL PAIN

Disorders causing acute abdominal pain may be categorized as intestinal, biliary, vascular, pancreatic, urinary, peritoneal and retroperitoneal, gynaecological and medical. See Table 7.9 for a complete list.

ACUTE APPENDICITIS

DIAGNOSIS

(1) Acute appendicitis causes poorly localized central abdominal pain, worse on coughing or moving, which classically shifts to the right iliac fossa. There is associated anorexia, nausea, vomiting, and diarrhoea or constipation.

(2) Low-grade pyrexia, localized abdominal tenderness, rebound and guarding are found.

(3) A rectal examination is commonly performed to help diagnose a retrocaecal or pelvic appendix, but really has little true discriminatory value.

(4) Always perform a urinalysis to look for glycosuria, white cells, and a beta-HCG pregnancy test. Even if positive, none of these rules out appendicitis.

(5) Gain i.v. access.
  (i) The FBC is frequently performed, but rarely influences decision making alone.

(6) Request an ultrasound in females to rule out pelvic pathology, or a CT scan for doubtful cases only.

(7) Diagnosis is most difficult in very young, elderly or pregnant patients.

MANAGEMENT

(1) Commence a normal saline infusion and administer i.v. analgesia.
(2) Keep the patient nil by mouth. Give gentamicin 5 mg/kg i.v., ampicillin 1 g i.v. q.d.s. and metronidazole 500 mg i.v. t.d.s. if rupture is suspected with peritonitis.
(3) Admit all patients under the Surgical team, whether the diagnosis appears clear or is just suspected in atypical cases, such as confused elderly patients, infants with diarrhoea, or older children that are off their food, all of whom could still have appendicitis.

Table 7.9 Causes of acute abdominal pain

Intestinal disorders	Acute appendicitis
	Intestinal obstruction
	Intussusception
	Perforation of a viscus
	Diverticulitis
	Inflammatory bowel disease
Biliary disorders	Biliary colic
	Acute cholecystitis
Vascular disorders	Ruptured aortic aneurysm
	Ischaemic colitis
	Mesenteric infarction
	Ruptured spleen
Pancreatic disorder	Acute pancreatitis
Urinary disorders	Renal and ureteric colic
	Pyelonephritis
	Acute urinary retention
	Acute epididymo-orchitis
	Acute testicular torsion
Peritoneal/retroperitoneal disorders	Primary peritonitis
	Retroperitoneal haemorrhage
Gynaecological disorders	
Medical disorders presenting with acute abdominal pain	

INTESTINAL OBSTRUCTION

DIAGNOSIS
(1) The causes are many, including an obstructed hernia, adhesions, diverticulitis, volvulus, intussusception, carcinoma, mesenteric infarction, and Crohn's disease.
(2) Intermittent colicky abdominal pain occurs with abdominal distension and vomiting in high obstruction, and constipation with failure to pass flatus in low obstruction.
(3) Visible peristalsis may be seen, associated with tinkling bowel sounds and signs of dehydration.
(4) The pain becomes more continuous and generalized if strangulation occurs (most common with a femoral hernia), associated with tachycardia and signs of shock.
(5) Always examine the hernial orifices and perform a rectal examination.
(6) Gain i.v. access and send blood for FBC, U&Es, lipase and blood sugar.
(7) Request erect and supine abdominal X-rays and look for the following features:
  (i) Small bowel obstruction:
    (a) X-rays show dilated loops of small bowel and a colon devoid of air
    (b) small bowel is usually central in distribution with regular transverse bands (*valvulae conniventes*) extending across the entire diameter of the bowel
    (c) fluid levels, which may also occur in gastroenteritis. Over five fluid levels are considered significant.
  (ii) Large bowel obstruction:
    (a) X-rays show dilated large bowel, with a peripheral distribution, irregular haustral folds and faecal mass content.

MANAGEMENT
(1) Commence an infusion of normal saline to correct dehydration from vomiting and fluid loss into the bowel.
(2) Pass a nasogastric tube, administer analgesia, and refer the patient to the Surgical team.

INTUSSUSCEPTION

DIAGNOSIS

(1) This is caused by telescoping or prolapse of one portion of bowel into an immediately adjacent segment. It usually occurs in children aged 3–18 months and is characterized by intermittent abdominal pain with sudden screaming and pallor, followed by vomiting.

(2) Abdominal distension and a mass may be felt, with blood-stained mucus ('redcurrant jelly') found on rectal examination in 50%.

(3) Send blood for FBC, U&Es and blood sugar.

(4) Request erect and supine AXRs, which may be normal in the early stages, or reveal signs of intestinal obstruction.

    (i) Look for evidence of a soft-tissue mass surrounded by a crescent of air ('doughnut sign') or free air from perforation of a viscus.

MANAGEMENT

(1) Insert an i.v. cannula and commence careful i.v. rehydration.

(2) Refer immediately to the Surgical team and arrange a contrast or air enema, which is diagnostic in 95% of cases and will result in therapeutic reduction in 75% of cases.

PERFORATION OF A VISCUS

DIAGNOSIS

(1) Perforation may occur anywhere in the gastrointestinal tract. Common sites are a peptic ulcer, the appendix, or a colonic diverticulum.

    (i) There may be an antecedent history of alcohol or NSAID ingestion, dyspepsia, or lower abdominal pain, but perforation can occur *de novo*.

(2) It presents with severe pain and signs of generalized peritonitis with board-like rigidity. Shock soon supervenes.

(3) Gain i.v. access and send blood for FBC, U&Es, blood sugar and lipase/amylase.

(4) Request an erect CXR to look for gas under the diaphragm, seen in over 70% of cases.

MANAGEMENT

(1) Treat shock with i.v. normal saline, administer i.v. analgesia with morphine in 2.5–5 mg increments and pass a nasogastric tube.

(2) Commence broad-spectrum antibiotics such as gentamicin 5 mg/kg once daily, ampicillin 1 g i.v. q.d.s. and metronidazole 500 mg i.v. t.d.s.

(3) Refer the patient immediately to the Surgical team.

DIVERTICULITIS

DIAGNOSIS

(1) This follows inflammation of one or more colonic diverticulae.

(2) It causes lower abdominal pain radiating to the left iliac fossa, and bloody diarrhoea, sometimes with sudden profuse rectal bleeding.

(3) Look for a low-grade fever, abdominal tenderness, and guarding on the left with a palpable mass.

(4) Complications of perforation, severe bleeding, fistula formation and bowel obstruction may occur.

(5) Gain i.v. access and send blood for FBC, U&Es, blood sugar and G&S.

(6) Perform an ECG and request an erect CXR if perforation is suspected.

MANAGEMENT

(1) Commence an i.v. infusion to treat dehydration or shock.

(2) Refer the patient to the Surgical team for analgesia and antibiotics such as gentamicin 5 mg/kg once daily, ampicillin 1 g i.v. q.d.s. and metronidazole 500 mg i.v. t.d.s., or for surgery if bowel obstruction or a pelvic abscess is suspected.

INFLAMMATORY BOWEL DISEASE

DIAGNOSIS

(1) Ulcerative colitis associated with bouts of diarrhoea with blood-stained mucus may present as a fulminating attack with fever, tachycardia and hypotension.

(2) Crohn's disease, associated with recurrent abdominal pain, diarrhoea, malaise and perianal fistulae or abscesses, may present acutely with obstruction, perforation or right iliac fossa pain. This can mimic acute appendicitis.

(3) Gain i.v. access and send blood for FBC, U&Es, blood sugar, lipase/amylase, and blood culture.

(4) Request a plain AXR to look particularly for the following:

(i) Ulcerative colitis: extensive mucosal ulceration may leave normal mucosal islands (pseudopolyps) visible on plain film. Dilation of the transverse colon greater than 6 cm indicates the presence of toxic megacolon. Perforation is common.

(ii) Crohn's disease: free air associated with perforation may be seen. Stenotic regions of small bowel are best visualized with barium follow-through studies, or on colonoscopy.

MANAGEMENT

(1) Commence an i.v. infusion and treat pain with i.v. analgesia.

(2) Refer all cases with shock, fever, peritonitis, severe bleeding and a dilated megacolon or obstructed bowel immediately to the Surgical team.

BILIARY COLIC

DIAGNOSIS

(1) This presents with discrete episodes of colicky pain in the right hypochondrium, referred to the scapula.

(2) Look for right upper quadrant tenderness on examination. The patient may be jaundiced if the common bile duct is obstructed, with yellow sclera, and bilirubin in the urine.

(3) Gain i.v. access and send blood for FBC, U&Es, LFTs and lipase/amylase.

(4) Request an upper abdominal ultrasound.

MANAGEMENT

(1) Treat pain with i.v. analgesia such as morphine 0.1 mg/kg i.v. with an antiemetic such as metoclopramide 10 mg i.v.

(2) Refer the patient to the Surgical team if the pain is severe or acute cholecystitis is suspected.

(3) Otherwise, advise patients to eat a diet low in saturated fats and refer the patient to the GP or Surgical outpatients for follow-up.

ACUTE CHOLECYSTITIS

DIAGNOSIS

(1) This causes acute, constant right upper quadrant pain referred to the scapula, with anorexia, nausea and vomiting.

(2) Look for localized tenderness, with involuntary guarding and

rebound tenderness. Painful splinting of respiration on deep inspiration and right upper quadrant palpation is frequent (Murphy's sign). Fever is common.

(3) Occasionally a palpable gall bladder may be felt in association with jaundice, although more commonly the gall bladder is not felt as it is shrunken and contracted.

(4) Gain i.v. access and send blood for FBC, U&Es, blood sugar, LFTs, lipase/amylase, and blood culture.

(5) Request an upper abdominal ultrasound.

MANAGEMENT

(1) Commence an i.v. infusion of saline.

(2) Give gentamicin 5 mg/kg i.v., ampicillin 1 g i.v. q.d.s. and analgesia such as morphine 0.1 mg/kg i.v. with an antiemetic such as metoclopramide 10 mg i.v.

(3) Refer the patient to the Surgical team for bed rest, analgesia, antibiotics and cholecystectomy.

RUPTURED ABDOMINAL AORTIC ANEURYSM (AAA)

DIAGNOSIS

(1) This classically presents with sudden abdominal pain radiating to the back or groin, syncope, collapse, or unexplained shock. Tachycardia and hypotension occur in 50% of cases.

(2) Feel for a tender mass with expansile pulsation on examination, or a vague fullness with discomfort to the left of the umbilicus.

(3) Always consider this diagnosis in men over 45 years in particular, even when only one feature of the 'classic triad' of abdominal or back pain, shock, and a pulsatile or tender abdominal mass is present.

    (i) Also consider a ruptured AAA first in the older patient with apparent 'ureteric colic'.

(4) Gain large-bore i.v. access in both arms and send blood for FBC, U&Es, blood sugar, lipase/amylase and cross-match up to 10 units of blood.

(5) Catheterize the bladder.

(6) Record the ECG because ischaemic heart disease is usually associated with or exacerbated by the hypotension.

(7) Request a CXR if there is time.

(8) Perform a rapid bedside ultrasound scan to confirm the presence of an abdominal aneurysm if the patient is haemodynamically

unstable and the diagnosis is uncertain. Or proceed directly to theatre if the patient is moribund.

(9) Only request a CT scan if the patient is haemodynamically stable. Remember to modify the dose of i.v. contrast depending on the renal function.

MANAGEMENT

(1) Give the patient high-flow oxygen by face mask and commence a slow i.v. infusion only.

(2) Give minimal amounts of normal saline or Hartmann's (compound sodium lactate) aiming for a systolic blood pressure of no more than 90–100 mmHg.

   (i) Avoid giving massive fluid replacement, as this leads to coagulopathy, hypothermia, increases the bleeding and causes a higher mortality.

(3) Refer the patient urgently to the vascular Surgical team for immediate laparotomy. Contact the duty anaesthetist, alert theatre, and inform ICU.

ISCHAEMIC COLITIS

DIAGNOSIS

(1) This usually occurs in an elderly patient with recurrent abdominal pain, progressing to episodes of bloody diarrhoea or intestinal obstruction from stricture formation.

(2) Gain i.v. access and send blood for FBC, coagulation profile, ELFTs, blood sugar, lipase/amylase, a lactate and G&S.

(3) Record an ECG.

(4) Request a plain AXR that may reveal 'thumb-printing' of the colonic wall, or proximal colon dilation, intramural gas, and the most ominous sign of gas within the portal vein.

(5) Alternatively request a CT scan with i.v. contrast that may show free fluid and colonic-wall oedema or air, although many of the features are non-specific.

MANAGEMENT

(1) Commence an i.v. infusion of normal saline.

(2) Give analgesia and keep the patient nil by mouth.

(3) Refer the patient to the Surgical team.

MESENTERIC INFARCTION

DIAGNOSIS

(1) This may be due to embolism from atrial fibrillation or a myocardial infarction, or due to arterial or venous thrombosis, or arterial occlusion such as following an aortic dissection.

(2) There is sudden onset of severe, diffuse abdominal pain, usually in an elderly patient, associated with vomiting and bloody diarrhoea.

(3) Abdominal examination reveals distension, generalized tenderness, absent bowel sounds, and fresh rectal blood.

(4) Gain i.v. access and send blood for FBC, U&Es, LFTs, lipase/amylase, blood sugar and cross-match 2–4 units of blood. Send a lactate as a marker of lactic acidosis.

(5) Record the ECG.

MANAGEMENT

(1) Commence an i.v. infusion of normal saline or Hartmann's (compound sodium lactate) to treat shock.

(2) Refer the patient to the Surgical team, who will determine the need for angiography to confirm the diagnosis. However, the prognosis is poor.

RUPTURED SPLEEN

DIAGNOSIS

(1) Left lower rib injuries following blunt trauma are associated with splenic damage in up to 20% of cases. Occasionally, trivial injury to an enlarged spleen from glandular fever, malaria or leukaemia may cause rupture.

(2) The timing of the splenic rupture may be:
   (i) *Acute*: causing tachycardia, hypotension and abdominal tenderness with referred pain to the left shoulder.
   (ii) *Delayed*: occurring up to 2 weeks or more after an episode of trauma. Initial localized discomfort and referred shoulder-tip pain give way to signs of intra-abdominal haemorrhage.

(3) Gain large-bore i.v. access and send blood for a FBC and cross-match 6 units of blood for an acutely ruptured spleen.

(4) Request a CXR to look for fractured left lower ribs and a basal pleural effusion, especially in delayed splenic rupture.
   (i) AXR is unhelpful, with non-specific features such as a displaced stomach bubble to the right and an enlarged

soft-tissue shadow in the splenic area.

(5) Arrange an urgent upper abdominal ultrasound if the patient is unstable, or a CT scan with i.v. contrast if the patient is stable.

MANAGEMENT

(1) Commence an infusion of normal saline and refer the patient immediately to the Surgical team.

ACUTE PANCREATITIS

DIAGNOSIS

(1) Predisposing factors include alcohol abuse, gallstones, trauma and vasculitis.

(2) Acute pancreatitis presents with sudden, severe abdominal pain radiating to the back, that is eased by sitting forward, associated with repeated vomiting or retching.

(3) Vital signs may reveal a low-grade fever and tachycardia with hypotension.

(4) Look for epigastric tenderness, guarding, and decreased or absent bowel sounds on abdominal examination.

(5) Insert a large-bore i.v. cannula and send blood for FBC, U&Es, LFTs, blood sugar, calcium, lipase/amylase, and G&S. Check an arterial blood gas.

(6) Record the ECG, which may show diffuse T wave inversion, in the absence of myocardial ischaemia.

(7) Request an erect CXR to exclude viscus perforation or lobar pneumonia as a cause of the pain. An abdominal film may reveal pancreatic calcification or a sentinel loop, but is often normal.

(8) Perform a CT scan of the abdomen in severe cases that provides both diagnostic and prognostic information.

MANAGEMENT

(1) Commence an i.v. infusion of normal saline and pass a nasogastric tube. Give morphine 5–10 mg i.v. with an antiemetic such as metoclopramide 10 mg i.v.

(2) Refer the patient to the Surgical team.

(3) Admit patients with hypoxia and shock to ICU.

RENAL AND URETERIC COLIC

DIAGNOSIS

(1) Renal and ureteric calculi may cause pain, haematuria, obstruction or infection.

(2) Symptoms are caused by obstruction of one or more calyces, the renal pelvis or ureter.

(3) Characteristically these include sudden, severe colicky pain radiating from the loin to the genitalia, restlessness, vomiting and sweating. There may also be urinary frequency and haematuria.

(4) Look for loin tenderness in the costovertebral angle, and remember to consider a possible ruptured abdominal aortic aneurysm in men over 45 years, especially with a first episode of renal colic, and/or if haematuria is absent (see p. 261).

(5) Gain i.v. access and send blood for FBC, U&Es, LFTs, lipase/amylase, calcium and uric acid.

(6) Perform a bedside urinalysis for macroscopic or microscopic haematuria, which occurs in 90%. Send a formal MSU for microscopy and culture.

(7) Request a plain AXR KUB (kidneys, ureters, bladder), as most renal calculi are radio-opaque. It is of more use in subsequently tracking the course of a calculus.

(8) Request a non-contrast abdominal CT scan of the renal tract in all patients over 40 years with acute flank pain, to rule out other retroperitoneal pathology at the same time.

   (i) CT can determine the presence of calculi, their size, degree of ureteric obstruction and exclude other important differential diagnoses particularly an AAA.

(9) Alternatively request a renal ultrasound, particularly in patients with impaired renal function or for recurrent colic.

   (i) The intravenous pyelogram may be performed in younger patients, but is best reserved for post complex urological surgery.

MANAGEMENT

(1) Start analgesia:

   (i) Give morphine 0.1 mg/kg i.v. with an antiemetic such as metoclopramide 10 mg i.v. particularly if the pain is intense and incapacitating.

   (ii) Alternatively, use diclofenac 75 mg i.m. or indomethacin 100 mg p.r.

(iii) NSAIDs are as effective as opiates, but are not controlled drugs, and will also discourage those who are simply 'seeking' narcotics.

(2) Admit all patients with resistant pain, urinary infection, or stones greater than 6 mm in diameter with an obstructed kidney, as these are unlikely to pass spontaneously.

    (i) An infected obstructed kidney is a urological emergency needing immediate drainage. Call the Urology team urgently.

(3) Discharge the remainder to their GP or Urology outpatients for follow-up, and recommend a reduced sodium and low-protein diet, to reduce the likelihood of recurrent calcium-based stones.

PYELONEPHRITIS

DIAGNOSIS

(1) Typically symptom onset is rapid and characterized by frequency, dysuria, malaise, nausea, vomiting and sometimes rigors.

(2) Raised temperature, renal-angle tenderness, and vague low abdominal pain are found.

(3) Dipstick urinalysis shows blood and protein.

(4) Insert an i.v. cannula and send blood for FBC, U&Es, blood sugar and blood cultures in any patient who is significantly ill.

(5) Send an MSU to look for bacteria, leucocytes and red blood cells on microscopy and for culture.

MANAGEMENT

(1) Significantly ill patients.

    (i) These include those with vomiting, dehydration, or prostration; those who are pregnant, very young or old; and those who are known to have urinary tract abnormalities, e.g. a duplex system, horseshoe kidney or renal/ureteric stones.

    (ii) Commence i.v. fluids. Give gentamicin 5 mg/kg i.v. and ampicillin 1 g i.v. q.d.s. Refer these patients to the Medical team for admission.

(2) Otherwise, if the symptoms are mild and consistent with predominant cystitis, commence an oral antibiotic such as ciprofloxacin 500 mg b.d. for 7 days, amoxicillin 500 mg with clavulanic acid 125 mg one tablet orally t.d.s. for 14 days, or trimethoprim 300 mg once daily, depending on local prescribing policy.

(3) Return the patient to the GP with a letter requesting the GP to organize a repeat urine culture after the completion of a full antibiotic course, to ensure that the infection has been eradicated.

(4) Arrange a renal ultrasound in any male with a proven UTI and refer to Urology outpatients for follow-up.

ACUTE URINARY RETENTION

DIAGNOSIS

(1) Predisposing factors include prostatic hypertrophy, urethral stricture, pelvic neoplasm, anticholinergic drugs, pregnancy, local painful conditions such as genital herpes and constipation in the elderly.

(2) Occasionally, retention is due to a neurogenic cause such as multiple sclerosis.

(3) The enlarged bladder is easily palpable, dull to percussion and is usually painful, although in the semi-conscious patient it may manifest as restlessness.

(4) Always perform a rectal examination and assess perineal sensation and leg reflexes in all patients.

(5) Send blood for FBC, ELFTs and blood sugar.

MANAGEMENT

(1) Carefully pass a urethral catheter as a strict aseptic procedure, and send a specimen of urine for microscopy and culture.

(2) Refer the patient to the Surgical team or Gynaecology as appropriate.

ACUTE EPIDIDYMO-ORCHITIS

DIAGNOSIS

(1) This occurs in sexually active men with a preceding history of urethritis, or following urinary tract infection or instrumentation including catheterization.

(2) Pain begins gradually and is usually localized to the epididymis or testis, associated with a low-grade fever.

(3) Send an FBC to look for a neutrophilia and request a urine microscopy to look for leucocytes.

MANAGEMENT

(1) *Never* diagnose epididymo-orchitis in a patient under 25 years old without considering testicular torsion first (see below).

(2) Give the patient a scrotal support if torsion has been excluded, analgesics such as paracetamol 500 mg and codeine phosphate 8 mg two tablets q.d.s., and an antibiotic.

(3) The choice of antibiotic depends on the suspected aetiology:

(i) *Bacterial cystitis with epididymitis*: give amoxicillin 500 mg with clavulanic acid 125 mg one tablet orally t.d.s. or trimethoprim 300 mg orally once daily or 200 mg orally b.d. for 2 weeks and refer to the Urology clinic.

(ii) *Non-specific urethritis with epididymitis*: give doxycycline 100 mg orally b.d. for 7 days and follow-up in a Genitourinary Medicine clinic.

(iii) *Suspected gonococcal urethritis with epididymitis*: ideally, this should be treated from the outset by a Genitourinary Medicine clinic. If this is not possible, give ceftriaxone 250 mg i.m.

ACUTE TESTICULAR TORSION

DIAGNOSIS

(1) Suspect this diagnosis in any male under 25 years old with sudden pain in a testicle, which may radiate to the lower abdomen. There may be associated nausea and vomiting.

(2) The testicle lies horizontally and high in the scrotum, and is very tender. There may be a small hydrocoele.

(3) Urinalysis is typically negative and WCC normal.

MANAGEMENT

(1) Always refer all suspected cases urgently to the Urology team, as the testicle becomes non-viable after 6 hours of torsion.

(2) Still refer the patient for surgery even if more than 6 hours have elapsed, as orchidopexy is required on the other side to prevent subsequent torsion there.

(3) Scrotal ultrasound to assess blood supply and to look for an alternative diagnosis must *never* delay urgent urological assessment.

PRIMARY PERITONITIS

DIAGNOSIS AND MANAGEMENT

(1) Primary bacterial peritonitis occurs almost exclusively in patients with ascites, particularly due to cirrhosis or the nephrotic syndrome.

(2) Look for fever, abdominal pain and tenderness.

(3) Send blood for FBC, U&Es, LFTs, blood sugar and blood cultures. Check a urinalysis.

(4) Refer the patient to the Medical team for a diagnostic peritoneal tap and culture, to exclude *Mycobacterium tuberculosis* and to distinguish bacterial peritonitis from familial Mediterranean fever.

RETROPERITONEAL HAEMORRHAGE

DIAGNOSIS

(1) This may occur following trauma to the pelvis, kidney or back, or from aortic aneurysm rupture, or from trivial trauma – even spontaneously in those with a bleeding tendency or on anticoagulants.

(2) It presents with hypovolaemic shock following trauma, in the absence of an obvious external or internal thoracic or abdominal source for haemorrhage. A paralytic ileus may develop.

(3) Insert a wide-bore i.v. cannula and send blood for FBC, coagulation profile, ELFTs, blood sugar, lipase/amylase, and cross-match blood according to the degree of shock. Check the urine for blood.

(4) Plain abdominal X-ray is not helpful. It may show loss of the psoas shadow or possibly fractures of the vertebral transverse processes in traumatic cases, but a CT is indicated.

(5) Request a CT scan of the abdomen to localize the bleeding.

MANAGEMENT

(1) Commence an infusion of normal saline.

(2) Refer to the Surgical team for admission.

GYNAECOLOGICAL CAUSES

The following causes are discussed in *Section XI Obstetric and Gynaecological Emergencies.*

- Ruptured ectopic pregnancy (see p. 381)
- Pelvic inflammatory disease (acute salpingitis) (see p. 383)
- Ruptured ovarian cyst (see p. 384)
- Torsion of an ovarian tumour (see p. 385)
- Endometriosis (see p. 385)

MEDICAL DISORDERS PRESENTING WITH ACUTE ABDOMINAL PAIN

It is rare for non-surgical disorders causing acute abdominal pain to present without other symptoms or signs suggesting their true medical origin. Always remember diabetic ketoacidosis (DKA) and perform a urinalysis in every patient with abdominal pain. DKA is suggested by finding glycosuria and ketonuria (see p. 52).

DIAGNOSIS
Medical disorders presenting with acute abdominal pain include:
(1) *Thoracic origin*
  (i)   Myocardial infarction, pericarditis.
  (ii) Pulmonary embolus, pleurisy, pneumonia.
  (iii) Aortic dissection.
(2) *Abdominal origin*
  (i)   Hepatic congestion from hepatitis or right heart failure.
  (ii) Infection, including gastroenteritis, pyelonephritis and primary peritonitis.
  (iii) Intestinal ischaemia from atheroma or sickle cell disease, vasculitis and Henoch–Schönlein purpura.
  (iv) Irritable bowel syndrome.

> **(!)** **Warning:** constipation, particularly in the elderly, should be regarded as a symptom and *not* a diagnosis, until other more significant underlying conditions such as bowel obstruction, diverticular disease, a tumour, hypercalcaemia or neurological disease have been actively excluded first.

(3) *Endocrine and metabolic origin*
  (i)   Diabetic ketoacidosis.
  (ii) Addison's disease.
  (iii) Hypercalcaemia – 'stones, bones and abdominal groans'.
  (iv) Lead poisoning, paracetamol or iron poisoning.

(v) Porphyria (acute intermittent).

(4) *Neurogenic origin*

(i) Herpes zoster.

(ii) Radiculitis from spinal cord degeneration or malignancy.

(iii) Tabes dorsalis.

(5) *Thoracolumbar spine origin*

Collapsed vertebra due to osteoporosis, neoplasm or infection, e.g. tuberculosis (see p. 336).

(6) *Psychiatric*

Münchausen syndrome or 'hospital hopper':

(i) Be suspicious of patients presenting with acute abdominal pain or renal colic, who usually don't live locally, and with no GP, who may have multiple abdominal scars from operations 'at another hospital'.

(ii) Their aim is to gain narcotic analgesia or hospital admission by feigning illness.

(iii) Ask for a previous hospital number or admission details, so you can 'go and verify their story'. Seek advice from the senior ED doctor, unless this prompts them to leave of their own accord.

(7) Take a careful history in every case, do a thorough examination, and send blood for FBC, U&Es, LFTs, blood sugar and lipase/amylase.

(8) Request a urinalysis, perform an ECG and request a CXR and AXR to avoid missing the more serious diagnoses.

MANAGEMENT

(1) Discuss the case with the senior ED doctor. Admit the patient as appropriate according to the underlying diagnosis.

FURTHER READING

American Heart Association (2005) Guidelines for cardiopulmonary resuscitation and emergency cardiovascular care. Part 10.7: Cardiac arrest associated with trauma. *Circulation* **112**:IV-146–49.

American Heart Association. http://www.circulationaha.org/ (CPR and ECC guidelines 2005).

European Resuscitation Council (2005) Guidelines for resuscitation. Section 7: Cardiac arrest in special circumstances. *Resuscitation* **67**(**Suppl 1**):S135–70.

European Resuscitation Council. http://www.erc.edu/ (CPR and ECC guidelines 2005).

Health Protection Agency. http://www.phls.co.uk/ (injuries).

National Electronic Library for Health. http://www.nelh.nhs.uk

National Institute for Health and Clinical Excellence. http://www.nice.org.uk/ (head injury).

Patel HC, Bouamra O, Woodford M (on behalf of the Trauma Audit and Research Network) (2005) Trends in head injury outcome from 1989 to 2003 and the effect of neurosurgical care: an observational study. *Lancet* **366**:1538–44.

Resuscitation Council (UK). http://www.resus.org.uk/ (resuscitation guidelines 2005).

Trauma.Org. http://www.trauma.org/ (trauma education and resources).

ORTHOPAEDIC EMERGENCIES

FRACTURES OF THE CLAVICLE

DIAGNOSIS

(1) These fractures are usually due to direct violence or to transmitted force from a fall on to the outstretched hand.

(2) A greenstick fracture is common in children. A fracture between the middle and outer thirds is common in adults.

(3) The patient experiences pain on movement of the shoulder and examination reveals tenderness over the clavicle associated with local deformity.

(4) An anteroposterior X-ray of the shoulder usually shows the fracture clearly.

MANAGEMENT

(1) Support the weight of the arm in a triangular sling, and give an analgesic such as paracetamol 500 mg and codeine phosphate 8 mg two tablets q.d.s.

    (i) The traditional figure-of-eight bandage has generally been abandoned, as it is uncomfortable and difficult to keep tight.

(2) Refer the patient to the next Fracture clinic.

(3) Rarely, comminuted fractures or fractures causing compression of underlying nerves or vessels may be treated operatively. Refer these immediately to the Orthopaedic team.

ACROMIOCLAVICULAR DISLOCATION

DIAGNOSIS

(1) Acromioclavicular injuries usually occur following a fall on to the apex of the shoulder with the arm held in adduction.

(2) A fall on to the shoulder that tears the acromioclavicular ligament results in subluxation, but if the strong coracoclavicular ligaments are torn as well, dislocation occurs, with the clavicle losing all connection with the scapula.

(3) Subluxation causes local tenderness to palpation with minimal deformity. Full dislocation causes a prominent outer end of the clavicle and drooping of the shoulder, with pain on movement.

(4) Assess the clavicle and scapula for associated fractures.

(5) X-ray the acromioclavicular joint with the patient standing to show the displacement of the clavicle. This is highlighted by comparing the shoulders when the patient is holding a weight in each hand.

MANAGEMENT
(1) Treat minor subluxations with ice, oral analgesics, sling immobilization, daily range of motion exercises, and refer to the next Fracture clinic.
(2) Give complete dislocations the same supportive treatment, but discuss with the Orthopaedic team for consideration of operative intervention.

STERNOCLAVICULAR DISLOCATION

DIAGNOSIS
(1) This dislocation is rare and is caused by either:
   (i) A direct blow to the anteromedial aspect of the clavicle forcing the clavicle backwards resulting in a posterior dislocation.
   Or:
   (ii) Transmission of indirect forces from the anterolateral or posterolateral shoulder displacing the clavicle either forwards or backwards.
(2) Patients commonly complain of chest and shoulder pain exacerbated by arm movements particularly when supine.
(3) Anterior displacement results in local tenderness and asymmetry of the medial ends of the clavicles.
(4) Posterior displacement may impinge on the trachea or great vessels and present with dyspnoea, dysphagia and arm paraesthesiae.
(5) On examination the affected shoulder appears shortened and thrust forward, and the medial aspect of the sternoclavicular joint is painful to palpate.
(6) X-rays are not easy to interpret, although anteroposterior and oblique views should be requested.
(7) A CT scan is often required, particularly in posterior displacements.

MANAGEMENT
(1) Treat subluxations with a triangular sling, oral analgesics and refer to the next Fracture clinic.
(2) Refer posterior dislocations with pressure symptoms immediately

to the Orthopaedic team.

(3) Discuss full anterior dislocations with the Orthopaedic team; as with acromioclavicular dislocations, once reduced they are difficult to hold in place.

FRACTURES OF THE SCAPULA

DIAGNOSIS

(1) These can be divided into fractures of the neck, body, spine, acromion and coracoid, and are usually due to direct trauma.

(2) Their importance is that they indicate considerable trauma has been applied to the area. Check for associated rib, pulmonary, spinal column and shoulder injuries.

(3) Request an anteroposterior shoulder view and lateral scapula view for adequate visualization of the majority of scapula injuries. A CT scan is helpful for delineating associated glenoid and coracoid fractures.

MANAGEMENT

(1) Treat the associated injuries as a priority.

(2) The majority of isolated undisplaced scapula fractures respond well to ice, sling immobilization, oral analgesics, and early range of motion exercises. Refer to the next Fracture clinic.

(3) Displaced fractures of the glenoid and scapula neck may be associated with significant shoulder soft-tissue trauma and may require surgical reduction. Refer these to the Orthopaedic team.

ANTERIOR DISLOCATION OF THE SHOULDER

DIAGNOSIS

(1) This dislocation is caused by forced abduction and external rotation of the shoulder relative to the trunk. It is commonest in young adults from sports or traffic crashes, or in the elderly from a fall.

(2) It tends to become recurrent, when dislocation may occur with a trivial injury, with movement, or even spontaneously in bed.

(3) Patients generally complain of severe shoulder pain and limited range of movement.

(4) The arm appears slightly abducted and the shoulder looks 'squared off' with loss of the deltoid contour and with a prominent acromion.

(5) Look for the following complications before any attempt at manipulation is made:
   (i) *Axillary (circumflex) nerve damage*. Assess for pinprick sensory loss over the 'regimental badge' area on the upper lateral aspect of the deltoid (testing for shoulder movement by the deltoid is too painful to be meaningful).
   (ii) *Posterior cord of the brachial plexus*. Test wrist extension by the radial nerve. Rarely other parts of the brachial plexus are damaged.
   (iii) *Axillary artery damage*. Palpate the radial pulse. Prompt reduction usually restores the circulation.
   (iv) *Fracture of the upper humerus*. Look specifically for this on the X-ray.
(6) Always X-ray the shoulder, even if you are sure of the diagnosis, to avoid missing an associated humeral head fracture. Look for the following features:
   (i) The humeral head is displaced medially and anteriorly with loss of contact with the glenoid fossa on the anteroposterior view.
   (ii) Look at the lateral 'Y' view in doubtful cases. The humeral head lies anterior to the 'Y' in anterior dislocation.
   (iii) Humeral head fracture:
      (a) fracture of the greater tuberosity does not influence the initial reduction
      (b) refer a fracture through the humeral head, neck, or upper humerus directly to the Orthopaedic team. *Do not* attempt reduction.

MANAGEMENT
(1) Give the patient morphine 2.5–5 mg i.v. with an antiemetic such as metoclopramide 10 mg i.v. if there is severe pain (unusual in recurrent dislocations). Reduce the dose of morphine in elderly patients.
(2) Perform the reduction using conscious sedation with diazepam 5–10 mg i.v. or midazolam 2.5–5 mg i.v., provided that monitoring and resuscitation equipment are available, and dentures, rings, etc. have been removed.
(3) There are many different methods of reduction:
   (i) *Kocher's manoeuvre*
      (a) hold the arm in adduction with the elbow flexed

    (b) apply gentle traction and external rotation until resistance is felt

    (c) the shoulder may 'clunk' back during external rotation. If it does not, when 90 degrees is reached, adduct the arm across the chest and internally rotate it.

  (ii) *Hippocratic method.* Apply traction to the straight arm gently adducted over countertraction from the physician's stockinged foot placed in the axilla.

(4) Place the arm in a sling strapped to the body after reduction, or enclosed under the patient's clothes, to prevent external rotation and a recurrent dislocation. Repeat the shoulder X-ray to confirm the reduction.

(5) Test again for neurovascular damage.

(6) Give the patient an oral analgesic, instructions to keep the arm adducted and internally rotated, and refer to the next Fracture clinic.

POSTERIOR DISLOCATION OF THE SHOULDER

DIAGNOSIS

(1) This condition is uncommon, occurring classically during electrocution or seizures or from a direct blow (e.g. in boxing), and is easily missed.

(2) The arm is held adducted and internally rotated, and the greater tuberosity of the humerus feels prominent. Any external rotation is severely limited and painful.

(3) X-rays of the shoulder must include two views, as the anteroposterior view may appear normal.

    (i) Look for the 'light bulb' sign on the anteroposterior view, due to the internally rotated humerus displaying a globular head, and for an irregular, reduced glenohumeral joint space.

  (ii) Look for the humeral head lying behind the glenoid on the lateral scapular 'Y' view.

MANAGEMENT

(1) Give the patient morphine 2.5–5 mg i.v. with an antiemetic such as metoclopramide 10 mg i.v.

(2) Perform the reduction using conscious sedation with diazepam 5–10 mg i.v. or midazolam 2.5–5 mg i.v., provided that monitoring and resuscitation equipment are available.

(i) Apply traction to the arm abducted to 90 degrees.

(ii) Gently externally rotate the arm.

(3) Place the arm in a sling and repeat the shoulder X-ray to confirm reduction. Occasionally, the reduction may be unstable and immediate orthopaedic referral will be required.

(4) Give the patient an analgesic and refer to the next Fracture clinic.

FRACTURES OF THE UPPER HUMERUS

DIAGNOSIS

(1) These fractures usually occur in elderly patients and may involve the greater tuberosity, the lesser tuberosity, the anatomical neck or most commonly the surgical neck of the humerus.

(2) There is localized pain and loss of movement, often with dramatic bruising gravitating down the arm.

(3) Complications include:

(i) Dislocation of the humeral head.

(ii) Complete distraction of the humeral head from the shaft.

(iii) Axillary (circumflex) nerve damage causing anaesthesia over the upper, lateral aspect of the upper arm and loss of deltoid movement.

(iv) Axillary vessel damage with compromised blood supply to the humeral head or distal arm.

(4) Confirm proximal head fracture and associated humeral head distraction or comminution with plain X-rays of the shoulder.

MANAGEMENT

(1) Immediately refer to the orthopaedic team patients with:

(i) Gross angulation or total distraction of the humeral head.

(ii) Fractures associated with a dislocation.

(iii) Associated neurovascular damage.

(2) Otherwise, use a collar and cuff to allow gravity to exert gentle traction. Give the patient an analgesic such as paracetamol 500 mg and codeine phosphate 8 mg two tablets q.d.s.

(3) Remember that the elderly patient may now need social services support in the form of 'meals on wheels', a home help, and possibly a community nurse. Inform the GP by fax and letter so he or she may visit the patient.

(4) Refer the patient to the Fracture clinic for follow-up.

FRACTURES OF THE SHAFT OF THE HUMERUS

DIAGNOSIS

(1) These fractures are caused by direct trauma or a fall on to the outstretched hand.

(2) Upper-third fractures tend to result in the proximal fragment being adducted by the pectoralis major, whereas in middle-third fractures the proximal fragment is abducted by the deltoid.

(3) Clinically the diagnosis is usually evident, with obvious local deformity and loss of function of the arm. Examine the affected arm for neurovascular complications, which are common.

(4) Complications are usually seen in middle-third fractures, including:

  (i) Compound injury.

  (ii) Radial nerve damage in the spiral groove, causing weak wrist extension and sensory loss over the dorsum of the thumb.

(5) Always include views of the shoulder and elbow, remembering the old adage to X-ray the joint above and the joint below any fracture.

MANAGEMENT

(1) Immediately refer to the Orthopaedic team patients with:

  (i) Grossly angulated or comminuted fractures.

  (ii) Compound fractures.

  (iii) Radial nerve palsy.

(2) Otherwise, support the arm for comfort in a U-slab plaster or hanging cast. This should not require analgesia to apply.

  (i) Pad the arm well with cotton-wool and apply a 10–15-cm wide plaster slab medially under the axilla, around the elbow, and up over the lateral aspect of the upper arm on to the shoulder.

  (ii) Hold the slab in place with a crêpe bandage, and support the arm in a sling.

(3) Give the patient analgesics and review in the next Fracture clinic. Social services support is needed for the elderly, who may require admission if they are unable to cope.

INJURIES TO THE ELBOW AND FOREARM

SUPRACONDYLAR FRACTURE OF THE HUMERUS

DIAGNOSIS

(1) This fracture occurs most commonly in children from a fall on to the outstretched hand, although it is also seen in adults.

(2) There is tenderness and swelling over the distal humerus, but the olecranon and two epicondyles remain in their usual 'equilateral triangle' relationship (which is lost in dislocation of the elbow).

(3) Test for median nerve damage and look for any signs of arterial occlusion, such as pain, pallor, paralysis, paraesthesiae, and pulselessness.

(4) Complications include:

   (i) Brachial artery damage – compression, intimal damage or division can be caused by posterior displacement of the lower end of the proximal humeral fragment.

   (ii) Median nerve damage – associated with sensory loss over the radial three-and-a-half fingers and weakness of abductor pollicis.

   (iii) Local tissue swelling – tense and rapidly progressive swelling may cause vascular compromise to the distal forearm.

   (iv) Volkmann's ischaemic contracture – a late but devastating complication resulting from tissue necrosis secondary to distal forearm arterial compromise.

(5) X-ray will show any displacement, although one-third of fractures are undisplaced, some merely greenstick.

   (i) Request comparison views of the other normal elbow if there is difficulty in interpreting the radiographs, especially in children with epiphyseal growth plates.

MANAGEMENT

(1) Refer the patient immediately to the Orthopaedic team if arterial occlusion is suspected, for manipulation under general anaesthesia.

(2) Refer displaced, comminuted, or severely angulated fractures also to the Orthopaedic team, even if there is no arterial damage.

(3) Manage undisplaced and greenstick fractures conservatively with analgesics, collar and cuff with the forearm flexed to 80 degrees and arrange Orthopaedic outpatient follow-up. A plaster backslab is not essential.

CONDYLAR AND EPICONDYLAR FRACTURES OF THE HUMERUS

DIAGNOSIS

(1) The lateral condyle is usually fractured in children, and the medial epicondyle at any age, due to direct violence or forced contraction of the forearm flexors that attach to it.

(2) There is pain, swelling (which may be minimal) and loss of full elbow extension if the medial epicondyle is trapped in the joint, usually following dislocation of the elbow.

(3) Test for ulnar nerve damage, causing sensory loss over the medial one-and-a-half digits and weakness of the finger adductors and abductors.

(4) X-rays are often difficult to interpret in children, as many of the structures are still cartilaginous. Helpful clues to look for are:

   (i) The posterior fat-pad sign (see Fig. 8.1). This indicates a joint effusion, and is indirect evidence of significant trauma. It is also typically seen with radial head fractures.

   (ii) Comparison with the normal elbow placed in a similar anatomical position. Look for any differences between the two sides.

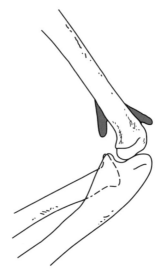

Figure 8.1 Line-drawing of a lateral elbow X-ray showing an anterior and posterior fat-pad sign (shaded areas are abnormal and indicate a joint effusion)

(iii) Suspect displacement from injury if an epiphysis that should be visible by age is missing.

(a) the capitellum epiphysis is visible by age 1 year, the medial epicondyle epiphysis by age 6 years, and the lateral epicondyle epiphysis by age 11 years.

MANAGEMENT

(1) Refer all these fractures to the Orthopaedic team. The fractures are always more extensive than they appear on the X-ray, because the structures are mainly cartilaginous.

DISLOCATION OF THE ELBOW

DIAGNOSIS

(1) This is caused by a fall on to the outstretched hand driving the olecranon posteriorly. Rarely anterior, medial, or lateral displacement occurs.

(2) The normal 'equilateral triangle' between the olecranon and two epicondyles is disrupted (unlike in the supracondylar fracture).

(3) Look for the following complications:

(i) Ulnar nerve damage, causing sensory loss over the medial one-and-a-half fingers and weakness of the finger adductors, with the fingers held straight.

(ii) Median nerve damage, causing sensory loss over the radial three-and-a-half fingers and weakness of the abductor pollicis.

(iii) Brachial artery damage, causing loss of the radial pulse with pain, pallor, paralysis, paraesthesiae and feeling cold.

(4) Request an X-ray that usually shows the dislocation clearly. Look for associated fractures of the coronoid process of the ulna or radial head in adults, and of the humeral epicondyles or lateral condyle in children.

MANAGEMENT

(1) Support the elbow in a comfortable sling and give morphine 2.5–5 mg i.v. with an antiemetic such as metoclopramide 10 mg i.v.

(2) Call a senior ED doctor to help perform the reduction under conscious sedation with diazepam 5–10 mg i.v. or midazolam 2.5–5 mg i.v., provided monitoring and resuscitation equipment are available.

(3) Apply axial traction to the elbow in 30 degrees of extension, and

push the olecranon with the thumbs. Perform a post-reduction X-ray and refer all cases to the Orthopaedic team for neurovascular observation.

(4) Refer complicated cases, which involve comminuted fractures of the radial head, humeral epicondyles or coronoid process, or that are unable to be reduced by closed methods in the Emergency Department, to the Orthopaedic team.

PULLED ELBOW

DIAGNOSIS

(1) This is common in children aged 2–6 years and usually follows axial traction applied to an extended arm, for example when pulling a child's hand to prevent a fall or to put on a sweater.

(2) The radial head is subluxed out of the annular ligament, causing local pain and loss of use of the arm, particularly supination.

(3) Examination reveals an anxious child protecting the affected arm, which is held by the side, with the elbow semi-flexed and pronated. There is no neurovascular compromise and motor activity is normal.

(4) X-rays are usually not necessary, but should be performed to exclude a fracture if there is extensive swelling over the elbow, or reduction is not successful after two or three attempts.

MANAGEMENT

(1) Fix the elbow and apply pressure to the region of the radial head with one hand. Applying axial compression at the wrist, supinate the forearm and gently flex the elbow with the other hand.
   (i) The radial head is felt to click back in the majority of cases.

(2) The child is often still reluctant to use the arm for the first 15–30 minutes following reduction, and so observe in the Emergency Department until adequate return of function has been demonstrated.

(3) No immobilization is required. Discharge the child with the parents following education to prevent recurrence.

FRACTURES OF THE OLECRANON

DIAGNOSIS

(1) These fractures follow a fall on to the point of the elbow or forced triceps contraction, which may then distract the olecranon, leaving

a palpable subcutaneous gap.
(2) Examine for local tenderness, swelling and loss of active elbow extension.
(3) Request an X-ray to confirm the diagnosis and to delineate the degree of fracture comminution, displacement or angulation.
  (i) Anterior dislocation of the elbow may accompany a displaced olecranon fracture.

MANAGEMENT
(1) Give the patient analgesics and a sling, and refer immediately to the Orthopaedic team for operative reduction if there is displacement of the olecranon, or an associated anterior dislocation of the elbow.
(2) Treat an undisplaced hairline fracture with a long-arm plaster, with the elbow flexed, and review at the next Fracture clinic.

FRACTURES OF THE RADIAL HEAD

DIAGNOSIS
(1) These fractures are caused by direct violence or by indirect force, such as falling on to the outstretched hand, when the radius is driven proximally against the capitellum.
(2) There is localized pain and tenderness over the radial head, discomfort on supination of the forearm, and a loss of full elbow extension.
(3) Unfortunately, this injury is commonly missed, usually because it is not thought of or because it is not seen on X-ray.
(4) Request an X-ray of the elbow. It may be difficult or impossible to see a fracture, but look for corroborating evidence of a posterior fat-pad sign (see Fig. 8.1). If there is doubt, ask specifically for additional radial head views.

MANAGEMENT
(1) Place non-displaced fractures in a collar and cuff, and refer the patient to the next Fracture clinic.
(2) Use a plaster elbow backslab for comfort and protection if there is severe localized pain.
(3) Refer the patient directly to the Orthopaedic team if the radial head is severely comminuted or grossly displaced, for consideration of operative intervention.

FRACTURES OF THE RADIAL AND ULNAR SHAFTS

These two bones tend to act as a unit, attached proximally at the radial head by the annular ligament, throughout their length by the interosseous membrane and distally by the radio-ulnar ligaments.

It is rare to fracture one bone in isolation and, as in humeral shaft fractures, it is vital to X-ray the joints above and below (here, the elbow and wrist).

DIAGNOSIS

(1) Injury is caused by direct trauma or by falling on to an outstretched hand, usually with an element of rotation fracturing both bones.

(2) There is localized tenderness, swelling and deformity. Compound injuries are more common with direct trauma.

(3) X-ray will demonstrate the fractures. Look closely for an associated dislocation injury if one bone is fractured and angulated, with no radiographic evidence of the other bone being broken.

(i) *Monteggia fracture*: fracture of the proximal ulna with dislocation of the radial head.

(ii) *Galeazzi fracture*: fracture of the distal radius with dislocation of the inferior radio-ulnar joint at the wrist.

MANAGEMENT

(1) Refer all these fractures to the Orthopaedic team for open reduction and internal fixation.

(2) Place the arm in a full-arm plaster cast in the rare instance of an isolated, undisplaced, single forearm bone fracture, from the metacarpal heads to the upper arm, with the elbow flexed at a right angle and the wrist in the mid-position.

(i) Refer the patient to the next Fracture clinic.

INJURIES TO THE WRIST AND HAND

COLLES' FRACTURE

DIAGNOSIS

(1) This is a fracture of the distal radius usually within 2.5 cm of the wrist. It is most common in elderly women with osteoporosis and usually associated with a fall on the outstretched hand.

(2) The classical 'dinner fork' deformity is due to dorsal angulation and dorsal displacement of the distal radial fragment, which may also be impacted and radially displaced.

(3) X-ray demonstrates the distal radial fracture, with an associated avulsion of the ulnar styloid process in up to 60% of cases.

(4) Delayed complications of Colles' fracture include malunion, post-traumatic reflex sympathetic dystrophy (Sudeck's atrophy), acute carpal tunnel syndrome, shoulder stiffness or a 'frozen shoulder' and delayed rupture of the extensor pollicis longus.

MANAGEMENT

(1) Treat undisplaced or minimally displaced fractures, particularly in the elderly, directly with a Colles' backslab, without manipulation.

(2) Displaced, angulated fractures with radial deviation require reduction to promote optimal return of function and to reduce the delayed complications.

(3) Options for reduction include a Bier's block, axillary block, general anaesthetic or haematoma block, according to departmental policy.

(4) *Bier's block technique* or *intravenous regional anaesthesia*

   (i) Two doctors are required, one to perform the manipulation and the other, with anaesthetic experience and previous training in the procedure, to perform the block.

     (a) at least one nurse attends to the patient, checks the blood pressure and assists the doctors

     (b) explain the technique to the patient, who should sign a written consent form.

   (ii) The technique is contraindicated in peripheral vascular disease, including Raynaud's disease, sickle cell disease, cellulitis, in uncooperative patients including children, in known local anaesthetic sensitivity, and hypertension with systolic blood pressure over 200 mmHg.

   (iii) ECG and blood pressure monitoring must be available in an area with full resuscitation facilities and a tipping trolley. Ideally the patient should be starved for 4 hours before the procedure.

   (iv) Use a specifically designed and properly maintained Bier's block cuff, checking first for leaks or malfunction. Apply the cuff to the upper arm over cotton-wool padding.

   (v) Insert a small i.v. cannula into the dorsum of the hand on the affected side and a second cannula into the other hand or wrist.

(vi) Elevate the affected arm for 2–3 minutes to empty the veins, in preference to using an Esmarch bandage, which is generally too painful.

(vii) Inflate the cuff to 100 mmHg above systolic blood pressure, keeping the arm elevated, but to no more than 300 mmHg. The radial pulse should no longer be palpable and the veins should remain empty.

(viii) Lower the arm and slowly inject 0.5% prilocaine 2.5 mg/kg (0.5 mL/kg, as 10 mL of 0.5% prilocaine contains 50 mg). Make a note of the time of injection.

(ix) Continuously monitor the cuff pressure for leakage. Keep the cuff inflated for a minimum of 20 minutes to ensure the prilocaine is fully tissue bound, and for a maximum of 45 minutes.

(x) Wait at least 5 minutes before performing the manipulation after confirming the adequacy of block. Request a check X-ray and repeat the manipulation immediately if reduction is unsatisfactory.

(xi) If satisfactory, deflate the cuff then re-inflate for 2 minutes observing for signs of local anaesthetic toxicity – although the maximum safe dosage of prilocaine is 6 mg/kg (over double the amount used in the block) so toxicity is rare.

(xii) Signs of local anaesthetic toxicity are:
   (a) restlessness, perioral tingling, dizziness, and slurred speech
   (b) loss of consciousness, seizures, bradycardia and hypotension are potential sequelae, but are virtually unknown with prilocaine.

(xiii) Rest the patient then for at least 2 hours while regular observations are made. Allow home with an accompanying adult if the plaster is comfortable and the patient feels well.

(5) *Colles' reduction and immobilization*
   (i) Prepare a 20-cm width plaster slab measured from the metacarpal heads to the angle of the elbow. Cut a slot for the thumb and remove a triangle to accommodate the final ulnar deviation (see Fig. 8.2 (a) and 8.2 (b)).

   (ii) Disimpact the fracture by firm traction on the thumb and fingers, and by hyperextending the wrist in the direction of deformity. An assistant should provide countertraction to the upper arm, with the elbow kept flexed at 90 degrees.

   (iii) Next, extend the elbow and then use your thenar eminence to

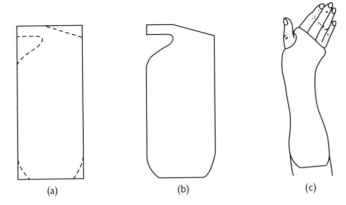

Figure 8.2 The Colles' Plaster of Paris backslab
(a) and (b) the backslab is prepared by trimming to permit thumb movements, full elbow flexion and to allow for the final ulnar deviation of the wrist; (c) the backslab in position.

reduce the dorsal displacement and to rotate back the dorsal angulation, with the heel of your other hand acting as a fulcrum.

(iv) Alter your grip to push the distal fragment towards the ulna to correct radial displacement.

(v) Finally, hold the hand pronated in full ulnar deviation with the wrist slightly flexed. Pad the forearm with cotton-wool and apply the backslab to the radial side of the forearm (see Fig. 8.2 (c)).

(vi) Hold the backslab in place with a crêpe bandage, and take a check X-ray to assess the adequacy of the reduction before terminating the anaesthetic.
   (a) reduction should be near perfect in a young person
   (b) up to 10 degrees of residual dorsal angulation can be accepted, i.e. neutral position in an elderly person.

(6) Give the patient a sling, with instructions to keep the shoulder and fingers moving, and review in the next Fracture clinic.

(7) Remember to check that the elderly patient will be able to manage at home, particularly if they already rely on a walking frame. Social services help may be needed. Inform the GP by fax and letter.

SMITH'S FRACTURE

DIAGNOSIS

(1) This fracture is caused by a fall on to the dorsum of the hand, a hyperflexion or a hypersupination injury. It results in a distal radial fracture with volar displacement and is often termed a reversed Colles' fracture.

(2) Examine for localized swelling and a classical 'garden spade' deformity. The patient is unable to extend the wrist and has pain on supination and pronation.

    (i) Assess for damage to the median nerve (see p. 283).

MANAGEMENT

(1) Reduce the fracture under a Bier's block, axillary block or general anaesthetic, according to departmental policy.

(2) *Smith's reduction and immobilization*

    (i) Disimpact the fracture by firm traction to the forearm in supination, with an assistant providing countertraction to the upper arm.

    (ii) Apply pressure with the heel of the hand to reduce the distal fragment dorsally.

    (iii) Place a long-arm plaster to hold the reduced fracture in position.

        (a) position the affected arm with the elbow in 90 degrees flexion, the forearm in full supination, and the wrist dorsiflexed (extended)

        (b) mould an anterior slab around the radius with a slot cut for the thumb

        (c) extend the plaster above the elbow, kept at a right angle.

    (iv) Take a check X-ray to assess the adequacy of reduction before terminating the anaesthetic. If reduction fails, internal fixation may be necessary.

(3) Give the patient a sling and analgesics, and review in the next Fracture clinic.

    (i) As the fracture is often unstable, it is prone to slipping and the patient usually requires weekly X-ray follow-up to ensure continued fracture reduction.

BARTON'S FRACTURE–DISLOCATION

DIAGNOSIS
(1) This is an intra-articular fracture of the distal radius with associated subluxation of the carpus and wrist, which move in a volar or dorsal direction.
(2) The volar Barton fracture has a similar mechanism of injury to the Smiths' fracture, and the intra-articular distal radius fracture is angulated in a palmar direction.
(3) The dorsal Barton fracture is caused by a fall on to the outstretched hand with the wrist extended and forearm pronated. The axial load causes the dorsal rim of the distal radius to fracture with anterior displacement.

MANAGEMENT
(1) Refer the patient immediately to the Orthopaedic team as this injury is unstable and open reduction with internal fixation is required.

DISTAL RADIAL FRACTURES IN CHILDREN

DIAGNOSIS
(1) These represent the commonest paediatric fractures.
(2) They are associated with marked local tenderness, sometimes with deformity.
(3) Request an X-ray to reveal the nature of the fracture:
   (i) Plastic deformation: most commonly associated with the ulnar.
   (ii) Greenstick fracture: occurs when one side of a bone breaks as the opposing side, usually where the force is directly applied, is bent.
   (iii) Buckle or 'Torus' fracture: compressive forces cause one side of the bone to 'buckle' under pressure as the opposing side is bent.
   (iv) Complete fracture: involves the entire bone and both cortical surfaces.
   (v) Epiphyseal fracture: involves the growth plate and is classified using the Salter–Harris system. The radial epiphysis may displace dorsally, often in adolescents, to mimic a Colles' deformity.

MANAGEMENT

(1) Refer all angulated fractures and displaced radial epiphyses to the Orthopaedic team for reduction under general anaesthesia.

(2) Place the arm in a Colles'-type plaster backslab otherwise, for a minimally buckled cortex that may be difficult to even see on an X-ray, and refer the patient to the next Fracture clinic.

FRACTURES OF THE SCAPHOID

DIAGNOSIS

(1) The scaphoid is the most commonly fractured carpal bone, usually caused by a fall on to the outstretched hand. Consider this in any patient presenting with a 'sprained wrist', particularly after a sporting injury.

(2) There is pain on dorsiflexion or ulnar deviation of the wrist, as well as pain and weakness of pinch grip.

(3) Look for localized pain and tenderness by:
   (i) Compressive pressure along the thumb metacarpal.
   (ii) Palpation in the anatomical 'snuff box' between extensor pollicis longus and abductor pollicis longus.
   (iii) Palpation of the scaphoid tubercle.

(4) Ask specifically for scaphoid views as well as for anteroposterior and lateral wrist X-ray views. Unless the fracture is complete, it may be difficult to detect in the acute phase.

(5) Repeat X-ray in 10–14 days allows time for decalcification to occur at the fracture site and for the fracture to become visible.

MANAGEMENT

(1) Place the wrist in a removable splint if the X-rays are normal and pain or tenderness are minor, or a double-elasticated stockinet bandage and a high-arm sling.
   (i) Review all patients in either the Emergency Department or Orthopaedic clinic within 10 days of injury depending on local policy.
   (ii) Repeat the X-ray if pain persists.

(2) Otherwise, if a fracture is confirmed on X-ray, or there is marked pain and tenderness particularly on moving the thumb or wrist, place the forearm in a scaphoid plaster.

(3) *Scaphoid plaster* (see Fig. 8.3).

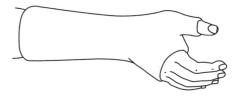

Figure 8.3 The scaphoid plaster
This extends from the angle of the elbow to the metacarpal heads, and around the
base of the thumb to below the interphalangeal joint.

    (i)   The wrist should be fully pronated, radially deviated and
partially dorsiflexed, and the thumb held in mid-abduction.

  (ii)   Apply the plaster from the mid-shaft of the forearm to the
metacarpal heads, to include the base of the thumb proximal
to the interphalangeal joint.

(4)   Give the patient a high-arm sling and refer to the next Fracture clinic.

(5)   The scaphoid holds a unique position in the proximal carpal row
and is important in maintaining radiocarpal stability.

    (i)   Delayed complications of scaphoid fracture include avascular
necrosis, non-union and osteoarthritis, which result in
disruption of carpal function.

  (ii)   Orthopaedic review is essential to reduce complications and
potential loss of function, as well as to exclude possible missed
injuries such as scapholunate dissociation, or even a Bennett's
fracture of the base of the thumb metacarpal.

DISLOCATIONS OF THE CARPUS

DIAGNOSIS

(1)   Dislocations of the carpus are uncommon, and are caused by a fall
on the outstretched hand. Two important types are seen:

    (i)   *Dislocation of the lunate*: the distal carpal bones and hand
maintain their normal alignment with the radius, but the
lunate is squeezed out anteriorly, like a pip.

  (ii)   *Perilunate dislocation of the carpus*: the lunate maintains its
alignment with the radius, but the distal carpal bones and the
hand are driven dorsally.

       (a) a displaced fracture through the scaphoid is often present.

(2) Test for median nerve compression in dislocation of the lunate, causing loss of sensation in the radial three-and-a-half digits and weakness of abductor pollicis.

(3) Request X-rays, but recognize that they are easy to misinterpret as normal in lunate dislocation, but particularly look for:

(i) The normal curved joint space between the distal radius and the scaphoid and lunate is disrupted on the anteroposterior view, so the lunate looks triangular instead of quadrilateral.

(ii) The dislocated lunate lies anteriorly on the lateral view, in the shape of the letter 'C'.

MANAGEMENT

(1) Refer all cases immediately to the Orthopaedic team, particularly if median nerve compression is found.

FRACTURES OF THE OTHER CARPAL BONES

DIAGNOSIS

(1) These fractures are rare, and include fractures of the capitate, triquetral, hook of hamate and pisiform bones.

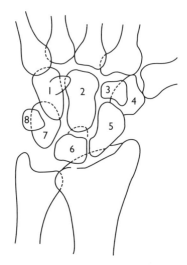

Figure 8.4 The two rows of carpal bones
(1) hamate, (2) capitate, (3) trapezoid, (4) trapezium, (5) scaphoid, (6) lunate, (7) triquetral, (8) pisiform.

(2) There is localized tenderness from direct trauma, sometimes with an associated ulnar nerve palsy affecting the deep branch that supplies most of the intrinsic hand muscles.

(3) A common problem on X-ray is to remember the names of the eight carpal bones.

   (i) Try remembering that the 'trapezium is at the base of the thumb' and use the mnemonic: Hamlet came to town shouting loudly to Polonius', which corresponds to the hamate, capitate, trapezoid, trapezium, scaphoid, lunate, triquetral and pisiform bones (see Fig. 8.4).

MANAGEMENT

(1) Place all these fractures in a scaphoid plaster and refer to the next Fracture clinic.

FRACTURES OF THE THUMB METACARPAL

DIAGNOSIS

(1) Injury usually results from forced thumb abduction, causing localized pain and tenderness.

(2) Always X-ray to distinguish stable from unstable injuries.

   (i) Stable injuries include transverse shaft and greenstick fractures.

   (ii) Unstable injuries include oblique shaft and comminuted fractures, and the fracture–dislocation of the base of the thumb (Bennett's fracture).

   (iii) *Bennett's fracture*

      (a) this is an oblique fracture through the base of the thumb metacarpal involving the joint with the trapezium, with subluxation of the rest of the thumb radially

      (b) look for swelling of the thenar eminence, sometimes with local palmar bruising

      (c) make sure the X-ray includes the base of the thumb to avoid missing this injury.

MANAGEMENT

(1) Splint stable fractures with a scaphoid plaster and refer the patient to the next Fracture clinic.

(2) Refer unstable fractures (including Bennett's) to the Orthopaedic team for possible open reduction and internal fixation.

DISLOCATION OF THE THUMB METACARPAL

DIAGNOSIS

(1) This may occur in motorcycle, skiing and football accidents, from forced thumb abduction or hyperextension.

(2) Request an X-ray to exclude an associated fracture.

MANAGEMENT

(1) Reduce under a general anaesthetic, a local Bier's block or under conscious sedation using an i.v. analgesic and sedative combination.

    (i) Apply traction to the thumb with pressure over the metacarpal head. After the manipulation, repeat the X-ray to confirm the reduction.

    (ii) Place the forearm in a scaphoid plaster with plenty of cotton-wool padding, and refer the patient to the next Fracture clinic.

(2) Refer the patient immediately to the Orthopaedic team if the reduction fails. The metacarpal head may have 'button-holed' through the joint capsule between tendons, and require open reduction.

RUPTURE OF THE ULNAR COLLATERAL LIGAMENT

DIAGNOSIS

(1) This condition ('gamekeeper's thumb', which referred to a chronic lesion) is caused by forced thumb abduction, typically in skiing accidents.

(2) It is often missed and must be suspected whenever pain and swelling are seen around the metacarpophalangeal (MCP) joint of the thumb, after an abduction injury.

(3) Look for tenderness over the ulnar aspect of the MCP joint.

    (i) Test for laxity of the ulnar collateral ligament by applying a gentle abduction stress to the proximal phalanx, which reproduces the pain and demonstrates movement at the MCP joint.

    (ii) Pinch grip and power are lost.

(4) X-ray may show an avulsion fracture of the proximal phalanx or a degree of MCP joint subluxation.

MANAGEMENT

(1) Immobilize the thumb in a thumb spica cast or splint, and refer to the Orthopaedic team, as permanent disability may follow missed or untreated ruptures.

FRACTURES OF THE OTHER METACARPALS

DIAGNOSIS

(1) These are caused by direct trauma and may be multiple. The classical, isolated, little-finger metacarpal neck fracture or 'boxer's fracture' is due to punching a hard object.

(2) Examine all cases for any rotational deformity. On flexing the fingers into the palm, the fingertips should point to the scaphoid. If not, a rotational deformity of that finger exists.

(3) Obtain anteroposterior, lateral and oblique X-rays of the hand.

MANAGEMENT

(1) Refer multiple fractures, rotated fractures, compound fractures, and fractures associated with marked soft-tissue swelling from crushing to the Orthopaedic team.

(2) Otherwise, for undisplaced, isolated fractures, give the patient a high-arm sling, an analgesic such as paracetamol 500 mg and codeine phosphate 8 mg and either a padded crêpe bandage, or a Plaster of Paris volar slab with the hand in the 'position of safe splintage'.

(3) *Position of safe splintage*

   (i) Pad well with cotton-wool, and extend the volar slab over the flexor aspect of the forearm, on to the palm of the hand to the fingertips.

   (ii) Hold the wrist extended, the MCP joints flexed, the interphalangeal joints extended, and the thumb abducted with the slab, which is kept in place with a crêpe bandage.

   (iii) Instruct the patient to keep the hand elevated.

   (iv) Refer all patients to the next Fracture clinic.

(4) *Isolated, little-finger knuckle 'boxer's injury'*

   (i) Many different methods of reduction and splintage have been tried. Simple 'buddy-strapping' of the little finger to the ring finger, a padded crêpe bandage, a sling and analgesia are as effective as any.

   (ii) Remember that if the knuckle struck a tooth and the skin has been broken, this is a potentially serious injury. It may involve underlying tendons or penetration of the joint capsule and there is high risk of infection.

(a) explore the wound in both the neutral position and with the fist clenched. If there is any suggestion of penetration into the joint space or tendon, refer the patient immediately to the Orthopaedic team for surgical exploration and debridement. Give flucloxacillin 2 g i.v.

(b) otherwise, take a wound swab for bacterial culture and irrigate the wound with normal saline. Give the patient amoxicillin 500 mg and clavulanic acid 125 mg, one tablet t.d.s. for 5 days and tetanus prophylaxis

(c) review the wound within 24 hours.

FRACTURES OF THE PROXIMAL AND MIDDLE PHALANGES

DIAGNOSIS

(1) Similar mechanisms of injury and rules of management apply, as described previously for metacarpal fractures.

(2) Examine all cases for rotational deformity. Check that on flexing the fingers into the palm, the tips point to the scaphoid.

(3) X-ray all injuries to look for fractures, dislocations, subluxations and radio-opaque foreign bodies.

MANAGEMENT

(1) Refer all multiple, compound, angulated or rotated fractures, and those associated with marked soft-tissue damage or involving a joint surface, to the Orthopaedic team.

(2) Otherwise, buddy-strap the finger, give the patient a high-arm sling to prevent oedema, and give an analgesic such as paracetamol 500 mg and codeine phosphate 8 mg. Refer to the next Fracture clinic.

FRACTURES OF THE DISTAL PHALANGES

DIAGNOSIS

(1) These fractures are usually caused by a crushing injury resulting in a comminuted fracture of the bone.

(2) The main problem is the associated soft-tissue injury to the nail and pulp space.

MANAGEMENT

(1) Provide adequate protection by using a plastic mallet-finger splint, elevate the hand and give analgesics.

(2) Fingernail injuries.
 (i) Cover the exposed bed with soft paraffin gauze if the nail is avulsed, and give tetanus prophylaxis and flucloxacillin 500 mg orally q.d.s. for 5 days.
 (ii) If the nail is partially avulsed from the base:
  (a) administer a ring block and remove the nail to exclude an underlying nail-bed injury
  (b) debride and clean the area, then replace the nail as a splint to the nail matrix, and as a dressing to the nail bed
  (c) reposition the nail bed with one or two fine sutures inserted into the sides of the tip of the finger, *not* into the nail bed. Dress the area, give tetanus prophylaxis and antibiotics, and elevate the hand in a high-arm sling.

(3) *Subungual haematoma*: Relieve this by trephining the nail with a red-hot paper clip to release the blood under tension. This is a painless procedure bringing instant relief.

DISLOCATION OF THE PHALANGES

DIAGNOSIS AND MANAGEMENT

(1) Dislocations of the phalanges result from hyperextension injuries and must be X-rayed to exclude an associated fracture. They almost always displace dorsally or to one side.

(2) Reduce under a ring block by traction applied to the finger, followed by a repeat X-ray to confirm adequate reduction.

(3) Immobilize by buddy-strapping and encourage active finger movements. Refer the patient to the next Fracture clinic.

(4) Complications include:
 (i) Rupture of the middle slip of the extensor tendon following proximal interphalangeal joint dislocation.
 (ii) Avulsion of the volar plate.
 (iii) Rupture of one or both collateral ligaments. Accompanying small avulsion flake fractures may be seen on X-ray.
 (iv) Button-holing of the head of the phalanx through the volar plate, necessitating open operation for a failed reduction.

FLEXOR TENDON INJURIES IN THE HAND

DIAGNOSIS
(1) These injuries occur from direct laceration or blunt injury.
(2) Assess for a flexor tendon injury:
    (i) *Flexor digitorum profundus* causes flexion at the distal interphalangeal joint.
    (ii) *Flexor digitorum superficialis* causes flexion of the finger at the proximal interphalangeal joint, while the neighbouring fingers are held extended.
    (iii) Suspect a partial tendon division from pain or reduced function against resistance.

MANAGEMENT
(1) Refer all suspected flexor tendon injuries directly to the Orthopaedic team.
(2) Give tetanus prophylaxis for any penetrating wounds.

EXTENSOR TENDON INJURIES IN THE HAND

DIAGNOSIS
(1) Injury can occur by:
    (i) Direct laceration.
    (ii) Avulsion of the middle slip of the extensor tendon that inserts onto the middle phalanx.
    (iii) Avulsion of the distal slip of the extensor tendon that inserts onto the distal phalanx.
(2) Assess for an extensor tendon injury:
    (i) Avulsion of the distal insertion causes a 'mallet-finger' deformity. The patient is unable to extend the distal interphalangeal joint with the middle phalanx held.
    (ii) Avulsion of the middle slip that inserts onto the middle phalanx may be missed.
        (a) initially, the proximal interphalangeal joint can be extended by the two lateral bands, but as they displace in a volar direction, they then begin to act as flexors
        (b) finally, the proximal interphalangeal joint becomes flexed and the distal interphalangeal joint hyperextended, resulting in the *boutonnière* deformity.
(3) Request an X-ray to show an associated flake fracture of avulsed bone.

MANAGEMENT
(1) Refer a lacerated tendon or middle slip avulsion immediately to the Orthopaedic team.
(2) Also refer patients to the Orthopaedic team for consideration of open reduction and internal fixation, if more than one-third of the articular surface of the distal phalanx has been avulsed.
(3) Manage a mallet-finger deformity in a plastic mallet-finger extension splint for 6 weeks, and refer the patient to the Fracture clinic.

DIGITAL NERVE INJURIES

DIAGNOSIS
(1) It is mandatory to test for digital nerve function before using any local anaesthetic blocks.
(2) Sensory loss, paraesthesiae or dryness of the skin from absent sweating, demonstrated along either side of a digit, indicate digital nerve injury.

MANAGEMENT
(1) Refer immediately to the Orthopaedic team nerve injuries that are:
   (i)   Proximal to the proximal interphalangeal joint.
   (ii) Along the ulnar border of the little finger.
   (iii) Along the radial border of the index finger.
   (iv) Affecting the thumb.
(2) Injuries distal to the proximal interphalangeal joint rarely justify repair unless local departmental policy differs.

FINGERTIP INJURIES

MANAGEMENT
(1) Clean and debride injuries of the distal fingertip that are less than 1 cm in diameter and that do not involve fracture of the terminal phalanx.
(2) Leave to granulate under a soft paraffin gauze dressing changed after 2 days.
(3) Give tetanus prophylaxis.
(4) Refer injuries involving substantial soft-tissue loss, distal phalanx exposure or a degloving directly to the Orthopaedic team.

CERVICAL SPINE INJURIES

See p. 211.

THORACIC AND LUMBAR SPINE INJURIES

See p. 233.

PELVIC INJURIES

See p. 229.

INJURIES TO THE HIP AND UPPER FEMUR

DISLOCATION OF THE HIP

DIAGNOSIS

(1) Dislocation of the hip occurs in violent trauma such as a traffic crash, a fall from a height or sometimes a direct fall on to the hip.

(2) The hip joint is inherently stable so always look for associated injuries, as considerable force is required to produce dislocation.

(3) The most common direction to dislocate is posteriorly (85%), such as when the knee strikes the dashboard of a car.

   (i) Other associated injuries from this particular accident are a fractured femoral shaft and a fractured patella.

(4) Less common are the central dislocation, fracturing through the acetabulum, or the rare anterior dislocation.

(5) Note on examination that in a posterior dislocation the hip is held slightly flexed, adducted and internally rotated, whereas in an anterior dislocation the hip is abducted and externally rotated.

(6) Check for sciatic nerve damage in posterior dislocation of the hip, particularly if an acetabular rim fracture is present.

   (i) Assess dorsiflexion (L5) and plantar flexion (S1) of the ankle, and sensation over the medial side of the ankle (L5) and the lateral border of the foot (S1).

(7) Gain i.v. access and send blood for FBC, U&Es, blood sugar and G&S.

(8) X-ray the pelvis, hip and the shaft of the femur in all cases.

(9) Complications are more common with posterior dislocations and include:

    (i) Avascular necrosis of the head of the femur. The risk of avascular necrosis developing is directly proportional to the length of time the hip remains dislocated and increases dramatically after 6 hours

    (ii) Sciatic nerve neurapraxia may occur in 15% and is usually relieved by reduction.

    (iii) Missed knee injuries occur in up to 15% of cases.

MANAGEMENT

(1) Commence an infusion of normal saline.

(2) Give morphine 5–10 mg i.v. and an antiemetic such as metoclopramide 10 mg i.v.

(3) Refer all cases to the Orthopaedic team for immediate reduction under general anaesthesia.

FRACTURES OF THE NECK OF THE FEMUR

DIAGNOSIS

(1) These fractures are most common in elderly women following a fall, and may be divided into two groups:

    (i) *Intracapsular*

        (a) subcapital – may be displaced or non-displaced

        (b) femoral head – rare and normally associated with hip dislocation.

    (ii) *Extracapsular*

        (a) intertrochanteric

        (b) pertrochanteric

        (c) subtrochanteric.

(2) Typically, after a fall the patient is unable to bear weight, and the leg is shortened and externally rotated.

(3) Occasionally the patient may be able to limp if the fracture impacts, and examination reveals localized tenderness and pain on rotating the hip.

(4) Gain i.v. access and send blood for FBC, U&Es, blood sugar and G&S.

(5) Record an ECG.

(6) Request X-rays and include the pelvis, as well as anteroposterior and lateral views of the hip.

(i)   Request a CXR in addition as a pre-operative aid for the anaesthetist.

(ii) Look carefully for a fractured pubic ramus on the pelvic X-ray if no femoral neck fracture is seen, because this also presents with hip pain and a limp.

MANAGEMENT

(1) Commence i.v. fluid resuscitation, because comminuted extracapsular neck of femur fractures may be associated with up to 1.5 L blood loss.

(2) Give i.v. analgesia titrated to response.

(3) Consider a femoral nerve block (see below) for proximal neck of femur fractures, especially in the elderly when opiates must be given with caution.

(4) Keep the patient fasted until consultation with the orthopaedic team.

FRACTURES OF THE SHAFT OF THE FEMUR

DIAGNOSIS

(1) These fractures are due to considerable violence, as in a traffic crash, crushing injury or fall from a height.

(2) They may be associated with a hip dislocation, pelvic fracture or fracture of the patella, and may cause concealed haemorrhage of 1–2 L in a closed injury (more if compound).

(3) Rarely there is damage to the femoral vessels or sciatic nerve.

(4) Gain large-bore i.v. access and send blood for FBC, U&Es, blood sugar and cross-match 4 units of blood.

(5) X-ray the pelvis, hip and knee, as well as the shaft of femur, to avoid missing other injuries.

MANAGEMENT

(1) Give high-flow oxygen by face mask.

(2) Commence an infusion of normal saline or Hartmann's (compound sodium lactate).

(3) Perform a femoral nerve block to help relieve the pain:

(i)   Prepare local anaesthetic in a 20-mL syringe. Mix 1% lignocaine (lidocaine) 10 mL (a total of 100 mg: maximum safe dosage 3 mg/kg) with 0.5% bupivacaine 10 mL (a total of 50 mg: maximum safe dosage 2 mg/kg).

(ii) Palpate the femoral artery and insert a 21-gauge needle with syringe perpendicular to the skin, lateral to the artery and just below the inguinal ligament.

(iii) Withdraw slightly if paraesthesia is elicited down the leg,
indicating proximity of the needle to the femoral nerve.
Aspirate to exclude vessel puncture, and inject 15–20 mL of
the mixed solution of local anaesthetic.

(iv) Alternatively, a characteristic loss of resistance may be felt as
the needle passes through the fascia lata then fascia iliaca:

(a) aspirate to exclude vessel puncture

(b) inject 15–20 mL of the mixed solution of local anaesthetic
fan-wise, moving outwards up to 3 cm lateral to the artery.

(4) Supplement the femoral nerve block with morphine 5–10 mg i.v.
and an antiemetic such as metoclopramide 10 mg i.v. as required.

(5) Apply traction as quickly as possible to reduce the pain and blood
loss, and to facilitate movement of the patient during X-ray, which
should *not* be done until after the splint is in place.

(i) Use a commercially available Donway or Hare traction splint,
or alternatively use a traditional skin traction device such as
the Thomas splint.

(ii) Get help to apply the splint, which cannot easily be placed alone.

(6) Reassess lower limb neurovascular status after the traction splint
has been applied.

(7) Refer the patient to the Orthopaedic team.

INJURIES TO THE LOWER FEMUR, KNEE AND UPPER TIBIA

SUPRACONDYLAR AND CONDYLAR FRACTURES OF THE FEMUR

DIAGNOSIS AND MANAGEMENT

(1) These injuries are caused by direct trauma or a fall in an elderly
person with osteoporotic bones.

(2) Rarely the popliteal artery is damaged by supracondylar fractures,
although condylar fractures often cause a tense haemarthrosis.

(3) Give the patient analgesics and refer immediately to the
orthopaedic team for aspiration of any tense haemarthrosis and
operative fixation in certain cases.

FRACTURES OF THE PATELLA AND INJURY TO THE QUADRICEPS APPARATUS

DIAGNOSIS

(1) Damage is caused by direct trauma as in a traffic crash or fall, or by indirect force from violent quadriceps contraction.

(2) Patients typically present with acute knee pain, swelling, bruising and loss of function. There is inability to extend the knee in most cases associated with the local pain.

(3) Remember always to examine the shaft of femur and the hip at the same time.

(4) There may be a palpable defect in the suprapatellar region if the quadriceps mechanism is torn, and a low-lying patella.

(5) Request an X-ray to demonstrate the patella fracture.
   (i) Confusion may arise from congenital bipartite or tripartite patellae, although these are often bilateral, unlike fractures, so if in doubt X-ray the other knee.
   (ii) Look for a lipohaemarthrosis causing a horizontal line fluid level on the lateral X-ray view of the knee, which is a useful indicator of an intra-articular fracture.
   (iii) Request a 'skyline' X-ray view in subtle patellar fractures.
   (iv) Consider a CT scan when a suspected fracture is not visible on plain X-ray.

MANAGEMENT

(1) Refer distracted or comminuted patella fractures, and patients with disruption of the knee extensor mechanism directly to the Oorthopaedic team.

(2) Otherwise, place the leg in a padded plaster cylinder from the thigh to the ankle if there is a stable, undisplaced fracture of the patella, and refer the patient to the next Fracture clinic.

(3) Aspirate a tense haemarthrosis first, before applying the plaster cylinder.

(4) *Aspiration of the knee*
   (i) Use a strict aseptic technique. Clean the skin with chlorhexidine and inject 2% lignocaine (lidocaine) 2–3 mL into the skin, subcutaneous tissue and synovium.
   (ii) Insert a large-bore, 14-gauge cannula at the midpoint of the superior portion of the patella 1 cm lateral to the anterolateral edge.
   (iii) Aim the cannula between the posterior surface of the patella

and the intercondylar femoral notch.

(iv) Withdraw the needle and attach a 50-mL syringe with three-way tap to the remaining catheter. Aspirate to dryness.

    (a) gently squeeze the suprapatellar region to 'milk' any residual fluid

    (b) up to 70 mL or more of blood-stained fluid may be removed

    (c) look for evidence of fat globules floating on the surface of the blood dispelled into a kidney dish, because they indicate an intra-articular fracture.

DISLOCATION OF THE PATELLA

DIAGNOSIS

(1) The patella usually dislocates laterally in teenage girls and may become recurrent. It is most commonly associated with a direct blow to the anterior or medial surface of the patella.

(2) Patients complain of the knee suddenly giving way, and inability to weight-bear or extend the knee and are often in considerable pain.

(3) Examine for an anterior defect, the laterally deviated patella, and swelling and medial joint line tenderness of the partly-flexed knee.

(4) Sometimes, spontaneous reduction occurs and the patient then presents with a tender knee, particularly along the medial border of the patella.

    (i) A careful history and a positive 'patella apprehension' test (moving the patella laterally causes pain) suggest the original injury.

MANAGEMENT

(1) Reduce under nitrous oxide with oxygen (Entonox™) analgesia by pushing the patella medially with firm pressure, whilst extending the knee.

(2) Request a skyline patellar X-ray after the reduction to exclude an associated osteochondral fracture.

(3) Place the leg in a padded plaster cylinder and refer the patient to the next Fracture clinic.

(4) Use a pressure bandage instead of a plaster cylinder if the dislocation is recurrent.

SOFT-TISSUE INJURIES OF THE KNEE

A careful history of the mechanism of injury and the subsequent events is crucial, as knee examination is often difficult or impossible immediately afterwards due to acute pain. Always lie the patient on an examination trolley and undressed properly.

DIAGNOSIS

(1) Rapid swelling of the knee suggests a haemarthrosis, usually due to an anterior cruciate tear, peripheral meniscal tear, or intra-articular fracture.
    (i) Delayed swelling, occurring after several hours, is more likely to be due to a serous effusion.

(2) Injuries may be deduced from the direction of force.
    (i) Sideways stresses will rupture the collateral ligaments or joint capsule.
    (ii) A twisting injury will damage one of the menisci, usually the medial.
    (iii) Combinations may be seen. A severe, twisting lateral blow to the knee, e.g. from a car bumper, will rupture the medial collateral ligament, tear the medial meniscus, and rupture the anterior cruciate ligament (O'Donoghue's 'unhappy triad').

(3) Always undress the patient, examine on a trolley and include the hip and spine, as the pain may be referred, particularly in children. Include the following in every knee examination:
    (i) Observe the size and extent of knee swelling and the location of bruising.
    (ii) Look at the position of the knee.
        (a) meniscal tears may result in 'locking' of the knee with inability to extend the knee fully.
    (iii) Palpate the knee to elicit the area of maximum pain.
    (iv) Assess the medial and lateral collateral ligaments by stressing each side with the knee slightly flexed.
    (v) Assess the cruciate ligaments.
        (a) with the knee flexed, attempt to move the tibia backwards (posterior cruciate tear) or abnormally forwards (anterior cruciate tear)
        (b) note that a posterior cruciate tear allows the head of the tibia to slip backwards on posterior stressing, which then moves forwards into a correct anatomical position on anterior stressing

(c) this forwards movement does not indicate an anterior cruciate tear; only movement into an *abnormally* forwards position indicates this.

> ⚠ **Warning:** passive and active movements of the knee are restricted by the pain and swelling in the setting of acute injury and are difficult to evaluate accurately.

(4) X-ray all patients and look for associated fractures, such as:
   (i) Tibial condyle fracture.
   (ii) Avulsion fracture of the tibial spines in cruciate ligament tears.
   (iii) Flake fractures of the lateral or medial femoral condyles in collateral ligament tears.
   (iv) Vertical avulsion fracture off the lateral tibia from the lateral capsular ligament attachment (Segond fracture).
   (v) Avulsion of the tibial tubercle (Osgood–Schlatter's disease) due to traction apophysitis, more common in young male teenagers.

MANAGEMENT
(1) Refer the following to the Orthopaedic team having given adequate analgesics:
   (i) A tense effusion, including all suspected haemarthroses with an associated fracture.
   (ii) A 'locked' knee with sudden loss of ability to extend the knee fully.
   (iii) A suspected torn cruciate ligament.
   (iv) Any penetrating wound of the knee suggested by air or foreign material in the joint on X-ray (these may be absent).
(2) Otherwise, if there is only moderate swelling, a good range of joint movement and no ligamentous laxity:
   (i) Apply a double-elasticated stockinet bandage to the knee or a proprietary Velcro™-fitted knee splint.
   (ii) Give the patient anti-inflammatory analgesics such as ibuprofen 200–400 mg orally t.d.s. or naproxen 250 mg orally t.d.s.
   (iii) Lend the patient crutches to use until the acute symptoms settle.
   (iv) Review the patient within 5 days.

DISLOCATION OF THE KNEE

DIAGNOSIS AND MANAGEMENT

(1) This is a severe injury and an orthopaedic emergency.

(2) It is associated with up to 30% incidence of damage to the popliteal vessels and lateral popliteal nerve, so requires urgent reduction.

(3) Insert an i.v. cannula, administer opiate analgesia, check the distal pulses, X-ray and refer immediately to the Orthopaedic team.

FRACTURES OF THE TIBIAL CONDYLES

DIAGNOSIS

(1) These fractures are caused by falls from a height, or severe lateral or medial stresses, which in addition may rupture the knee ligaments.

(2) A tense haemarthrosis is usual and precludes further detailed examination of the knee due to pain.

(3) Always check for vascular damage by palpating the foot pulses.

(4) Check for a lateral popliteal nerve palsy by testing for active foot dorsiflexion and eversion, and sensation over the lateral aspect of the calf.

(5) Request an X-ray to show the tibial condyle fracture either laterally or (rarely) on the medial side, although sometimes they are subtle and difficult to see.

   (i) Look for a horizontal line fluid level in the suprapatellar pouch on the lateral view due to a lipohaemarthrosis, indicating an intra-articular fracture, and request a CT scan.

MANAGEMENT

(1) Give the patient analgesics and refer immediately to the Orthopaedic team.

INJURIES TO THE LOWER TIBIA, ANKLE AND FOOT

FRACTURES OF THE SHAFT OF THE TIBIA

DIAGNOSIS

(1) These injuries are often compound and associated with direct trauma.

(2) Greenstick fractures in children and stress fractures in athletes are also seen.

(3) X-rays should always include the knee and ankle, as well as the shaft of the tibia.

(4) Gain i.v. access and send blood for FBC, U&Es, blood sugar, and cross-match 2 units of blood in compound injuries.

MANAGEMENT

(1) *Compound injuries*

    (i) Commence an i.v. infusion of normal saline or Hartmann's (compound sodium lactate).

    (ii) Give the patient morphine 5–10 mg i.v. with an antiemetic such as metoclopramide 10 mg i.v.

    (iii) Restore anatomical alignment.

    (iv) Cover the exposed area with a sterile dressing.

    (v) Give flucloxacillin 2 g or cefuroxime 750 mg i.v. and tetanus prophylaxis.

    (vi) Apply a temporary plastic adjustable splint or a long-leg Plaster of Paris backslab from thigh to foot, with the ankle placed at a right-angle, especially when there are other injuries to the chest or abdomen requiring more urgent care.

    (vii) Refer the patient immediately to the Orthopaedic team.

(2) Refer all other tibial shaft fractures to the Orthopaedic team, after giving the patient analgesia and applying a long-leg Plaster of Paris backslab with the knee slightly flexed, and the ankle at a right-angle.

ISOLATED FRACTURES OF THE FIBULA

DIAGNOSIS AND MANAGEMENT

(1) Associated with a direct blow to the lateral aspect of the lower leg, typically when playing football.

(2) Patients present with local pain, swelling and difficulty walking.

(3) Perform a neurovascular assessment especially for isolated proximal fractures to exclude damage to the common peroneal nerve causing foot drop.

(4) Request full-length anteroposterior and lateral X-rays of the tibia and fibula, including the ankle and knee joints.

(5) Provided there is definitely no injury to the ankle, and no tibial fracture at another level, apply *either*

    (i) A firm crêpe bandage with cotton-wool padding.

    or

(ii) A below-knee walking plaster, which affords more protection.

(6) Refer the patient to the next Fracture clinic.

INVERSION ANKLE INJURIES

DIAGNOSIS

(1) These injuries are common following sports or tripping on a staircase or on uneven ground.

(2) The aim of clinical examination is to distinguish ligament tears from bony injury, and to assess the stability of the ankle.

(3) Immediate swelling and inability to weight bear suggest a fracture or serious ligament tear.

    (i) Examine the ankle for evidence of pain over the following specific sites:

        (a) distal fibula and lateral malleolus

        (b) distal tibia and medial malleolus

        (c) medial (deltoid) ligament and lateral ligament (anterior talofibular, middle calcaneofibular and posterior talofibular portions) of the ankle

        (d) anterior tibiofibular ligament

        (e) base of the fifth metatarsal, navicular and calcaneus

        (f) proximal fibula head (for the uncommon but serious Maisonneuve fracture).

(4) *Ottawa ankle rules*

These are prospectively validated clinical decision rules, which aim to reduce the number of ankle X-rays requested, without missing clinically significant fractures. Request an anteroposterior and lateral X-ray of the ankle based on these Ottawa criteria, if there is pain in the malleolar area and any one of the following:

    (i) Inability to bear weight (e.g. unable to take four steps without assistance, regardless of limping) both within the first hour of injury and in the Emergency Department.

    (ii) Bone tenderness over the posterior edge or tip of the distal 6 cm of the medial malleolus.

    (iii) Bone tenderness over the posterior edge or tip of the distal 6 cm of the lateral malleolus.

(5) *Ottawa foot rules*

Request additional foot X-rays only when there is pain in the mid-foot and any one of the following:

    (i) Inability to bear weight both immediately and in the

Emergency Department.

(ii) Bone tenderness over the base of the fifth metatarsal.

(iii) Bone tenderness over the navicular.

MANAGEMENT

(1) Refer the following injuries immediately to the Orthopaedic team, after giving suitable analgesia and applying a below-knee plaster backslab (see below):

(i) Compound ankle injury.

(ii) Displaced lateral malleolar or medial malleolar fractures, with widening or diastasis of the ankle mortice.

(iii) Bimalleolar and trimalleolar ankle fractures.

(2) Treat conservatively in a below-knee plaster stable ankle fractures such as undisplaced lateral malleolar fractures or malleolar avulsion fractures.

Below-knee plaster slab

(i) Apply this from the metatarsal heads to below the tibial tubercle, with the ankle at a right-angle (*not* in equinus).

(ii) Repeat the ankle X-ray after application of the plaster.

(iii) Refer the patient to the next Fracture clinic, with instructions to keep the leg elevated as much as possible.

(3) Patients able to bear weight, with minimal swelling and with no fracture seen on X-ray:

(i) Apply a double-elasticated stockinet bandage, give the patient crutches or a walking frame, and give an anti-inflammatory analgesic such as ibuprofen 200–400 mg orally t.d.s. or naproxen 250 mg orally t.d.s.

(ii) Recommend initial elevation, no weight-bearing, and a cold compress (e.g. a bag of frozen peas) at home, followed by gradual mobilization.

(iii) Warn patients that they will not be fully fit for active sports for at least 3–4 weeks, and recommend Physiotherapy if available.

(iv) Review the patient after 5–10 days and refer to Physiotherapy when there is persisting disability, if not already attending.

OTHER ANKLE INJURIES

DIAGNOSIS

(1) Eversion injuries damaging the medial malleolus and medial deltoid ligament, hyperflexion injuries or rotational injuries tend to

cause more complicated damage.

(2) Examine the ankle as before to localize the maximum area of tenderness.

   (i) Palpate the upper fibula for a high, oblique fracture (Maisonneuve) in addition, associated with tibiofibular diastasis tearing the syndesmosis and a widened ankle mortice.

(3) X-ray all patients meeting the Ottawa criteria on p. 312, and include the upper tibia and fibula if there is proximal bony tenderness.

MANAGEMENT

(1) Refer all fractures, a widened ankle mortice, or patients who are totally unable to bear weight to the Orthopaedic team.

(2) Otherwise treat as in point (3) on page 313.

DISLOCATION OF THE ANKLE

DIAGNOSIS AND MANAGEMENT

(1) This dislocation is most commonly posterior and is clinically obvious. Reduce urgently to prevent ischaemic pressure necrosis of skin stretched across the malleolus.

(2) Give the patient morphine 5 mg i.v. and metoclopramide 10 mg i.v. and X-ray immediately.

(3) Then use conscious sedation with diazepam 5–10 mg i.v. or midazolam 2.5–5 mg i.v. in a monitored area with resuscitation equipment available.

(4) Reduce the ankle dislocation by steady traction on the heel, applying gentle dorsiflexion to the foot.

(5) After the reduction, re-examine the neurovascular status, and support the lower leg in a plastic splint or padded plaster backslab, before sending the patient for post-reduction X-rays.

(6) Refer the patient to the Orthopaedic team.

FRACTURES AND DISLOCATION OF THE TALUS

DIAGNOSIS

(1) The talus articulates in three joints: the ankle joint with the tibia and fibula, the subtalar joint with the calcaneus, and the mid-tarsal joint with the navicular (along with the calcaneus and cuboid).

(2) Injuries result from falls from a height or sudden violence to the foot, as from the pedal of a car being forced upwards in a car crash.

(3) There is pain and swelling. Request an X-ray to define the injuries.

(4) Complications of talar injuries include avascular necrosis and persistent pain and disability from osteoarthrosis, particularly if the injury is missed.

MANAGEMENT

(1) Refer all fractures including the osteochondral dome fracture immediately to the Orthopaedic team.

(2) The only exception is an avulsion flake fracture of the neck of the talus from a ligamentous or capsular insertion.
   (i) Treat this in a below-knee plaster and refer to the next Fracture clinic.

(3) Occasionally, the talus dislocates completely and lies laterally in front of the ankle joint.
   (i) Refer the patient for urgent manipulation to avoid overlying skin necrosis, similar to the dislocated ankle.

FRACTURES OF THE CALCANEUS

DIAGNOSIS AND MANAGEMENT

(1) These are usually due to a fall from a height, and are bilateral in 20% of cases.

(2) Falls from a height are associated with a characteristic collection of injuries, which includes fractures to the:
   (i) Calcaneus.
   (ii) Ankle.
   (iii) Tibial plateau.
   (iv) Femoral head or hip.
   (v) Thoracolumbar vertebrae.
   (vi) Atlas and base of the skull.

(3) Look specifically for each of these in turn, and X-ray any tender areas found.

(4) The heel tends to flatten following a calcaneal fracture, and is locally tender with bruising spreading to the sole and even up the calf.

(5) Request an anteroposterior and lateral ankle X-ray with an additional tangential (axial) calcaneal view to avoid missing the calcaneal fracture.

(6) A CT scan may be necessary to demonstrate involvement of the subtalar joint.

(7) Elevate the foot and give analgesia.

(8) Refer all fractures to the Orthopaedic team.

RUPTURE OF THE TENDO ACHILLIS

DIAGNOSIS

(1) This injury is most common in middle-aged men following abrupt muscular activity. There is pain and weakness of plantar flexion, although some is still possible by the long toe flexors. However, the patient is unable to walk on tiptoe.

(2) Feel for a palpable gap in the tendon, although this rapidly fills with blood and may then disappear.

(3) Perform the 'calf squeeze' test. This demonstrates reduced or absent foot plantar flexion compared with the uninjured side.

    (i) It is best performed with the patient kneeling on a chair with both feet hanging free over the edge.

    (ii) Squeeze the unaffected calf just distal to its maximal girth, and compare the normal plantar flexion response elicited with the reduced flexion response in the affected leg.

MANAGEMENT

(1) Give the patient analgesics and refer to the Orthopaedic team for operative repair or conservative treatment.

MID-TARSAL DISLOCATIONS

DIAGNOSIS

(1) These follow a twisting injury to the forefoot, causing pain and swelling around the talonavicular and calcaneocuboid mid-tarsal joint.

(2) Request a foot X-ray to show disruption of the mid-tarsal joint, often associated with fractures of the navicular, cuboid, talus or calcaneus. These may merely be avulsion flake fractures.

(3) A CT scan is usually required to evaluate these injuries further.

MANAGEMENT

(1) Give the patient analgesics, elevate the foot, and refer to the Orthopaedic team.

METATARSAL INJURIES AND TARSOMETATARSAL DISLOCATIONS

DIAGNOSIS

(1) These are caused by direct trauma, crushing or twisting.

(2) A transverse avulsion fracture of the base of the fifth metatarsal often accompanies an ankle inversion injury, at the site of insertion of peroneus brevis.

(3) A stress fracture may occur, usually in the neck of the second metatarsal, known as the 'march fracture' after repetitive use.

(4) Tarsometatarsal fracture–dislocation (Lisfranc fracture) is uncommon and usually involves multiple bones, resulting in widening of the gap between the base of the hallux and the second metatarsal, with lateral shift of the remaining metatarsals.

   (i) It is easy to miss, as the significance of the foot swelling is not appreciated and interpretation of the X-ray is difficult.

   (ii) Look carefully for any signs of circulatory impairment in the forefoot.

MANAGEMENT

(1) Refer immediately to the Orthopaedic team all compound, displaced or multiple fractures, fractures of the first metatarsal, tarsometatarsal fracture–dislocations, injuries associated with crushing or marked oedema and any signs of circulatory impairment.

(2) Treat an avulsion fracture of the base of the fifth metatarsal as for an ankle sprain, and a 'march fracture' in a support bandage, or rarely a below-knee plaster if the pain is severe.

FRACTURES OF THE PHALANGES OF THE FOOT

DIAGNOSIS AND MANAGEMENT

(1) These fractures are usually caused by direct trauma.

(2) Clean all the wounds and release any subungual haematoma by trephining.

(3) Otherwise, give an analgesic and a support bandage after buddy-strapping the damaged toe.

(4) Apply a below-knee plaster with a toe platform extension if pain is severe, particularly with injury to the great toe.

(5) Refer all patients to the next Fracture clinic.

DISLOCATIONS OF THE PHALANGES OF THE FOOT

DIAGNOSIS AND MANAGEMENT

(1) These occur by direct trauma, usually to bare or unprotected feet.
(2) Insert a ring block (see p. 320).
(3) Request an X-ray, to exclude an associated fracture.
(4) Reduce by restoring normal anatomical alignment, with axial traction.
(5) Buddy-strap and refer to the next Fracture clinic.

FURTHER READING

McRae R, Esser M (2002) *Practical Fracture Treatment*, 4th edn. Churchill Livingstone, Edinburgh.

Stiell IG, McKnight RD, Greenberg GH, *et al.* (1994) Implementation of the Ottawa ankle rules. *J Amer Med Assoc* **271**:827–32.

MUSCULOSKELETAL AND SOFT-TISSUE EMERGENCIES

SOFT-TISSUE INJURIES

The so-called 'minor injury' is of major importance to the patient and may lead to serious problems if managed incorrectly. Therefore, adopt a consistent, careful approach to every patient presenting with a soft-tissue injury.

GENERAL MANAGEMENT OF A SOFT-TISSUE INJURY
(1) Assessment.
  (i) Obtain a history of:
    (a) the nature of the injury, and when and where it was sustained
    (b) the possibility of a foreign body, wound contamination, and damage to deeper structures
    (c) any crushing injury
    (d) current medical conditions and drug therapy
    (e) antibiotic allergy and tetanus immunization status.
  (ii) Examine nerves and tendons for evidence of damage, before infiltrating with local anaesthetic.
  (iii) Send the patient for X-rays before exploring the wound, if a radio-opaque foreign body (metal or glass) is suspected. Inform the radiographer of the nature of the foreign body.
(2) Wound preparation.
  (i) When assessing and preparing the wound:
    (a) always lie the patient down on a trolley
    (b) wash hands thoroughly before and after wound review
    (c) wear sterile gloves and prepare a sterile field.
  (ii) Remove all the dirt and debris from around the edges of the wound prior to anaesthetic infiltration, using normal saline or a disinfectant, e.g. chlorhexidine with gentle swabbing.
  (iii) Only trim adjacent hair for 3–5 mm if absolutely necessary, but *never* shave the eyebrows or eyelashes.
(3) Local anaesthetic infiltration.
  (i) Simple laceration. Infiltrate 1% lignocaine (lidocaine) along the edge of the wound using a 25-gauge orange needle.
  (ii) *Ring block*
    Use 2% plain lignocaine (lidocaine) without adrenaline

(epinephrine) to ring block wounds around the nail, fingertip, distal finger and toes.

    (a) a ring block is contraindicated in patients with peripheral vascular disease, Raynaud's phenomenon and local sepsis at the base of the digit

    (b) do not use a tourniquet due to the risk of creating high pressures locally and occluding the digital vessels

    (c) clean the base of the finger first with antiseptic

    (d) insert a 25-gauge orange needle into the side of the base of the finger, and angle at 45 degrees from the vertical injecting up to 1.5 mL of 2% plain lignocaine (lidocaine) (without adrenaline/epinephrine) into the lateral palmar aspect of the finger

    (e) remove the needle until subcutaneous, and rotate until it is pointing to the extensor surface of the finger. Inject 0.5 mL into the lateral extensor aspect of the finger

    (f) perform the same procedure on the other side of the finger

    (g) allow at least 5–10 minutes for the ring block to take effect.

(iii) The maximum safe dose of lignocaine (lidocaine) is 3 mg/kg. A 1% solution contains 10 mg/mL. Therefore, the maximum safe amounts allowed in a 67-kg patient are:

    (a) 20 mL of a 1% solution containing 200 mg lignocaine (lidocaine), or

    (b) 10 mL of a 2% solution again containing 200 mg lignocaine (lidocaine).

(iv) Signs of lignocaine (lidocaine) (or other local anaesthetic) toxicity include:

    (a) perioral tingling, a metallic taste, restlessness, dizziness and slurred speech

    (b) confusion, seizures and coma

    (c) bradycardia, hypotension and circulatory collapse.

(v) Treat seizures with lorazepam, diazepam or midazolam i.v., and circulatory collapse with inotropes or by commencing cardiopulmonary resuscitation if needed (see p. 2).

(4) Exploration, irrigation, debridement and haemostasis.

(i) Look carefully for evidence of foreign bodies, and severed tendons, vessels or nerves within the wound. Seek assistance from the senior ED doctor if the latter are found.

(ii) Irrigate the wound using a 20-mL syringe filled with saline and fitted with a 23-gauge blue needle to provide a high-pressure jet. Repeat this procedure until the wound is clear of debris.

    (a) use protective eyewear to prevent eye splash contamination with body fluids.

(iii) Excise any dead or contaminated tissue and remove local dirt on the skin by swabbing briskly. Make certain all ingrained gravel and grit is removed to avoid permanent tattooing of the skin. A general anaesthetic may be required.

(iv) Achieve haemostasis by local pressure. Avoid using mosquito forceps to clamp a bleeding area, as this may cause further local tissue damage.

(5) Sutures.

   (i) The aim is to appose the edges of the wound without tension using interrupted sutures, starting in the middle of the wound and halving the remaining distance each time.

  (ii) The choice of suture material depends on the type of tissue being repaired and local practice.

    (a) use an absorbable suture such as polydioxanone or polyglactin when closing deep wounds, to close the deep space first, and bury the knot at the depth of the wound

    (b) silk was traditionally most popular for skin closure, although it is more likely to cause micro-abscess formation with scarring

    (c) use non-absorbable synthetic monofilament sutures such as nylon or polypropylene instead. Although harder to tie, requiring an initial double throw and multiple knots, they cause much less of a foreign-body reaction.

(iii) Use the smallest practical suture size:

    (a) limb laceration: 4/0 synthetic monofilament sutures removed at 7–10 days

    (b) scalp: 2/0 or 3/0 synthetic monofilament sutures removed at 7 days

    (c) face: 5/0 or 6/0 synthetic monofilament sutures removed at 4 days.

(iv) Cover the wound with a non-adherent dressing. There is no need to keep the area dry in the first 24 hours.

  (v) Arrange an appointment for removal of the sutures in the Emergency Department or with the GP.

(vi) Make a record in the notes of the size and nature of the wound, the deep structures involved, and the number of sutures used to close it.

(6) Antibiotics.

Do not use antibiotics indiscriminately. They are secondary to thorough surgical toilet in preventing infection, and are best reserved for:

(i) *Cellulitis*

    (a) this is usually due to a beta-haemolytic *Streptococcus* or *Staphylococcus aureus* if associated with a wound. Send a swab first

    (b) give 1 week of phenoxymethylpenicillin (penicillin V) 500 mg orally q.d.s., or flucloxacillin 500 mg orally q.d.s. if staphylococcal infection is suspected.

(iii) *Dirty, contaminated wound*

    Give flucloxacillin 2 g i.v., gentamicin 5 mg/kg i.v. and metronidazole 500 mg i.v.

(iii) *Bites*

    (a) clean, debride and irrigate with copious normal saline. Do not suture, except on the face

    (b) give amoxicillin 500 mg and clavulanic acid 125 mg one tablet orally t.d.s. for 5 days, unless just a trivial scratch. If penicillin-allergic, use doxycycline 100 mg once daily orally and metronidazole 400 mg orally t.d.s. Give erythromycin if pregnant or breastfeeding, and in children

    (c) give tetanus prophylaxis

    (d) consider rabies prophylaxis if the patient was bitten abroad by a dog, or by a bat in Australia. Discuss this with a local Infectious Diseases expert.

(iv) *Compound fractures*

    (a) give flucloxacillin 2 g i.v. or cefuroxime 750 mg i.v.

    (b) remember tetanus prophylaxis.

(7) Tetanus prophylaxis.

See below.

TETANUS PROPHYLAXIS

DIAGNOSIS

(1) Routine tetanus immunization was progressively introduced into the UK and Australasia after the Second World War, so elderly people are now the most likely to be non-immune.

(2) Virtually any wound can become contaminated, however trivial.

(3) Meticulous wound toilet is an essential part of tetanus prophylaxis, rather than simply relying on tetanus immunization or antibiotics.

(4) Treat patients according to their immune status and the type of wound (see Table 9.1):

   (i) *Tetanus-prone wound* – wounds at significant risk of developing tetanus include:

      (a) wounds or burns requiring surgical intervention that is delayed more than 6 hours

      (b) wounds or burns with significant devitalized tissue, or puncture-type injury particularly in contact with soil or manure

      (c) wounds containing foreign bodies especially wood splinters

      (d) compound fracture

      (e) wounds or burns in patients who have systemic sepsis.

   (ii) *Clean minor wound* – any wound that is clean, incised or superficial, i.e. does not fulfil any of the criteria of the tetanus-prone wound.

Table 9.1 Tetanus immunization prophylaxis

Immune status category	Treatment	
	Tetanus-prone wound	Clean minor wound
Fully immunized[a]	None	None
Primary immunization complete, or boosters[b] incomplete but up to date	None (unless convenient to give booster now)	None (unless convenient to give booster now)
Primary immunization incomplete, or boosters not up to date	Toxoid booster + complete course[a] + HTIG[c]	Toxoid + complete course[a]
Not immunized, or state of immunity unknown/uncertain	Complete course of toxoid[a] + HTIG[c]	Complete course of toxoid[a]

[a]A total of 5 doses of a tetanus-containing vaccine i.m. at appropriate intervals, e.g. given on day 1, at 4 weeks, and at 2 months, plus boosters at 3–5 years and at 10 years.
[b]A booster is a subsequent injection of adsorbed tetanus toxoid i.m.
[c]HTIG is human tetanus immunoglobulin 250 IU given i.m. at a different site to the toxoid, increased to 500 IU if over 24 hours have elapsed or there is heavy contamination.

(5) Tetanus vaccines and immunoglobulin:
  (i) Active tetanus toxoid immunization in the UK from 2006 is recommended given combined with diphtheria, pertussis, *Haemophilus influenzae* type B (HiB) and inactivated polio vaccines up to age 10 years, then combined with diphtheria and inactivated polio thereafter.
  (ii) Tetanus toxoid in Australia is combined with diphtheria and pertussis up to age 17 years, and thereafter combined with diphtheria alone.
      (a) administer by deep i.m. injection into upper arm or anterolateral thigh
      (b) contraindications to tetanus vaccine include prior anaphylaxis to tetanus toxoid, neomycin, streptomycin or polymyxin B (all these are extremely rare).
  (ii) Confer additional passive protection immediately by administering human tetanus immunoglobulin (HTIG) when indicated (see Table 9.1):
      (a) give 250 IU by deep i.m. injection, or 500 IU if the wound is heavily contaminated or more than 24 hours old, at a site distant from the tetanus toxoid combined vaccines.

MANAGEMENT

(1) Tetanus immunization schedule (see Table 9.1).
  (i) Clean minor wounds:
      (a) patients fully immunized and with boosters up to date require no immunization
      (b) give patients with an incomplete tetanus immunization schedule a tetanus toxoid combined-vaccine booster, and arrange completion of a full tetanus course with the GP
      (c) give non-immune patients an initial dose of tetanus toxoid combined-vaccine followed by a full course of the tetanus vaccine.
  (ii) Tetanus-prone wounds:
      (a) administer human tetanus immunoglobulin to patients who are non-immune, immunocompromised, or have not completed a full tetanus immunization programme
      (b) give fully immunized patients human tetanus immunoglobulin only if the risk of infection is particularly high.
(2) Tetanus itself is rare, but worldwide it is a frequent cause of death in parts of Asia, Africa and South America.

(i) The incubation time from injury to first symptoms ranges from 4 to 21 days (usually about 7 days).

(ii) The most common symptoms are jaw stiffness (trismus), dysphagia, and abdominal and back pain. Hypertonia is found on examination.

(iii) Localized or generalized painful spasms follow within 24–72 hours, becoming more severe and prolonged from minimal stimuli.

(iv) Death may occur from laryngospasm, respiratory failure, or autonomic dysfunction.

(v) There is no rapid diagnostic test to prove the diagnosis, therefore admit suspected cases immediately to ICU.

CRUSH INJURIES AND COMPARTMENT SYNDROME

DIAGNOSIS

(1) Crush injuries may be caused by a roller or wringer injury, a direct blow or a vehicle wheel passing over a limb.

(2) With severe soft-tissue injury there may be little to see initially.

(3) Test for tendon, nerve or vessel damage.

  (i) Loss of skin blanching on digital pressure indicates shearing of capillaries, which may subsequently lead to extensive soft-tissue necrosis.

(4) *Compartment syndrome*

  (i) Tissue capillary perfusion pressure is compromised due to raised pressures locally within closed anatomic spaces or compartments.

  (a) this is most commonly seen associated with the lower leg, and forearm volar compartments.

  (ii) Causes include crush injuries, external compression from a tight plaster, fractures (especially tibial), constricting burns, local haemorrhage, vigorous exercise and prolonged immoblization in coma, e.g. following acute poisoning.

  (iii) Always consider compartment syndrome if there is marked pain particularly on passive stretching of muscles, associated with paraesthesiae and loss of motor and sensory nerve function.

  (iv) The entire area within the closed fascial compartment feels tense. However, arterial pulses and even skin perfusion may initially remain deceptively normal.

(5) Send blood for FBC, ELFTs, CK and dipstick the urine for myoglobinuria.

(6) Perform an ECG particularly if hyperkalaemia is suspected.

(7) Request X-rays to exclude underlying fractures.

MANAGEMENT

(1) Gain i.v. access and give normal saline 20–40 mL/kg i.v. to improve hypoperfusion, and give morphine 0.1 mg/kg i.v. and metoclopramide 10 mg i.v.

(2) Place the affected limb at the level of the heart. Excessive elevation reduces arterial flow and may worsen the ischaemia.

(3) Eliminate any external constricting factors such as a tight bandage or plaster by cutting, or bivalving a cast.

(4) Refer all severe crush injuries involving a limb, hand or foot to the Orthopaedic team, including patients suspected of having a compartment syndrome.

    (i) Management will include consideration of compartment pressure monitoring, the use of vasodilator agents, mannitol and sodium bicarbonate, or operative fasciotomy.

(5) Otherwise, clean and debride isolated finger or toe injuries without suturing, elevate the limb to the level of the heart, and give the patient analgesics.

    (i) Review within 3 days for consideration of delayed primary suture.

PUNCTURE INJURIES

DIAGNOSIS

(1) This type of injury is caused by treading on a nail or pin, by penetration of a sewing-machine needle, or through industrial accidents including nailguns or high-pressure guns for grease, paint, water or oil.

(2) Needlestick and sharps incidents are covered on p. 138.

MANAGEMENT

(1) Refer all high-pressure gun injuries immediately to the Orthopaedic team, even if no apparent damage is seen initially. They will require extensive debridement.

(2) Otherwise, clean the wound with antiseptic, give tetanus prophylaxis, and consider the need for antibiotics.

(3) Treat a rusty nail injury to the foot by soaking in betadine for 30 minutes and give amoxicillin 500 mg and clavulanic acid 125 mg one tablet orally t.d.s. for 5 days.

(4) Instruct the patient to return immediately if signs of infection or gross oedema supervene.

HAND INFECTIONS

DIAGNOSIS AND MANAGEMENT

(1) *Paronychia*
   (i) This is pus formation adjacent to the nail, with throbbing pain.
   (ii) Make a longitudinal incision parallel to the nail edge across the nail fold to release the pus, under a ring-block anaesthetic (see p. 320). Mop out the cavity with pledgets of cotton-wool.
   (iii) Dress the finger with paraffin-impregnated gauze tucked into the cavity, and apply a plain viscose stockinet tubular bandage without tension. Use a high-arm sling for 24 hours, and review the dressing after 2 days.

(2) *Pulp space infection*
   (i) This is pus formation in the distal fat pad of the finger.
   (ii) Make a central longitudinal incision using a ring block, over the middle of the abscess. Take care not to cross the flexion crease of the distal interphalangeal joint, and mop out the cavity of pus.
   (iii) Dress and review as for paronychia.
   (iv) The flexor tendon sheath is in danger in more extensive infections when swelling approaches the distal interphalangeal joint. Refer the patient directly to the Orthopaedic team, after an X-ray to exclude osteomyelitis.

(3) *Suppurative tenosynovitis of the flexor tendons*
   (i) The original wound may have been forgotten, but intense discomfort, swelling and tenderness develop along the line of the flexor tendon, with characteristically severe pain on all passive finger movements.
   (ii) Refer the patient directly to the Orthopaedic team for operative debridement and i.v. antibiotics.

(4) *Deep palmar and web space infections*
   (i) These cause pain, swelling and loss of function with localized

tenderness and the development of a 'flipper' hand, from pronounced swelling on to the dorsum of the hand.

(ii) Refer the patient directly to the Orthopaedic team.

PRE-TIBIAL LACERATIONS

DIAGNOSIS

(1) These are most common in elderly patients, often from trivial trauma tearing a flap of skin.

MANAGEMENT

(1) Clean the wound, remove blood clots, trim obviously necrotic tissue and unfurl the rolled edges of the wound to determine actual skin loss.

(2) Refer the patient immediately to the Surgical team if there is significant skin loss or marked skin retraction preventing alignment of the skin edges, for consideration of early skin grafting.

(3) Otherwise, lay the flap back over the wound and hold it in place with adhesive skin-closure strips (Steristrips™). Cover the wound with a single layer of paraffin-impregnated gauze and a cotton-wool and gauze combine pad.

(4) Then apply a firm crêpe bandage and instruct the patient to keep the leg elevated whenever possible.

(5) Enquire about tetanus immunization status.

(6) Review the patient after 5 days, removing the dressing but leaving the Steristrips™ in place.

(i) Refer the patient to the surgical team for skin grafting if the skin is now obviously non-viable.

(ii) Otherwise, review the patient weekly if healing is taking place, or discharge to the care of the GP and community nurse.

INGROWING TOENAILS

DIAGNOSIS AND MANAGEMENT

(1) These are common, and associated with tight-fitting footwear or socks, poor foot hygiene, and trimming off the corners of the nail. They usually afflict young people.

(2) Medical treatment.

(i) Insert a pledget of cotton-wool under the nail edge with a pair of forceps, and cauterize the granulation tissue with a silver nitrate stick.

(a) advise the patient to wear loose shoes and on the importance of cutting the nail straight across in future

(b) ask the patient to repeat the cotton-wool insertion and silver nitrate cautery once or twice a day at home. This method is effective, cheap and requires no special apparatus, provided the patient is motivated and careful.

(ii) An alternative is liquid nitrogen cryotherapy, although this requires special equipment that may not be available.

(3) Consider surgical treatment by wedge resection or total nail-bed ablation in resistant cases.

NON-ARTICULAR RHEUMATISM

Joint pain, swelling and tenderness that mimics arthritis may be due to inflammation of periarticular structures. Most patients can be treated with NSAID analgesics such as ibuprofen 200–400 mg orally t.d.s. or naproxen 250 mg orally t.d.s. and then be referred to Outpatients or back to their GP.

Leave joint aspiration and steroid injection to the experts, as complications such as septic arthritis and joint destruction do occur.

Conditions include:

- Torticollis (wry neck)
- Frozen shoulder
- Rotator cuff tear: supraspinatus rupture
- Supraspinatus tendonitis
- Subacromial bursitis
- Tennis and golfer's elbow
- Olecranon bursitis
- de Quervain's stenosing tenosynovitis
- Carpal tunnel syndrome
- Housemaid's knee

TORTICOLLIS (WRY NECK)

DIAGNOSIS AND MANAGEMENT

(1) Torticollis is abnormal involuntary contraction of the neck

musculature lateralizing to one side, resulting in the neck being held in a twisted or bent position.

(2) Ask the patient about recent trauma, particularly if elderly.

(3) Direct the physical examination to identifying an underlying aetiology, as well as documenting the degree of neck movement.

(4) Look specifically for local sepsis such as tonsillitis, quinsy, and a submandibular abscess, or for sensory or motor signs suggesting a cervical disc prolapse.

(5) Remember to exclude drug-induced dystonia with an oculogyric crisis due to metoclopramide, phenothiazines, or butyrophenones such as haloperidol.

    (i) Give benzatropine 1–2 mg i.v. followed by 2 mg orally once daily for 3 days if dystonia is likely.

(6) Request a plain X-ray of the cervical spine if bony trauma or cervical pathology is suspected.

(7) Manipulate the neck into the neutral position in the absence of the alternative causes suggested above, and immobilize in a soft collar. Try diazepam 2–5 mg orally if muscular spasm is severe.

(8) Give an analgesic such as paracetamol 500 mg and codeine phosphate 8 mg two tablets orally q.d.s. and/or an NSAID such as ibuprofen 200–400 mg orally t.d.s. or naproxen 250 mg orally t.d.s. Return the patient to the care of the GP.

FROZEN SHOULDER

DIAGNOSIS AND MANAGEMENT

(1) This can occur spontaneously, following local trauma, or following disuse of the arm after a fracture, CVA, myocardial infarction or even shingles. It is more common in the elderly.

(2) There is pain and loss of all movement from an adhesive capsulitis.

(3) Encourage active shoulder movements following the conditions above to prevent the capsulitis in the first place.

(4) Otherwise, prescribe an anti-inflammatory analgesic and return the patient to the care of the GP.

(5) Physiotherapy may help, but although the pain subsides, the loss of movement tends to persist for months or even years.

ROTATOR CUFF TEAR: SUPRASPINATUS RUPTURE

DIAGNOSIS

(1) Sudden traction on the arm may tear the muscles that make up the rotator cuff. The onset may be insidious, but a traumatic incident may complete a tear causing sudden severe pain and reduced shoulder function.

(2) Evaluate full active and passive range of movement at the glenohumeral joint. There is reduction of active shoulder motion with inability to initiate abduction and weakness of external rotation of the shoulder.

(3) Tenderness is localized over the greater tuberosity and the subacromial bursa, particularly with supraspinatus rupture. Other muscles forming the rotator cuff may also tear but are difficult to differentiate clinically in the acute stage.

(4) Perform a shoulder X-ray that may reveal a decrease in the space between the head of the humerus and the acromion.

(5) Request an ultrasound, which is useful for characterizing the extent of full-thickness rotator cuff tears and biceps tendon dislocation. It is less sensitive for partial-thickness tears.

(6) MRI is highly sensitive and specific for delineating size, location and characteristics of rotator cuff pathology, when available.

MANAGEMENT

(1) Refer acute tears in young patients to the Orthopaedic team for consideration of operative repair, to ensure optimal return to a full range of movement and function.

(2) Give the elderly patient analgesics, an immobilizing sling and refer to the Physiotherapy Department for a physical therapy rehabilitation programme.

SUPRASPINATUS TENDONITIS

DIAGNOSIS AND MANAGEMENT

(1) This is one of the causes of the 'painful arc' between 60 and 120 degrees of shoulder abduction.

(2) Request X-ray which may show calcification in the supraspinatus tendon.

(3) Give an anti-inflammatory analgesic, and consider referral to the Orthopaedic or Rheumatology clinic for aspiration and local steroid injection.

SUBACROMIAL BURSITIS

DIAGNOSIS AND MANAGEMENT
(1) This may follow rupture of calcific material into the subacromial bursa, again causing a 'painful arc', or a constant severe pain.
(2) Treat as for supraspinatus tendonitis above.

TENNIS AND GOLFER'S ELBOW

DIAGNOSIS AND MANAGEMENT
(1) Tennis elbow causes pain over the lateral epicondyle of the humerus from a partial tear of the extensor origin of the forearm muscles used in repetitive movements (e.g. using a screwdriver or playing tennis).
(2) Advise the patient to avoid the activity causing the pain, and to rest the arm. Give an anti-inflammatory analgesic.
(3) Refer for local steroid injection if the pain is persistent.
(4) Golfer's elbow is a similar condition affecting the medial epicondyle and the flexor origin.

OLECRANON BURSITIS

DIAGNOSIS AND MANAGEMENT
(1) Painful swelling of this bursa is due to trauma, gout or infection, usually with *Staphylococcus aureus*.
(2) Aspirate under sterile conditions and send fluid for culture and polarizing light microscopy if the latter two conditions are likely.
(3) Refer the patient for drainage of the bursa under anaesthesia if significant infection is confirmed. Otherwise, give an NSAID analgesic and refer back to the GP.

DE QUERVAIN'S STENOSING TENOSYNOVITIS

DIAGNOSIS AND MANAGEMENT
(1) This causes tenderness over the radial styloid, a palpable nodule from thickening of the fibrous sheaths of the abductor pollicis

longus and extensor pollicis brevis tendons, and pain on moving the thumb.

(2) Treat by resting the thumb in a splint and by using an anti-inflammatory analgesic.

(3) This condition may require surgical release of the tendon sheaths if local injection of steroid fails.

CARPAL TUNNEL SYNDROME

DIAGNOSIS AND MANAGEMENT

(1) This is a compressive neuropathy of the median nerve at the wrist, most commonly affecting middle-aged females.

(2) Secondary causes include rheumatoid arthritis, post-trauma such as a Colles' fracture, pregnancy, and rarely myxoedema, acromegaly and amyloidosis. Most cases though are idiopathic or related to minor trauma.

(3) Patients complain of pain and paraesthesiae in the distribution of the median nerve in the hand, primarily the thumb, index, middle and lateral aspect of the ring finger. It is typically worse at night or following repetitive strain such as computer work.

(4) Test for reduced sensation over the palmar aspect of the affected digits and weakness of thumb abduction, associated with thenar muscle wasting in more chronic cases.

(5) Perform Phalen's test, by reproducing paraesthesiae in the distribution of the median nerve following 60-second wrist hyperflexion, or look for Tinel's sign eliciting median nerve paraesthesiae by tapping on the volar aspect of the wrist over the median nerve.

(6) Treat with an anti-inflammatory analgesic, and immobilize the wrist in a volar splint in the neutral position, particularly at night.

(7) Refer resistant cases to the Orthopaedic clinic for consideration of carpal tunnel decompression.

HOUSEMAID'S KNEE

DIAGNOSIS AND MANAGEMENT

(1) This is a pre-patellar bursitis due to friction or infection.

(2) Treat by giving an anti-inflammatory analgesic, avoiding further trauma and, if necessary, by aspiration and steroid injection by the GP or Outpatient clinic (orthopaedic or rheumatology).

(3) Refer the patient to the Orthopaedic team if infection is suspected.

BACK PAIN

This is a common problem that is considered under four headings:
- Direct back trauma
- Mechanical (indirect) back trauma
- Severe or atypical, non-traumatic back pain
- Mild to moderate, non-traumatic back pain

DIRECT BACK TRAUMA

Back pain that follows direct trauma is managed according to the principles in the appropriate section on multiple injuries (see p. 233).

MECHANICAL (INDIRECT) BACK TRAUMA

DIAGNOSIS
(1) Bending, lifting, straining, coughing or sneezing may precipitate acute, severe low back pain.
(2) There is intense muscle spasm, or even complete immobility. The normal lumbar lordosis is lost, with development of a scoliosis.
(3) Assess for any reduction in straight-leg raise (SLR), suggesting sciatic nerve-root irritation, with an inability to raise more than 30 degrees due to pain going down the leg being abnormal.
   (i) Remember that the ability to sit up in bed with the legs out straight is equivalent to a SLR of 90 degrees on both sides.
(4) Examine for neurological signs of nerve-root irritation or compression from an acute prolapsed intervertebral disc.
   (i) Look for motor loss occurring in the following myotomes:
      (a) L1, L2 – hip flexion (iliopsoas)
      (b) S1 – hip extension (gluteus maximus)
      (c) L5 – knee flexion (hamstrings)
      (d) L3, L4 – knee extension (quadriceps)
      (e) L5 – ankle dorsiflexion (extensor hallucis longus)
      (f) S1 – ankle plantar flexion (calf muscles).
   (ii) Check for reduced or absent reflexes:
      (a) L3, L4 – knee jerk
      (b) L5, S1 – ankle jerk.
   (iii) Assess for sensory loss in the following dermatomes:
      (a) L3 – medial lower thigh and knee

    (b) L4 – medial side of calf

    (c) L5 – lateral side of calf

    (d) S1 – lateral border of the foot and sole.

(5) Always look for any signs of a central disc prolapse causing cauda equina compression, with the following diagnostic features:

    (i)   History of difficulty emptying the bladder or bowels.

    (ii) Saddle-area anaesthesia over dermatomes S2, S3, S4 and S5.

    (iii) Weakness in both legs.

    (iv) Lax anal sphincter tone on p.r. exam.

MANAGEMENT

(1) Refer any patient with features of a central disc prolapse causing any signs of cauda equina compression immediately to the Orthopaedic team. It is an orthopaedic emergency.

    (i)   Arrange an urgent MRI to best demonstrate the cauda equina (or any spinal cord) compression.

(2) Also refer any patient who is completely unable to move or has signs of nerve-root compression, and those who fail a trial of mobilization within the Emergency Department, particularly if elderly or living alone.

(3) Discharge patients with moderate pain and with no nerve root signs.

    (i)   Give the patient a non-steroidal anti-inflammatory analgesic such as ibuprofen 200–400 mg orally t.d.s. or naproxen 250 mg orally t.d.s.

    (ii) Encourage early return to ordinary activities within the limits of the pain. Bed rest should be kept to a minimum.

    (iii) Request review and follow-up by a physiotherapist or the GP for back-care education including correct posture, abdominal and back exercises and safe lifting techniques.

SEVERE OR ATYPICAL, NON-TRAUMATIC BACK PAIN

DIAGNOSIS

(1) The aim is to look in particular for any underlying serious pathological causes, which vary according to the patient's age.

    (i)   Under 30 years:

        (a) ankylosing spondylitis

        (b) rheumatoid arthritis

        (c) osteomyelitis

(d) discitis

(e) extradural abscess.

(ii) Over 30 years:

(a) bony metastases

(b) myeloma

(c) lymphoma

(d) renal or pancreatic disease

(e) aortic aneurysm.

(iii) Over 60 years:

(a) as (ii) above

(b) osteoporosis

(c) Paget's disease

(d) osteoarthritis

(e) spinal stenosis.

(2) Therefore enquire specifically about previous back trouble, joint trouble, unremitting spinal symptoms particularly pain at night, fever, weight loss, associated abdominal symptoms and urinary tract symptoms.

(3) Perform a full examination including abdominal, rectal, neurological and breast examinations, and a urinalysis.

(4) X-ray the chest and thoracic and lumbosacral spine.

MANAGEMENT

(1) Refer the patient to the appropriate specialist team according to the most likely suspected aetiology.

MILD TO MODERATE, NON-TRAUMATIC BACK PAIN

DIAGNOSIS AND MANAGEMENT

(1) This nebulous group with no abnormal physical signs, apyrexial with a normal urinalysis may go home.

(2) Prescribe a non-steroidal anti-inflammatory analgesic such as ibuprofen 200–400 mg orally t.d.s. or naproxen 250 mg orally t.d.s.

(3) Give patients a letter for their GP to follow them up and to arrange physiotherapy, an abdominal and back exercise regimen, and behaviour modification, including weight reduction and safe lifting techniques, as appropriate.

FURTHER READING

Australian Department of Health and Ageing (2003) *The Australian Immunisation Handbook*, 8th edn.
http://immunise.health.gov.au/handbook.htm (tetanus).

Department of Health UK.
http://www.dh.gov.uk/PolicyAndGuidance/HealthAndSocialCareTopics/GreenBook/fs/en/ Immunization Against Infectious Diseases 2006 '*The Green Book*' (tetanus).

PAEDIATRIC EMERGENCIES

(1) It is essential to recognize the sick or seriously ill child and understand the key differences between adults and children.

(2) Knowing what is abnormal and identifying the sick child is impossible, unless the doctor is first able to recognize 'normal' paediatric developmental and physiological parameters (see Tables 10.1 and 10.2).

(3) Early recognition and immediate management of potential respiratory, circulatory or neurological failure will reduce mortality and secondary morbidity. Fig. 10.1 is a paediatric resuscitation chart from which all drug doses, endotracheal tube sizes and defibrillator settings can be read according to the age, weight or body length – whichever is known.

Table 10.1 Developmental milestones in early childhood

Age	Developmental milestones
Neonate	Symmetrical antigravity movement of four limbs Cries Looks at faces, responds to light Startles to loud noises
6 months	Sits erect with support Alert and interested Localizes sound
1 year	Crawls on all fours Walks holding onto furniture Understands simple commands Babbles Socially responsive
2 years	Runs, manages stairs Joins words: simple phrases Dry by day
3–4 years	Stands on one foot momentarily Speaks full (three-word) sentences Gives full name Dry by night
5 years	Skips/hops/stands on one foot Fluent speech Dresses self unaided

Table 10.2 Normal paediatric physiological parameters

Age	Weight (kg)		Height (cm)		Heart rate (beats/min)	Systolic BP (mmHg)	Circulating blood volume (mL)	Respiratory rate (breaths/min)
	Male	Female	Male	Female				
0–1 year	3.5–10.3	3.4–9.6	50–75	50–74	110–160	70–90	300–800	30–40
1–2 years	–	–	–	–	100–150	80–95	–	25–35
2–5 years	12.5–19	12–18.5	85–107	84–106	95–140	80–100	990–1390	25–30
5–12 years	19–38	18.5–40	107–147	106–149	80–120	90–110	1390–1700	20–25
12+ years	49–60	51–56	160–172	160–162	60–100	100–120	3500–4000	15–20
	For 1–10 years: weight (kg) = 2 × (age in years + 4)				SBP = 80 + 2 × (age in years) DBP = $\frac{2}{3}$ × SBP mmHg		80–85 mL/kg	Tidal volume = 5–7 mL/kg

DBP, diastolic blood pressure; SBP, systolic blood pressure.

(4) Most emergencies generate fear in children causing additional distress to the child and adding to parental anxiety.

(i) Allow parents to stay with the child at all times.

(ii) Use toys and picture books to placate the distressed infant.

(iii) Explain things as clearly as possible to both the child and the parent.

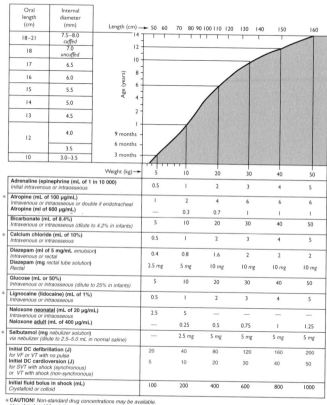

Figure 10.1 Paediatric resuscitation chart

Drug doses, endotracheal tube sizes and defibrillator settings are read off the chart according to the age, weight, or body length. DC, direct current; SVT, supraventricular tachycardia; VF, ventricular fibrillation; VT, ventricular tachycardia. Reproduced with kind permission from the BMJ Publishing Group.

(5) Commence the assessment from the first moment the child is seen, while the parent or child is giving the history or the child alone is talking. Even infants and children unable to talk will give non-verbal cues about illness or pain, such as facial expressions and posture.

(6) A complete examination of every child is guided by the clinical history, but should include:

  (i) Height, weight and head circumference measurements plotted on a percentile chart.

  (ii) An oral, rectal or tympanic temperature and full vital signs.

  (iii) Examination of the chest, eardrums, mouth, throat (not if epiglottitis suspected) and the skin.

  (iv) A urine sample for sugar, protein and microscopy.

(7) The child may present with non-specific symptoms and signs. Potentially serious illness may be present in children presenting with:

  (i) Respiratory distress, stridor, grunting or gasping respirations, nasal flaring or a silent chest.

  (ii) Pallor, reduced peripheral circulation, poor capillary refill and cyanosis.

  (iii) Altered level of consciousness, drowsiness and lethargy – particularly the floppy infant.

  (iv) Reduced fluid intake or urine output with decreased skin turgor and dry mucous membranes.

CARDIOPULMONARY RESUSCITATION

DIAGNOSIS

(1) Cardiac arrest in children is usually secondary to respiratory or circulatory failure rather than ventricular fibrillation triggered by myocardial ischaemia, as in adults.

(2) The outcome is poor and if hypoxia, hypovolaemia and acidosis are left untreated, bradycardia progressing to asystole is almost invariable. Early recognition and treatment of impending respiratory or circulatory failure is therefore essential to avoid cardiopulmonary arrest.

(3) Look for signs of respiratory failure:

  (i) Increased effort of breathing:

(a) respiratory rate outside normal range for age (too fast or too slow)

(b) intercostal, subcostal or sternal recession, stridor and wheeze

(c) grunting and gasping respiratory effort (signs of severe respiratory distress, especially in infants).

 Warning: decreased or minimal effort of breathing heralds pre-terminal respiratory failure as the child nears exhaustion.

(ii) Efficacy of breathing:

(a) reduced oxygen saturations as measured by pulse oximetry

(b) reduced chest expansion with reduced, asymmetrical or bronchial breath sounds.

Warning: the silent chest is an ominous sign in respiratory failure.

(iii) Effects of hypoxia:

(a) initial tachycardia, followed by pre-terminal bradycardia if prolonged hypoxia

(b) initial skin pallor with vasoconstriction. Cyanosis is a pre-terminal sign

(c) altered level of consciousness leading to loss of consciousness.

(4) Look for signs of circulatory failure:

(i) Increased heart rate (bradycardia is an ominous sign).

(ii) Decreased peripheral perfusion, poor capillary refill.

(iii) Decreased systemic blood pressure.

(iv) Decreased urine output.

MANAGEMENT

Similar principles and practice apply to those for adult resuscitation (see p. 2). Fig. 10.1 depicts drug doses, endotracheal tube sizes, and defibrillator settings, and Fig. 10.2 is the advanced life support (ALS) algorithm in children. Specific points relevant to paediatric resuscitation are outlined below:

(1) *Ventilation and oxygenation*

(i) Give high-flow oxygen.

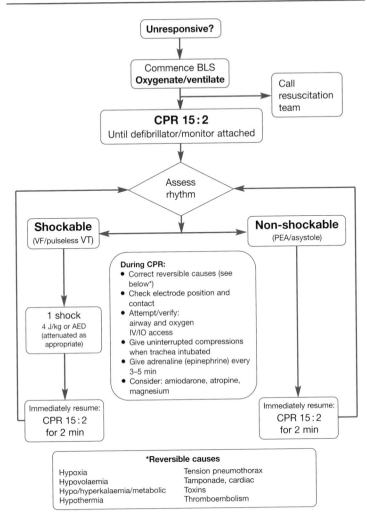

Figure 10.2 Paediatric advanced life support algorithm

AED, automatic external defibrillator; BLS, basic life support; CPR, cardiopulmonary resuscitation; IO, intraosseous; IV, intravenous; J, joules; PEA, pulseless electrical activity; VF, ventricular fibrillation; VT, ventricular tachycardia. Reproduced by kind permission. European Resuscitation Council (2005) European Resuscitation Council Guidelines for Resuscitation 2005. Section 6: Paediatric life support. *Resuscitation* **67(Suppl 1):**S97–133.

(ii) Clear the airway. If the airway is blocked by an inhaled foreign body:

    (a) hold the infant or small child prone and deliver up to five blows over the back, between the scapulae, followed by up to five chest thrusts

    (b) perform abdominal thrusts in an older child, if back blows do not relieve the obstruction.

(iii) Provide ventilatory assistance if respiratory effort is slow, shallow or absent:

    (a) position the head in a neutral position in infants under 1 year, as overextension of the head may actually occlude their airway

    (b) insert an oropharyngeal airway under direct vision, if the child is unconscious with no gag reflex and the tongue is occluding the airway. Measure this airway from the centre of the mouth to the angle of the jaw

    (c) perform bag–mask ventilation, which is preferable to inexperienced attempts at endotracheal intubation. Leave intubation to an airway-skilled doctor

      – use a face mask that fits closely over the nose and mouth. Soft circular plastic masks are ideal

      – attach a hand-ventilating device. Standard infant ventilating bags have a volume of 240 mL, require an oxygen flow rate of at least 4 L/min and are suitable for children up to 2 years. Standard child ventilating bags have a volume of 500 mL and are suitable for children up to 10 years. Inflate the chest at a faster rate than adults, up to 20 breaths/min.

    (d) have an endotracheal tube ready and both straight and curved-blade laryngoscopes for the airway-skilled doctor (see Table 10.3).

      – internal diameter of endotracheal tube (mm) = (age in years/4) + 4

      – oral endotracheal tube length (cm) = (age in years/2) + 12

      – nasotracheal tube length (cm) = (age in years/2) + 15

(2) *External cardiac massage*

    (i) Commence external cardiac massage with positive-pressure ventilation in the ratio of 15: 2 (30: 2 if lone rescuer) after opening the airway and administering 5 rescue breaths.

Table 10.3 Paediatric endotracheal tube sizes

Endotracheal tube (ET) size (formulae)		Age (years)									
		Birth	4/12	1	3	7	10	12	14	16	Adult
Internal diameter (mm): $\frac{age}{4} + 4$ Oral length (cm): $\frac{age}{2} + 12$	Internal diameter (mm)	3.0	3.5	4.0	5.0	6.0	6.5	7.0 (+ cuff)	7.5	8.0	9.0
Nasal length (cm): $\frac{age}{2} + 15$ Neonates: 3–3.5 mm ET tube	Oral length (cm)	9	10	12	13	16	17	18	21	22	23

(ii) Use two fingers in infants over the lower half of the sternum in the centre of the chest, and in a child, use a single hand.

(iii) Perform compressions at a rate of 100/min.

(3) *Vascular access*

(i) Vascular access will be difficult, but is needed to administer drugs and fluids and obtain blood samples. There is no advantage to central venous access over peripheral or intraosseous (i.o.) access in resuscitation.

(ii) *Venous access*

(a) insert a 20- or 22-gauge cannula into a familiar site such as the antecubital fossa, the back of the hand, external jugular or internal jugular vein

(b) perform intraosseous (bone marrow) vascular access, if venous access is not gained within 90 seconds or is likely to take longer than this.

(iii) *Intraosseous (i.o.) access*

(a) intraosseous access is rapid, safe and effective for administering drugs, fluids and blood products, and for drawing blood for cross-match, blood sugar and chemical analysis

(b) use in children up to the age of 6 years when alternate i.v. access has failed or will take over 90 seconds to perform

(c) insert the intraosseous needle into the anteromedial surface of the proximal tibia, 1–2 cm distal to the tuberosity. Advance the needle with a gentle twisting or boring motion until it gives on entering the marrow cavity, and remove the stylet

(d) aspirate blood and marrow contents to confirm correct placement

(e) flush each drug with a bolus of normal saline to ensure dispersal beyond the marrow cavity and to achieve faster central circulation distribution.

(iv) Connect an infusion of normal saline via a paediatric giving set slowed to a minimal rate to the vascular or venous access.

(a) give an initial fluid bolus of 20 mL/kg rapidly if hypovolaemia is suspected.

(v) Adrenaline (epinephrine), atropine and lignocaine (lidocaine) may be given via the endotracheal tube if venous or intraosseous access is delayed. Dilute solutions in 1–2 mL (infants) or 2–5 mL (small child) normal saline and follow with five ventilations:

(a) adrenaline (epinephrine) endotracheal dose is 100 µg/kg (ten times the initial i.v. dose)

(b) atropine endotracheal dose is 30 µg/kg

(c) lignocaine (lidocaine) endotracheal dose is 2 mg/kg (twice initial i.v. dose).

(4) *Drug administration*

(i) Recommended drug doses are shown in Table 10.4.

(5) *Defibrillation*

See Fig. 10.1.

(i) 'Time to defibrillation' is the main determinant of survival in ventricular fibrillation (VF) or pulseless ventricular tachycardia (VT), the so-called shockable rhythms, which are uncommon in children.

(ii) Perform immediate defibrillation in shockable rhythms VF and pulseless VT.

(a) place paddles or defibrillator pads one below the right clavicle, and the other in the left axilla

(b) administer defibrillation with 4 J/kg whether biphasic, or an older monophasic device

(c) resume CPR as soon as possible after each individual shock

(d) review rhythm every 2 minutes

(e) give further shocks at 4 J/kg if VF or pulseless VT persists.

Table 10.4 Paediatric emergency drugs

Drug		Dose and route of administration			
		Intravenous	Intraosseous	Intramuscular	Endotracheal
Adrenaline (epinephrine)	1 in 10 000	Initial: 0.1 mL/kg (10 µg/kg)	Initial: 0.1 mL/kg (10 µg/kg)	–	–
	1 in 1000	–	–	0.01 mL/kg (10 µg/kg)	0.1 mL/kg (100 µg/kg)
Atropine 0.6 mg/mL		IV or IO bolus over 1 min Birth–1 month: 15 µg/kg (0.025 mL/kg) 1 month–12 years: 20 µg/kg (0.033 mL/kg) (minimum 100 µg, maximum 600 µg)		–	0.05 mL/kg (30 µg/kg)
Sodium bicarbonate 8.4%		IV or IO 1 mmol/kg or 1.0 mL/kg		–	–
Calcium chloride 10%		Central line or large IV 0.2 mmol/kg (0.2 mL/kg) to maximum 10 mL	–	–	–
Dextrose	10%	IV bolus 10%: 5 mL/kg	–	–	–
	25%	IV bolus 25%: 2 mL/kg	–	–	–
Lignocaine (lidocaine) 2% (100 mg/5 mL)		IV or IO 1 mg/kg (0.05 mL/kg), then IV infusion 15–50 µg/kg per minute		–	2–3 mg/kg (0.1–0.15 mL/kg)
Lorazepam		IV or rectal or sublingual 0.1 mg/kg (maximum 4 mg) Give as a single dose (may be repeated once)	–	–	–

IO, intraosseous; IV, intravenous.

(6) *Heat loss*

Remember that in infants and small children, considerable heat loss may occur. Organize overhead heating, warming blankets or an incubator as appropriate, although paradoxically once CPR has been in progress, induced hypothermia may be beneficial (certainly it is in adults).

(7) *Parents in the resuscitation room*

Having parents present in the resus room has several advantages. They should be asked and encouraged to attend. A member of the resuscitation team explains the resuscitation processes with care and empathy:

(i) Parents can then witness that everything possible is being done to assist their child.

(ii) They have the opportunity to say goodbye to their child.

(iii) It reduces parental anxiety, subsequent depression, and facilitates the grieving process.

(8) *When to stop*

The senior ED physician or paediatric doctor will decide at which point further resuscitation attempts are futile. They will also be responsible for the distressing duty of telling the parents, who may have been present and watching.

(9) *Formal debrief*

The resuscitation of a child can be a highly emotional experience. It is important to set aside time to enable any concerns to be expressed and for the resuscitation team to reflect on their clinical practice in a supportive environment.

THE BREATHLESS CHILD

Disorders of the respiratory tract are common in childhood. Most respiratory illnesses are self-limiting minor infections, but a few present as potentially life-threatening emergencies. Important causes of a breathless child are:

- Asthma
- Anaphylaxis
- Bronchiolitis
- Pneumonia

ASTHMA

DIAGNOSIS

(1) This is reversible airways obstruction in children associated with infection (usually viral), allergy, atopy, exercise and emotion.

(2) It is one of the most common reasons for admission to hospital in childhood.

(3) Asthma presents wth dyspnoea, wheeze and cough. Obtain a history regarding treatments used, trigger factors, intercurrent illness and previous ICU admissions.

(4) Make a similar assessment as in adults. Include the heart rate, respiratory rate, oxygen saturation and peak flow prior to treatment (see p. 36).

(5) Look for tachycardia with a full pulse, tachypnoea with prolonged expiratory phase, nasal flaring, intercostal recession and expiratory wheeze on examination.

(6) Markers of severe asthma include any one of:
  (i) Oxygen saturation less than 92%.
  (ii) Peak expiratory flow rate 50% or less of predicted or best.
  (iii) Too breathless to talk or feed.
  (iv) Respiratory rate of 50 or more breaths/min if aged 2–5 years, or more than 30/min if over 5 years.
  (v) Tachycardia over 130 or more beats/min if aged 2–5 years, or more than 120/min if over 5 years.
  (vi) Altered level of consciousness (critical, life-threatening attack).
  (vii) Exhaustion (critical, life-threatening attack).
  (viii) Silent chest with absent wheeze on auscultation (critical, life-threatening attack).

(7) Send blood for FBC, U&Es and blood sugar levels only if the attack is severe. Hypokalaemia and hyperglycaemia are side effects of treatment.

(8) Perform a CXR only if the diagnosis is in doubt, infection is suspected, or there is sudden deterioration to exclude a pneumothorax.

MANAGEMENT

(1) Sit the child up and give oxygen, ideally with the parent in attendance to reassure the child. Attach a pulse oximeter, aiming for an oxygen saturation above 92%.

(2) Give a bronchodilator such as salbutamol:

(i) Use a metered-dose inhaler with spacer device (MDI spacer). Administer 6 puffs if less than 6 years of age and 12 puffs if older than 6 years, as a 'single dose'.

(ii) Review response after 10 minutes in mild cases.

(iii) Administer a burst of 3 doses over an hour and review in moderate to severe attacks.

(iv) The severity of the attack will determine the frequency of administration thereafter.

(3) Add ipratropium bromide (4 puffs if less than 6 years and 8 puffs if older than 6 years) to the MDI spacer every 20 minutes for the first hour of treatment in moderate to severe asthma, or if the response to salbutamol is ineffective.

(4) Give prednisolone 1–2 mg/kg orally to a maximum of 40 mg, or hydrocortisone 4 mg/kg i.v. if vomiting.

(5) Commence intravenous fluid administration if dehydration is present, but limit to 75% of maintenance requirements.

(6) Refer all severe cases to the paediatric team.

(7) Indications for ventilatory support and ICU admission:
   (i) Increasing exhaustion.
   (ii) Progressive clinical deterioration.
   (iii) Persistent hypoxaemia.
   (iv) Circulatory collapse.
   (v) Requires continuous salbutamol nebulizers for more than 1 hour.

(8) Discuss with the ICU staff administration of i.v. salbutamol, aminophylline or nebulized or i.v. magnesium.

ANAPHYLAXIS

DIAGNOSIS

(1) Anaphylaxis is an immune mediated reaction to ingested, inhaled, or topical substances such as antibiotics or nuts.

(2) Determine any history of atopy, the rapidity of symptom progression, previous reactions and prior response to medical management.

(3) Look for an urticarial rash, conjunctival injection, erythema, pallor, wheeze and cough.

(4) Symptoms and signs may rapidly progress to become potentially life-threatening, including stridor, severe wheeze, shock and altered conscious level.

MANAGEMENT

(1) Stop or remove precipitating agents such as antibiotics and contrast agents.

(2) Assess and secure the airway and give high-flow oxygen by face mask.

   (i) Call the senior ED doctor for assistance if signs of upper airway obstruction secondary to laryngeal oedema occur, for consideration of urgent endotracheal intubation.

(3) Prepare to give adrenaline (epinephrine).

   (i) Give 1 in 1000 adrenaline (epinephrine) 0.01 mg/kg (0.01 mL/kg) i.m. for significant reactions.

   (ii) Give 1 in 1000 adrenaline (epinephrine) 5 mL nebulized if the airway is obstructing, which can reduce laryngeal oedema.

   (iii) Intravenous adrenaline (epinephrine) is indicated in critical shock, when muscle blood flow is reduced. Call the senior ED doctor and begin adrenaline (epinephrine) i.v. after inserting a cannula.

      (a) put 0.15 mg/kg of 1 in 1000 adrenaline (epinephrine) (0.15 mL/kg) in 50 mL normal saline, and start at 1 mL/h equivalent to 0.05 μg/kg per minute, up to 100 mL/h in critical deterioration.

(4) Otherwise insert an i.v. cannula now and administer a fluid bolus of 10–20 mL/kg normal saline for tachycardia and hypotension.

(5) Give hydrocortisone 4 mg/kg i.v. for refractory bronchoconstriction and commence regular nebulized salbutamol 2.5 mg if under 5 years of age and 5 mg if over 5 years.

(6) Refer all these patients immediately to the paediatric team for admission, further investigations and follow-up.

BRONCHIOLITIS

DIAGNOSIS

(1) This is a viral lower respiratory tract infection, which occurs in seasonal epidemics and usually affects children under 1 year of age.

(2) The most common infecting organism is the respiratory syncytial virus. Although other viruses are implicated, a routine nasopharyngeal aspirate is *not* necessary in infants with a typical picture.

(3) It starts with fever and snuffles, but progresses rapidly to cough, irritability, fluid refusal, wheeze, chest hyperinflation and marked

tachypnoea. The illness usually peaks at day 2–3 and the wheeze and tachypnoea resolve by day 7. The cough may persist for weeks.

(4) Listen for expiratory rhonchi and fine crepitations. In severe cases, cyanosis develops with a raised respiratory rate and intercostal recession, or recurrent apnoeic episodes occur.

(5) Request a CXR. Hyperinflation, parahilar peribronchial thickening and patchy areas of atelectasis and collapse are the common abnormalities seen.

MANAGEMENT

(1) Attach a pulse oximeter and give the child oxygen if oxygen saturations are less than 90%.

(2) Treat mild cases where the child is well perfused, feeding well and has oxygen saturations above 90% expectantly, and discharge for GP review the next day.

(3) Admit moderate to severe cases with signs of lethargy, poor feeding, cyanosis, oxygen saturation less than 90%, or marked respiratory distress under the paediatric team.

   (i) Give oxygen, and commence i.v. fluids at 75% of maintenance.

   (ii) Include any infant with recurrent apnoea, pre-existing lung disease, congenital heart disease or immunodeficiency, who are at highest risk of respiratory failure.

PNEUMONIA

DIAGNOSIS

(1) Bronchopneumonia occurs in young children, or older children with chronic illness, e.g. cerebral palsy, and may be bacterial or viral. Up to 60% of pneumonias are caused by viruses.

(2) Bacterial pneumonias are more commonly associated with high fevers, localized findings on chest examination and lobar consolidation and pleural effusion on CXR.

(3) Lobar pneumonia typically presents with sudden illness, fever, breathlessness and pleuritic chest pain. Wheeze and hyperinflation are more commonly associated with asthma, bronchiolitis and croup.

(4) The presentation of pneumonia in younger children is often atypical. Consider this diagnosis in infants and children with:

   (i) Cough, fever and dyspnoea.

(ii) Abdominal pain, vomiting and diarrhoea.

(iii) Poor feeding, lethargy.

(iv) Persistent fever.

(5) Tachypnoea with nasal flaring and intercostal recession are typically associated with respiratory compromise in infants. Chest auscultation may be normal, especially in children under 12 months, or may reveal classic signs of bronchial breathing, crepitations and decreased breath sounds.

(6) Send bloods for FBC, U&Es, blood sugar and blood cultures in severe cases. Attach a pulse oximeter.

(7) Perform a CXR in all cases to confirm lung pathology such as lobar consolidation, empyema, or a pleural effusion, because clinical signs are unreliable.

MANAGEMENT

(1) Give oxygen to maintain oxygen saturations above 94%.

(2) Administer i.v. maintenance fluids to maintain hydration particularly if the child is hypotensive or has difficulty feeding secondary to dyspnoea.

(3) Administer antibiotic therapy according to local guidelines. Treatment regimens may include:

(i) Amoxycillin (amoxicillin) 40 mg/kg/day orally in three divided doses or ampicillin 50–100 mg/kg/day i.v. in four divided doses for uncomplicated community acquired pneumonia.

(ii) Cefuroxime 60 mg/kg/day i.v. in three divided doses for more severe community-acquired pneumonia.

(iii) Ceftriaxone 50 mg/kg once daily i.v. or cefotaxime 100–150 mg/kg daily i.v. in two to three doses for severe community-acquired pneumonia.

(iv) Flucloxacillin 500 mg i.v. q.d.s. if *Staphylococcus aureus* is suspected.

(v) Erythromycin 250 mg q.d.s. orally or 50 mg/kg/day i.v. in four divided doses for penicillin-allergic patients, and if *Chlamydia* or *Mycoplasma* are suspected.

(4) Admit any child for i.v. antibiotics with severe respiratory compromise, altered level of consciousness, lethargy, difficulty feeding, cyanosis, or oxygen saturation less than 90%.

STRIDOR

This is noise predominantly on inspiration originating from airway obstruction around and above the level of the larynx. There are three important causes:

- Croup (acute laryngotracheobronchitis)
- Epiglottitis
- Inhaled foreign body

CROUP (ACUTE LARYNGOTRACHEOBRONCHITIS)

DIAGNOSIS

(1) Croup is a viral infection primarily involving the larynx and subglottic area. It most commonly occurs in winter and mainly affects children aged between 1 and 3 years.

(2) It is characterized by a barking cough, harsh inspiratory stridor and hoarse voice. Symptoms often develop during the night and usually follow a mild upper respiratory tract infection.

(3) The child is febrile, irritable and tired, but lacks the drooling, dysphagia and toxic appearance of epiglottitis. Feeding and general activity is usually normal. In most cases of mild to moderate croup symptoms peak at 2–3 days and completely resolve within 1 week.

(4) Severe disease is indicated by:

(i) Harsh inspiratory *and* expiratory stridor.

(ii) Marked tachypnoea.

(iii) Sternal recession.

(iv) Accessory muscle use.

(v) Increasing agitation and restlessness.

(vi) Altered level of consciousness.

(5) Only attempt to examine the pharynx if the diagnosis is unclear and epiglottitis or bacterial tracheitis are not suspected.

(6) Croup is a clinical diagnosis and investigations are largely unhelpful.

MANAGEMENT

(1) Avoid distress, nurse in an upright position with parents present.

(2) Give nebulized 1 in 1000 adrenaline (epinephrine) 0.5 mL/kg to a maximum of 4 mL (4 mg) with oxygen in severe cases and call the senior ED doctor.

(3) Commence dexamethasone 0.15–0.3 mg/kg orally or i.m., nebulized budesonide 2 mg or prednisolone 1 mg/kg orally according to local policy.

(4) Admit for observation all patients with significant respiratory compromise, stridor at rest, patients who have required adrenaline (epinephrine) and patients presenting late at night.

EPIGLOTTITIS (SUPRAGLOTTITIS)

DIAGNOSIS

(1) This is a life-threatening infection of the supraglottic tissues usually caused by *Haemophilus influenzae* type B (HiB). It most commonly occurs in the winter months affecting children aged between 3 and 7 years, but has markedly declined with immunization.

(2) Onset of symptoms is rapid and occurs over 6–12 hours. These include:
   (i) High fever: usually the first symptom.
   (ii) Inspiratory stridor: softer than with croup.
   (iii) Severe sore throat: associated with dysphagia, inability to swallow saliva and drooling.
   (iv) Cough is usually absent and the voice is muffled.

(3) The child appears anxious and classically leans forwards with an open mouth that drools with saliva, and looks pale and extremely ill.

(4) Never place an instrument in the child's mouth to examine the pharynx.

(5) Only perform a lateral neck X-ray when the diagnosis is uncertain.

MANAGEMENT

(1) Keep the child calm and do not perform examinations or procedures that might cause undue distress to the child. Allow the child to be nursed on the parent's lap, sitting upright with an oxygen mask held near its face.

(2) Call the senior ED doctor, paediatric, anaesthetic and ENT teams to help, and warn ICU.

(3) Stay with the child until help arrives.

(4) Be prepared to attempt intubation with a small endotracheal tube and an introducer if sudden respiratory arrest occurs.
   (i) Or insert a large-bore i.v. cannula through the cricothyroid membrane if this fails, as an emergency airway (see p. 48).

INHALED FOREIGN BODY

DIAGNOSIS

(1) This is most common in toddlers aged 1–3 years, frequently involving food products and usually affects the right main bronchus.

(2) Children may present with upper airway obstruction, inspiratory stridor or with wheeze and a persistent cough following a sudden choking episode.

(3) All symptoms may disappear if the object passes into the lower airways. Later, wheeze, infection or obstructive emphysema supervene, causing localized rhonchi, crepitations and breathlessness.

(4) Request an anteroposterior and lateral CXR only in the stable child with lower respiratory tract features.

  (i) Although organic foreign bodies such as peanuts will not show, the secondary effects of compensatory hyperinflation on an expiratory film, collapse and consolidation will gradually appear.

MANAGEMENT

(1) *Complete airway obstruction*

  (i) Hold infants or small children head down and deliver up to five blows to the back between the shoulder blades, followed by up to five chest thrusts.

  (ii) Perform abdominal thrusts following back blows in an older child, but do not use in infants under 1 year.

  (iii) Attempt removal of the impacted object using a laryngoscope and a pair of long-handled forceps if the above two measures fail, and the patient is unconscious, or proceed directly to emergency cricothyroid puncture (see p. 48).

(2) *Stable airway obstruction:*
  Summon urgent anaesthetic and ENT help.

(3) *Disappearance of the symptoms of obstruction*

  (i) Consider the possibility that the foreign body has passed further into the lower airways.

  (ii) Refer the child to the paediatric team if the history is convincing, for consideration of rigid bronchoscopy even if the CXR appears normal.

ABDOMINAL PAIN, DIARRHOEA AND VOMITING

Abdominal pain may present acutely, or may become chronic and recurrent. Diarrhoea and vomiting are common problems that lead to dehydration.

ACUTE ABDOMINAL PAIN

DIAGNOSIS

(1) Abdominal pain is a common paediatric presentation with a large differential diagnosis including intra-abdominal and extra-abdominal pathologies.

(2) Accurate history taking is essential. Important points to ascertain include:

   (i) Onset, duration, radiation and nature of the pain.

   (ii) Children aged over 2 years should be able to indicate the site of their pain. In infants, pain may be inferred from spasms of crying, restlessness, drawing up of the knees and refusal to feed.

   (iii) Associated features such as vomiting, fever and rigors.

   (iv) Bowel motions: constipation, diarrhoea and the time of the last bowel motion or passage of flatus.

   (v) Significant features include pain for more than 3 hours, associated pyrexia and vomiting.

(3) Check the vital signs and perform a full general examination looking for a raised temperature, rash and upper respiratory tract infection.

   (i) Examine the abdomen for distension, palpable masses and signs of localized tenderness, guarding and rebound. Auscultate for bowel sounds and inspect the hernial orifices and genitalia.

(4) The common causes of abdominal pain may be considered in two groups:

   (i) Surgical:

      (a) appendicitis

      (b) Meckel's diverticulitis

      (c) peritonitis

      (d) intestinal obstruction: adhesions, malrotation, intussusception and mid-gut volvulus

  (e) inguinal hernia with incarceration or strangulation
  (f) testicular torsion
  (g) trauma, including child abuse.
 (ii) Medical:
  (a) mesenteric adenitis
  (b) gastroenteritis
  (c) constipation
  (d) urinary tract infection
  (e) hepatitis
  (f) Henoch–Schönlein purpura
  (g) diabetic ketoacidosis
  (h) pneumonia
  (i) tonsillitis
  (j) meningitis.
(5) Send bloods for U&Es if dehydrated, and FBC with blood cultures if septic or peritonitis is suspected.
(6) Always test the urine for glucose and, if urinary tract infection is suspected, send for microscopy and culture. White cells may be seen in the urine in peritonitis and appendicitis, as well as with a urinary tract infection.
(7) Only request erect and supine abdominal films for suspected intestinal obstruction.
(8) Request an ultrasound scan to demonstrate pyloric stenosis, intussusception and renal pathology.

MANAGEMENT
(1) Suspected surgical abdomen:
  (i) Establish i.v. access and administer a bolus of 20 mL/kg of normal saline i.v. for any hypotension and shock. Give morphine 0.1 mg/kg for severe pain.
  (ii) Place a nasogastric tube if bowel obstruction is present.
  (iii) Keep the patient fasted and refer for surgical review.
(2) Treat medical conditions accordingly.
(3) Arrange review within 24 hours for a well child allowed home.

DIARRHOEA, VOMITING AND DEHYDRATION

DIAGNOSIS
(1) Diarrhoea and vomiting are common problems that require investigation and treatment. Dehydration is a serious end result.

(2) Causes of diarrhoea include:
  (i) Gastroenteritis:
    (a) viral: most common cause, including rotavirus and adenovirus
    (b) bacterial: e.g. *Escherichia coli*, Salmonella or Campylobacter
    (c) protozoal: e.g. *Giardia lamblia*.
  (ii) Infection: septicaemia, urinary tract infection, pneumonia, tonsillitis, otitis media.
  (iii) Surgical conditions: appendicitis, intussusception and partial bowel obstruction.
  (iv) Drugs: particularly antibiotics such as ampicillin.
  (v) Chronic relapsing conditions such as ulcerative colitis, Crohn's disease.
(3) Vomiting is a common condition associated with a large number of causes:
  (i) Causes in the newborn:
    (a) infection: meningitis and urinary tract infection
    (b) intestinal obstruction from duodenal atresia, Hirschsprung's disease or meconium plug
    (c) cerebral haemorrhage or oedema
    (d) metabolic: galactosaemia and congenital adrenal hyperplasia.
  (ii) Causes in infants (up to 1 year):
    (a) pyloric stenosis, typically in males aged 3–8 weeks
    (b) infection: gastroenteritis, tonsillitis, otitis media, meningitis and urinary tract infection
    (c) intestinal obstruction from intussusception, or an obstructed hernia, etc.
    (d) gastro-oesophageal reflux and hiatus hernia
    (e) feeding problems secondary to overfeeding or excessive wind
    (f) poisoning.
  (iii) Causes after infancy:
    (a) infection: gastroenteritis, tonsillitis, otitis media, meningitis and urinary tract infection
    (b) intestinal obstruction or appendicitis
    (c) metabolic, such as ketoacidosis or uraemia
    (d) raised intracranial pressure or migraine
    (e) poisoning.
(4) Take a careful history because not all vomiting and diarrhoea in children is secondary to gastroenteritis. Examine to see if the child

has evidence of another cause and to determine the extent of dehydration. Features suggestive of an alternative diagnosis to 'viral gastroenteritis' include:

(i) Bloody diarrhoea.

(ii) Vomiting bile, blood or faecal material.

(iii) Systemic toxicity out of proportion to the degree of dehydration.

(iv) Severe abdominal pain with significant tenderness, distension or a palpable mass.

(5) *Assessment of dehydration*

Regardless of the suspected cause, assess and treat dehydration in its own right. Determine the degree of dehydration by clinical assessment and estimated percentage change in body weight.

(i) Mild dehydration (up to 5% body weight lost): there are no clinical signs and the child is in good general condition, but with increased thirst and mild oliguria.

(ii) Moderate dehydration (6–10% body weight lost): the child looks ill, is apathetic with sunken eyes and fontanel, has a dry mouth, decreased skin tissue turgor, tachycardia, marked thirst and oliguria.

(iii) Severe dehydration (10% or more body weight lost): the child is drowsy, cool, cyanosed, tachypnoeic, tachycardic, hypotensive and may become comatose. There is a risk of sudden death.

> **Warning:** beware not to miss the diagnosis of dehydration in an overweight baby presenting with tachycardia alone.

(6) Send blood for FBC, U&Es, blood sugar and arterial blood gases on patients with moderate to severe dehydration. Most children who can be orally rehydrated do not require blood tests.

(7) Send urine for microscopy culture and sensitivity if significantly dehydrated, febrile or in pre-school children with unexplained vomiting.

(8) Collect faecal samples only if the child has significant abdominal pain, persistent bloody diarrhoea or a history of recent overseas travel.

(9) Order CXR and AXR if there is clinical evidence of respiratory tract infection or intestinal obstruction.

MANAGEMENT

(1) The aims of management are to:
  (i) Restore and maintain fluid and electrolyte balance.
  (ii) Restore nutrition.
  (iii) Replace ongoing losses (diarrhoea and vomiting).

(2) Calculate the replacement fluids needed over the next 24 hours by adding together maintenance fluid requirements, estimated volume deficit and ongoing losses (see Table 10.5).

(3) *Maintenance fluid requirements* are:
  (i) 100 mL/kg per 24 hours for the first 10 kg of body weight (4 mL/kg per hour).
  (ii) 50 mL/kg per 24 hours for the next 10 kg of body weight (2 mL/kg per hour).
  (iii) 20 mL/kg per 24 hours for each remaining kg of body weight (1 mL/kg per hour).
  For example a 24-kg child has daily fluid maintenance requirements of:
  $(100 \text{ mL} \times 10) + (50 \text{ mL} \times 10) + (20 \text{ mL} \times 4) = 1580$ mL per 24 hours.

Table 10.5 Paediatric fluid and electrolyte requirements

Body weight	Fluid maintenance	
	mL/kg per hour	mL/kg per day
First 10 kg	4	100
Second 10 kg	2	50
Each subsequent kg	1	20
Potassium: maintenance	3 mmol/kg per 24 hours	
Fluid resuscitation: bolus	20 mL/kg crystalloid	
Deficit volume: estimation in dehydration (mL)	% body weight dehydration × weight (kg) × 10	
Burns: additional fluid requirement (mL per day)	% BSA burn × weight (kg) × 4	
Urine output: intended	Infants (< 2 years): 2 mL/kg per hour Children (> 2 years): 1 mL/kg per hour	

BSA, body surface area.

(4) *Estimation of volume deficit* in dehydration: base this on the estimated percentage dehydration (see earlier p. 362) multiplied by the body weight all multiplied by 10, that is:

percentage dehydration × body weight (kg) × 10 in mL.

   (i) For example, a 24-kg child thought to be 5% dehydrated has a fluid deficit of 5 × 24 × 10 = 1200 mL.

   (ii) Replace fluids over 24 hours if less than 5% dehydrated.

   (iii) Give half the fluids over the first 8 hours and the remaining half over the subsequent 16 hours if more than 5% dehydrated and the sodium is normal.

   (iv) Once the circulating volume has been corrected in the case of a shocked child, dehydration is then assumed to be a maximum of 10%, giving a maximum rehydration volume of 100 mL/kg.

(4) *Treatment of moderate or severe dehydration*

   (i) Give the shocked child immediate fluid resuscitation with 20 mL/kg normal saline boluses until the circulation is restored.

   (ii) Aim to replace the fluid deficit and maintenance requirements over 24 hours with half-normal 0.45% saline in 2.5% dextrose, if the sodium level is between 130 and 150 mmol/L and the circulation is restored.

   (iii) Replace fluid and electrolytes more slowly over 2–3 days if the sodium is less than 130 mmol/L or greater than 150 mmol/L. Refer the patient immediately to the paediatric admitting team.

   (iv) Give oral replacement therapy via a nasogastric tube if the child is not shocked, but has moderate dehydration. Replace the fluid deficit over the first 6 hours and daily maintenance fluids over the following 18 hours.

(5) *Treatment of mild dehydration*

Oral rehydration:

   (i) Continue milk and solid food during the diarrhoeal illness unless there is documented lactose intolerance. Continue breastfeeding, and supplement with extra water or glucose-electrolyte solution between feeds.

   (ii) Oral glucose-electrolyte solutions:

      (a) give 1–1.5 times the volume of their usual feed in infants

      (b) give 200 mL of solution after each loose motion in older children, or enough to quench the thirst, given in frequent small amounts

(c) aim to replace the normal maintenance fluid requirement plus deficit volume over 24 hours.

(iii) Discharge the child if they are tolerating oral fluids, have no clinical signs of dehydration, only occasional vomiting and a satisfactory social situation.

(a) give the parents a letter for the GP, and instruct them to return if the child's condition deteriorates.

THE FEBRILE CHILD

Fever is the most common 'emergency' presentation in childhood. The normal oral temperature is 37°C, and the normal rectal temperature is 37.5°C. A fever is defined as a rectal temperature above 38°C.

DIAGNOSIS

(1) A careful history and examination will identify the source of infection in the majority of cases. Look for the following common causes of fever in a child:

(i) Respiratory: upper and lower respiratory tract infection.

(ii) Abdominal: gastroenteritis, appendicitis, urinary tract infection.

(iii) ENT: otitis media, tonsillitis.

(iv) Exanthematous skin rash (see Table 1.6 on p. 96).

(2) No obvious focus of infection is found following preliminary history and examination in a small number of children presenting with fever; e.g. a '*fever without focus*'. Most will have a viral infection, but the potential for significant bacterial infection must be evaluated.

(3) The risk of significant bacterial infection in fever without focus is proportional to temperature and inversely proportional to age, with those most at risk aged less than 3 years. Common bacterial infections without localizing signs can include:

(i) Meningitis and septicaemia.

(ii) Bone and joint infections.

(iii) Urinary tract infection.

(iv) Pneumonia.

(v) Occult bacteraemia (usually non-toxic and appear well).

(4) Examine the child for signs of serious systemic compromise; i.e. that are potentially 'toxic':

    (i) Poor arousal, reduced activity and lethargy.

    (ii) Respiratory distress: nasal flaring, grunting respirations and tachypnoea.

    (iii) Circulatory impairment: poor peripheral perfusion, hypotension and tachycardia.

    (iv) Signs of dehydration, reduced oral intake and reduced urine output.

    (v) Sinister signs such as apnoea, cyanosis and convulsions.

(5) Send blood for FBC, blood sugar, U&Es and blood culture if clearly unwell.

(6) Collect a bag specimen urine sample, and if positive for leucocytes and/or nitrites, obtain a clean catch or catheter specimen of urine to send for urgent microscopy, culture and sensitivity, or perform a suprapubic aspirate.

(7) Request CXR in patients with respiratory distress, bradypnoea, abnormal breath sounds or oxygen saturations less than 95%.

(8) Indications to perform a lumbar puncture are based on clinical grounds and as part of the full sepsis workup of toxic infants less than 3 months of age. Only perform a lumbar puncture after consulting with the senior ED doctor.

MANAGEMENT

(1) Treat the toxic, unwell child symptomatically with oxygen via a face mask, an i.v. fluid bolus 10–20 mL/kg for hypotension and paracetamol 15 mg/kg orally or p.r. for pain or distress.

(2) *The febrile child with no focus of infection*

    (i) Admit the following who may need empiric antibiotics:

        (a) all febrile neonates less than 28 days old

        (b) all systemically unwell children less than 36 months old with no discernable focus of infection

        (c) infants and young children with any non-blanching rash, signs of meningism or irritability.

    (ii) Infants and young children displaying no overt toxic signs or symptoms:

        (a) most infants and small children under 36 months of age who appear well, have no systemic toxic findings and have normal lab results have a viral illness. Discharge these patients with appropriate advice and review after 24 hours in the Emergency Department

(b) up to 10% of these patients will turn out to have an *occult* bacteraemia, that is they return positive blood cultures, but negative urine and CSF culture:

– most patients with *Streptococcus pneumoniae* remain non-toxic and afebrile and will clear the organism themselves and require no further treatment. Advise parents to return if fever recurs within the first 7 days

– patients with *Neisseria meningitidis* on blood culture require admission and i.v. antibiotics.

(3) *The febrile child with a focus of infection*

(i) Manage children with an identified focus of infection according to the individual condition, its severity and the presence of systemic toxic signs.

(ii) Admit under the paediatric team if the child looks unwell, for management of the specific condition.

(iii) Discharge home if the child looks well with no toxic signs. Give symptomatic treatment and antibiotic therapy as indicated clinically.

(a) advise regular fluid intake 'little but often'

(b) give paracetamol 15 mg/kg orally 4–6-hourly and/or ibuprofen 10 mg/kg orally 8-hourly

(c) review within 24–48 hours in the Emergency Department or by the GP.

SEIZURES AND FEBRILE CONVULSIONS

SEIZURES

Seizures must be distinguished from other causes of brief loss of consciousness, such as syncope, pallid breath-holding, and cyanotic breath-holding.

DIAGNOSIS

The likely cause of a seizure may be related to the age of the child.

(1) *Newborn*

Seizures tend to be mere twitching of a limb, fluttering of an eyelid or conjugate eye deviation. Causes include:

(i) Hypoglycaemia.

(ii) Hypocalcaemia.

(iii) Hypoxia, especially from birth injury.

(iv) Cerebral haemorrhage and subdural haematoma.

(v) Infection.

(vi) Drug withdrawal.

(2) *Pre-school child*

The commonest cause is a febrile convulsion.

Other possibilities include:

(i) Idiopathic epilepsy.

(ii) Meningitis or encephalitis.

(iii) Head injury, including injury from child abuse.

(iv) Dehydration from gastroenteritis, etc.

(v) Hypoglycaemia.

(vi) Poisoning.

(vii) Sudden reduction in epilepsy medication.

(3) *Older child*

Causes include:

(i) Idiopathic epilepsy.

(ii) Sudden reduction in epilepsy medication.

(iii) Head injury.

(iv) Meningitis or encephalitis.

(v) Hypoglycaemia.

(vi) Poisoning, including theophylline, iron and tricyclic antidepressants.

MANAGEMENT

(1) Clear the airway, place the child on their side, and give oxygen via a face mask. Attach ECG monitoring and a pulse oximeter.

(2) Check for hypoglycaemia using a blood-glucose test strip. Give 10% dextrose 5 mL/kg i.v. if the reading is low, and send blood for formal laboratory evaluation.

(3) If the child has a further seizure or the seizure continues for up to 5 minutes:

(i) Gain i.v. access and give lorazepam 0.1 mg/kg i.v. or diazepam 0.1–0.2 mg/kg i.v. at 1 mg/min up to a maximum of 0.5 mg/kg. Monitor carefully for respiratory depression and record oxygen saturations every 2–5 minutes.

(ii) Give additional agents if seizures recur. Respiratory support may be needed and cardiac monitoring is essential:

(a) phenytoin 15–18 mg/kg i.v. at no faster than 1 mg/kg per minute, provided the child is not on oral phenytoin.

Or:

(b) phenobarbitone (phenobarbital) 15–20 mg/kg i.v. over 20 minutes if already on oral phenytoin.

(iii) Give rectal diazepam 0.5 mg/kg; or midazolam 0.5 mg/kg by the buccal route if i.v. access is impossible.

(iv) An alternative if venous access is still unavailable is paraldehyde: give 0.4 mL/kg rectally diluted 1 to 1 with olive oil or normal saline.

(4) Refer all children with a seizure to the Paediatric team for further investigation. Admit children who have not fully recovered from the seizure or have focal neurological signs.

(5) Advise parents that children allowed home should be supervised when bathing, swimming, riding a bike and climbing trees until fully assessed and stabilized as an outpatient.

FEBRILE CONVULSIONS

DIAGNOSIS

(1) These are common and occur in 2–5% of healthy pre-school children. They are benign with minimal morbidity and usually associated with a viral infection.

(2) Features that are consistent with the diagnosis of a febrile convulsion are:

(i) Age between 6 months and 6 years.

(ii) Brief generalized convulsion, less than 10 minutes in duration.

(iii) Febrile child (temperature over 38°C) with a prodromal illness.

(iv) No focal neurological deficit or residual weakness such as a Todd's palsy.

(v) No signs of meningitis or encephalitis.

(3) Do *not* label the episode a febrile convulsion when there are features different from those above.

(4) Following a 'simple' febrile convulsion the child will appear well. Focus the examination on looking for the source of the fever, including in the throat, ears, chest, abdomen, urine, skin, etc.

(5) Request a CXR, FBC and urinalysis, and consider a lumbar puncture if no focus of infection is identified, particularly if under 3 years.

MANAGEMENT

(1) Manage the convulsion:
  (i) Most convulsions are brief and do not require any specific treatment.
  (ii) Position the child on their side, ensure a patent airway and use oropharyngeal suction if required.
  (iii) Apply oxygen via face mask if the child is cyanosed.
  (iv) Manage as for generalized seizures if the seizure lasts longer than 5 minutes or is associated with focal neurology (see p. 367).
(2) Treat the fever:
  (i) Undress the child and reduce clothing to a minimum.
  (ii) Administer an antipyretic analgesic such as paracetamol 15 mg/kg orally or as a suppository, or ibuprofen 10 mg/kg.
  (iii) Treat appropriately if a focus is identified.
  (iv) Investigate and treat as for 'fever without focus' if no focus is identified (see p. 365).
(3) Consider other diagnoses if the child remains unwell or has an incomplete recovery, residual focal neurology, or prolonged or multiple seizures.
(4) Advise parents that:
  (i) A repeat febrile convulsion will occur in 10–15% of children during the same illness.
  (ii) The risk of developing further febrile convulsions during childhood is greater with younger children: in a 1-year-old 50%; in a 2-year-old 30%.
  (iii) Anticonvulsant treatment is not required.
  (iv) The potential for developing epilepsy is the same as in the general population (1%), unless risk factors are present such as a family history of epilepsy, atypical or prolonged febrile convulsion, or neurodevelopmental problems.

ACUTE POISONING

Most cases of acute poisoning in children are accidental, although rarely deliberate poisoning may occur as a form of child abuse, and adolescents may attempt suicide.

DIAGNOSIS

(1) Four categories of substances may be taken:
    (i) Proprietary tablets and syrups, often prescribed for the parents.
    (ii) Alcohol, solvents and other illicit substances.
    (iii) Household and garden chemicals.
    (iv) Leaves, berries, seeds and fungi.
(2) It is important to ascertain what was taken, how much and when. If possible, the container the poison was in, or an example of the flora ingested, should be brought with the child.
(3) Record baseline observations of temperature, pulse, blood pressure, respiratory rate, level of consciousness, and a blood glucose test stick for hypoglycaemia, particularly in alcohol and salicylate poisoning.
(4) Send blood for U&Es, blood sugar and a drug screen, which may include a paracetamol, iron, salicylate, theophylline or alcohol level as indicated clinically.

MANAGEMENT

(1) Clear the airway and give oxygen. Use a bag and mask if the gag reflex is absent, with an oropharyngeal airway, and call an airway-skilled doctor urgently to intubate the child.
(2) Give 10% dextrose 5 mL/kg i.v. if the blood sugar level is low.
(3) Give naloxone 10–40 µg/kg i.v., or i.m. if venous access is impossible, when there are pinpoint pupils and respiratory depression.
(4) Start an i.v. infusion of normal saline and give 10–20 mL/kg for hypotension.
(5) Give activated charcoal 1–2 g/kg to reduce the absorption of toxin.
    (i) Charcoal is unpalatable and difficult to administer in children, but may be given mixed with ice cream or via a nasogastric tube.
    (ii) It is of most benefit within 1–2 hours of ingestion, and is not effective against certain substances (see p. 150).
(6) Ipecacuanha should no longer be used in acute poisonings and gastric lavage is now rare, unless the child presents within 1 hour of ingesting a highly lethal drug, and/or is unconscious and has the airway protected.
(7) Advice and help is available from the various Poisons Information Centres and from local botanical departments for plant identification.
    (i) Specialist consultants are available for telephone advice in more complex clinical cases. A 24-hour number **0870 600 6266** will direct callers in the UK to the relevant local centre.

(ii) Obtain advice regarding toxic ingestions in Australia 24 hours a day from the Poisons Information Centres on **13 11 26**, and in New Zealand on **03 479 7248** (or **0800 764 766** within New Zealand only).

(8) Refer patients to the paediatric team for admission and observation if:
  (i) Symptomatic following significant ingestion.
  (ii) Presenting late at night and require overnight observation.
  (iii) Deliberate self-harm is suspected, for psychiatric assessment.

(9) Specific poisonings and their treatments are described on pp. 152–175 in the chapter on acute poisoning in adults.

THE LIMPING CHILD

DIFFERENTIAL DIAGNOSIS

(1) This diagnostic dilemma presents frequently to the Emergency Department. The causes of limp range from serious conditions such as bone tumours and septic arthritis to minor complaints including painful shoes or a plantar wart.

(2) Remember to consider the spine, pelvis, hip and lower limb as a potential source of pain or disability.

(3) Ask about the onset of symptoms, any history of trauma, localized pain and associated systemic symptoms such as fever or rigors.

(4) Check the vital signs, evaluate gait and perform a lower extremity neurological examination as the pain allows. Examine the full range of movement of all lower limb joints bilaterally.
  (i) Remember hip pain is often poorly localized and is commonly referred to the knee and vice versa, so always examine both.

(5) Typical causes specific to age are:
  (i) *Age 1–3 years*
      (a) infection: septic arthritis and osteomyelitis
      (b) congenital dysplasia or dislocation of the hip
      (c) trauma: Toddler's fracture, stress fracture, puncture wounds
      (d) transient synovitis 'irritable hip'
      (e) cerebral palsy, neuromuscular disease, tumours and congenital hypotonia.
  (ii) *Age 4–10 years*
      (a) trauma: fractures, dislocations and ligamentous injuries
      (b) Perthes' disease

(c) infection: septic arthritis and osteomyelitis

(d) rheumatoid disease and Still's disease

(e) leukaemia.

(iii) *Age 11–15 years*

(a) slipped capital femoral epiphysis

(b) trauma: overuse syndromes

(c) arthritis, including Still's disease, juvenile rheumatoid arthritis and ankylosing spondylitis

(d) infection: sexually transmitted disease (arthralgia and arthritis)

(e) neoplasia.

(6) Send blood for FBC, blood culture, ESR and CRP if infection is considered possible.

(7) Request plain X-rays of the affected limb.

(8) Arrange an ultrasound scan to demonstrate any hip effusion if the X-rays are normal and pain is localized to the hip region.

MANAGEMENT

(1) Examine and treat the patient on a trolley with the parents present to alleviate anxiety. Administer oral pain relief, and immobilize fractures and acute traumatic limb injuries with a splint.

(2) Disposition and further management is dependent on the underlying problem.

(3) Patients with constitutional symptoms, fever, leucocytosis and elevated ESR and CRP require joint aspiration under anaesthesia to exclude a septic arthritis.

(i) Refer these and traumatic fractures, slipped capital epiphysis, Perthes' disease and congenital dislocation or dysplasia of the hip to the orthopaedic team.

COT DEATH AND SUDDEN INFANT DEATH SYNDROME (SIDS)

DIAGNOSIS

(1) Cot death is the term used to describe the sudden and unexpected death of a baby, before an investigation has been carried out.

(2) The diagnosis of SIDS is attributed to those cot deaths where no specific cause of death is found even after a post-mortem examination.

(3) The cause of the syndrome is unknown, but is thought to be associated with respiratory failure. It accounts for 50% of cot deaths.

(4) It is more common during winter, with a peak age of 3 months. Higher rates are seen with bottle-fed males, parental smoking, and prone sleeping position.

MANAGEMENT

(1) Always continue in the resuscitation room if the child is brought in by ambulance with resuscitation in progress. Call the senior ED doctor and Paediatric team urgently (see *Cardiopulmonary Resuscitation* on p. 343).

(2) Examine the child carefully for any signs of trauma or infection, including evidence of asphyxia or petechiae. Check the temperature.

(3) Discuss the necessity for post-mortem blood tests for infection or a drug screen with the senior doctor. In addition, keep all clothes in a labelled hospital bag.

(4) Check that the parents have full access to the resuscitation area, and encourage them to attend the resus room if they wish. Provide a senior Emergency Department staff member to be with them at all times.

(5) The senior doctor should then speak in private to the parents, and encourage them to talk about the circumstances of the death and any recent illnesses in the child.

(6) Encourage the parents to see and hold their child in privacy afterwards. They may derive benefit from the presence of the hospital chaplain and social worker, and may like a photograph or a lock of the child's hair.

(7) Tell the parents that because the death is sudden, the coroner (or procurator fiscal in Scotland) will be informed, and a post mortem may be required.

(8) The coroner's officer or the police will then visit the parents later that day, and will take further details, possibly even removing the bedding for examination.

(9) Write down and give the parents the details and phone number of the local SIDS help group (in the UK the Foundation for the Study of Infant Deaths is http://www.sids.org.uk/and in Australia

the SIDS and Kids site is http://www.sidsandkids.org/home.html/).

(10) Make certain you also inform the following by telephone:

 (i) GP, to arrange for a home visit and to make sure all future clinic attendances for the deceased child are cancelled.

 (ii) Health visitor.

 (iii) Social Work department.

 (iv) Paediatric team, if they were not present at the resuscitation.

 (v) Community Child Health Service, to cancel immunization appointments, etc.

CHILD ABUSE (NON-ACCIDENTAL INJURY)

DIAGNOSIS

(1) Child abuse occurs when the adult responsible for the care of a child either harms the child, or fails to protect them from harm. It can manifest in different ways:

 (i) Physical abuse including striking, shaking and burning.

 (ii) Emotional abuse often associated with delayed emotional development.

 (iii) Sexual abuse.

 (iv) Neglect including failure to provide shelter, clothing and nourishment.

(2) Maintain a high index of suspicion in the following cases, especially if the child is less than 4 years old:

 (i) *History*

  (a) delay between the alleged injury and the presentation to the Emergency Department

  (b) inconsistency between the story and the actual injuries

  (c) abnormal parental behaviour, poor interaction with the child, and apparent lack of parental concern

  (d) frequent attendance in the Emergency Department by the child or a sibling, often for little apparent reason

  (e) previous injuries on different dates

  (f) failure to thrive, or clinical signs of neglect.

 (ii) *Examination*

  (a) examine the child with the consent of at least one parent or the child's legal guardian. Undress the child fully in stages, and carefully document all the findings

(b) measure bruises, scratches, burns and other skin marks with a ruler. Arrange clinical photographs detailed in the medical notes to provide contemporaneous evidence. Look specifically for:

- torn upper-lip frenulum, or palatal haemorrhage from a feeding bottle or even a fist thrust into the mouth to prevent the baby crying, or from a direct blow
- human bite marks, and bruising from a fist or slapping, which may rupture the tympanic membrane
- deep cigarette burns, or scalds limited to the buttocks and genitalia or both feet, suggesting immersion in hot water
- a fractured skull or long bone, particularly in a child not yet able to walk. A spiral fracture of a long bone is most suspicious, as are other healing fractures of differing ages on skeletal survey
- subconjunctival, vitreous or retinal haemorrhage, suggesting violent shaking, or from a direct blow
- signs of trauma to the genitalia or anus, perianal warts or other sexually transmitted diseases.

MANAGEMENT

(1) Inform the senior ED doctor and Paediatric team immediately if you have any suspicion of child abuse, and arrange for admission of the child.

(2) Check whether the child is on the Child Protection Register already and involve the ED social worker early.

(3) Do not confront the parents at this stage. Explain that you want a further opinion from a senior Paediatric doctor, which necessitates admitting the child.

(4) Make sure to accurately document in the medical notes the history, physical examination findings, timing and nature of consultations, and suspicions of child abuse.

(5) Contact the Social Work department and follow local procedural policy with respect to the timing and involvement of additional agencies such as the police and Social Services, if the parent refuses admission.

(6) Enlist the help of additional support groups such as the National Society for Prevention of Cruelty to Children (NSPCC) in the UK or the National Association for Prevention of Child Abuse and

Neglect (NAPCAN) in Australia, if further advice or help is requested.

> ✓ **Tip:** similar presentations are seen in osteogenesis imperfecta with multiple fractures, and idiopathic thrombocytopaenic purpura and leukaemia with widespread bruising and bleeding. However, these are rare compared with the genuine cases of child abuse.

FURTHER READING

Advanced Life Support Group (2005) *Advanced Paediatric Life Support,* 4th edn. Blackwell, Oxford.

American Heart Association (2005) Guidelines for cardiopulmonary resuscitation and emergency cardiovascular care. Part 11: Pediatric basic life support. *Circulation* **112**:IV-156–66.

American Heart Association (2005) Guidelines for cardiopulmonary resuscitation and emergency cardiovascular care. Part 12: Pediatric advanced life support. *Circulation* **112**:IV-167–87.

American Heart Association. http://www.circulationaha.org/ (CPR and ECC guidelines 2005).

Australian Resuscitation Council. http://www.resus.org.au/ (resuscitation guidelines 2006).

European Resuscitation Council (2005) Guidelines for resuscitation. Section 6: Paediatric life support. *Resuscitation* **67** (**Suppl 1**):S97–133.

European Resuscitation Council. http://www.erc.edu/ (ERC guidelines and resuscitation practice 2005).

Foundation for the Study of Infant Deaths. http://www.sids.org.uk/

Resuscitation Council UK. http://www.resus.org.uk/ (Resuscitation guidelines 2005).

Stillbirth and Neonatal Death Society. http://www.uk-sands.org/

OBSTETRIC AND GYNAECOLOGICAL EMERGENCIES

GYNAECOLOGICAL ASSESSMENT AND MANAGEMENT

All gynaecological emergencies that present with abdominal pain or vaginal bleeding require a thorough history and examination. Be delicate and empathic when taking the history of the presenting complaint and discussing the patient's sexual history.

Pay particular attention to the menstrual history, site of pain, presence of vaginal discharge, and urinary symptoms. Ascertain the patient's contraceptive history, her potential for being pregnant, and her gravida and parity. Also consider possible non-gynaecological conditions.

Perform a thorough examination including an abdominal examination, and vaginal examination with speculum and bimanual palpation. Allow the patient privacy to undress and *always* have a chaperone in attendance.

Send urgent blood samples to the laboratory, perform a urine or serum beta-HCG pregnancy test, and institute resuscitative procedures as necessary.

PRESCRIBING IN PREGNANCY

Consult the prescribing information first before giving any drug to a pregnant patient, or breastfeeding mother. Look in the local drug formularies such as the Appendix at the back of the *British National Formulary* (BNF) or in *MIMS*.

Ideally, avoid all drugs in the first trimester of pregnancy unless absolutely necessary. Therefore, always enquire about the possibility of pregnancy in every female of reproductive age.

This is also important when requesting X-rays. Most hospital Radiology Departments have their own guidelines to minimize the risk of irradiation in early pregnancy.

GYNAECOLOGICAL CAUSES OF ACUTE ABDOMINAL PAIN

The following conditions present with acute abdominal pain in females:
- Ruptured ectopic pregnancy
- Pelvic inflammatory disease (acute salpingitis)

- Ruptured ovarian cyst
- Torsion of an ovarian tumour
- Endometriosis

RUPTURED ECTOPIC PREGNANCY

DIAGNOSIS

(1) Ectopic pregnancy is more common in patients with a previous ectopic pregnancy, pelvic inflammatory disease, previous tubal surgery, IVF treatment, and in patients using an intrauterine contraceptive device (IUCD).

(i) However 50% occur with no predisposing risk factors.

(2) Ectopic pregnancy usually presents from the 5th to the 9th weeks of pregnancy. Patients may not realize they are pregnant, although they may give a history of breast tenderness, nausea, or recent unprotected intercourse.

(i) Consider an ectopic in every female patient with menstrual irregularities, vaginal bleeding, lower abdominal pain or collapse.

(3) The predominant feature on history is lower abdominal pain, which is present in over 90% of presentations. Vaginal bleeding is usually mild.

(4) Haemodynamically unstable patient:

(i) Unstable patients present with sudden abdominal pain, often referred to the shoulder tip, followed by scanty vaginal bleeding, proceeding to circulatory collapse and haemorrhagic shock.

(ii) On examination the patient is pale, collapsed and hypotensive with a tender, rigid silent abdomen.

(5) Haemodynamically stable patient:

(i) Stable patients present with a recent history of a missed period or sometimes erratic period, lower abdominal pain and slight vaginal bleeding that is typically dark brown ('prune juice'), although the bleeding can be fresh red.

(ii) There is localized lower abdominal tenderness and guarding to one side, with discomfort and swelling in that lateral fornix on vaginal examination, and a smaller uterus than expected for the duration of apparent amenorrhoea.

(6) Be gentle on pelvic examination to avoid the potential for traumatic tubal rupture.

(7) Insert one or two large-bore i.v. cannulae and send blood for FBC, U&Es, blood sugar and G&S. Note the rhesus status.

(8) Perform a pregnancy test.

    (i) A serum radioimmunoassay pregnancy test for beta-HCG in blood is highly sensitive, with a negative test ruling out a recent ectopic or miscarriage, although it takes time to do and may not be available after hours.

    (ii) Alternatively, test for urinary beta-HCG. This urine dipstick test can be done rapidly in the Emergency Department, and may be positive even before the first missed period. Again, a negative test virtually rules out an ectopic.

(9) Ultrasound scan:

    (i) Request a transabdominal (TA) ultrasound scan to demonstrate a gestational sac within the uterus, which effectively excludes an ectopic pregnancy.

        (a) the only exception to this rule is the rare heterotopic pregnancy, with an intrauterine *plus* an ectopic pregnancy, that occurs particularly in women undergoing assisted reproductive technology treatment such as IVF.

    (ii) Transvaginal (TV) ultrasound scan is more sensitive, and should show a gestational sac if the beta-HCG is greater than 1000 IU or the pregnancy is estimated at greater than 5 weeks. It should be able to identify most signs of the extrauterine pregnancy itself.

    (iii) Thus, ultrasound features suggesting an ectopic pregnancy include an empty uterus, intrauterine pseudosac, a tubal ring, adnexal mass and fluid in the pouch of Douglas.

> **Tip:** a patient presenting with a positive pregnancy test, abdominal pain, scanty vaginal bleeding and absence of intrauterine pregnancy on ultrasound scan has an ectopic pregnancy until proven otherwise.

MANAGEMENT

(1) Haemodynamically unstable ectopic pregnancy:

    (i) Give high-flow oxygen by face mask and organize urgent cross-match of 4 units of blood.

    (ii) Commence an infusion of crystalloid such as normal saline or Hartmann's, and refer the patient immediately to the gynaecology team. Inform theatre and the duty anaesthetist.

(2) Haemodynamically stable ectopic pregnancy:
   (i) Stratify these patients on the basis of the ultrasound and beta-HCG findings.
      (a) admit patients with a positive pregnancy test, empty uterus on TV ultrasound examination and clinical signs of an ectopic for a laparoscopy
      (b) follow patients with a positive pregnancy test, an empty uterus but no ultrasound signs of an ectopic with serial beta-HCG examinations every 48 hours.
   (ii) Therefore refer all cases to the Gynaecology team. Ultimately, a laparoscopy or laparotomy confirms the condition and allows definitive management.
(3) Give all rhesus-negative mothers anti-D immunoglobulin 250 units i.m. to prevent maternal formation of antibodies from isoimmunization.

PELVIC INFLAMMATORY DISEASE (ACUTE SALPINGITIS)

DIAGNOSIS
(1) Pelvic inflammatory disease (PID) includes any combination of endometritis, salpingitis, tubo-ovarian abscess, or pelvic peritonitis. It is usually a sexually transmitted disease caused principally by chlamydial or gonococcal infection.
   (i) It may also follow instrumentation of the cervix, or recent insertion of an IUCD.
   (ii) Recurrent infections are increasingly likely to cause infertility, and an increased risk of ectopic pregnancy.
(2) It presents acutely with fever, malaise, bilateral lower abdominal pain, dyspareunia, menstrual irregularities and vaginal discharge.
(3) On examination there is an elevated temperature with bilateral lower abdominal tenderness and guarding. Vaginal examination reveals a cervical discharge, adnexal tenderness and cervical excitation (pain on moving the cervix).
(4) Send an endocervical and urethral swab for gonococcal culture, and an endocervical swab for *Chlamydia* antigen, nucleic acid amplification by polymerase chain reaction (PCR) or culture.
(5) Send blood for FBC and blood culture. Perform a pregnancy test.
(6) Send an MSU for microscopy, culture and chlamydial PCR.

> **!** **Warning:** PID is a notoriously difficult diagnosis to make, being regularly missed or conversely diagnosed when not present. Seventy per cent of patients with pyrexia, abdominal tenderness, adnexal tenderness, cervical excitation, raised white cell count and negative pregnancy test will have salpingitis.

MANAGEMENT

(1) Remove an IUCD if present and send it for culture.

(2) Admit all patients who are systemically unwell, pregnant (unusual), intolerant to oral medication, have a confirmed tubo-ovarian abscess, or in whom the diagnosis is uncertain. Start parenteral antibiotics according to local guidelines.

(3) Discharge the patient if clinically well with a 14-day course of ofloxacin 400 mg b.d. orally *plus* metronidazole 400 mg b.d. orally; or give azithromycin 1 g orally with ceftriaxone 250 mg i.m. and then doxycycline 100 mg b.d. orally and metronidazole 400 mg b.d. orally for 14 days.

    (i) Arrange follow-up in Gynaecology outpatients, or a Genitourinary Medicine clinic to facilitate contact screening and treatment.

    (ii) Contact tracing of chlamydial- or gonococcal-positive patients is vital to prevent new and recurrent cases. Advise patients to abstain from sexual intercourse until the partner has been tested and treated.

RUPTURED OVARIAN CYST

DIAGNOSIS AND MANAGEMENT

(1) There is sudden, moderate, lower abdominal and pelvic pain without gastrointestinal symptoms.

(2) The patient is afebrile with localized tenderness, but no mass is felt.

(3) A pregnancy test is negative, and pelvic ultrasound confirms the diagnosis.

(4) Give analgesia as indicated and refer the patient to the Gynaecology team.

TORSION OF AN OVARIAN TUMOUR

DIAGNOSIS AND MANAGEMENT

(1) Fibroids or cysts that twist or suddenly distend from a bleed cause sudden lower abdominal pain, often with preceding episodes of milder pain.

(2) The patient may have nausea, a low-grade fever and localized abdominal tenderness with a palpable mass.

(3) Send blood for FBC, collect an MSU, and exclude pregnancy with a pregnancy test.

(4) Arrange a pelvic ultrasound, and refer the patient to the Gynaecology team for possible laparoscopy.

ENDOMETRIOSIS

DIAGNOSIS AND MANAGEMENT

(1) There is a preceding history of recurrent abdominal and flank pain, worse at the time of menstruation and immediately pre-menstrually. Other common symptoms include acquired dysmenorrhoea, dyspareunia, painful defecation, and infertility.

(2) This is a difficult diagnosis that requires review by the Gynaecology team and a laparoscopy, as there is poor correlation between symptoms and laparoscopic findings.

BLEEDING IN EARLY PREGNANCY

Two important causes are ectopic pregnancy (see p. 381) and spontaneous miscarriage. The old term 'spontaneous abortion' has now been replaced by the more appropriate terminology 'spontaneous miscarriage' to diminish negative self-perceptions of women experiencing early pregnancy fetal demise.

SPONTANEOUS MISCARRIAGE

Spontaneous miscarriage is the expulsion of the products of conception before the 24th week of pregnancy. It is most common in the first trimester and occurs in 10–20% of all early pregnancies. There are five recognized stages of spontaneous miscarriage.

DIAGNOSIS

(1) *Threatened miscarriage*

    (i) This is most common up to 14 weeks gestation, causing mild cramps and transient vaginal bleeding. These symptoms indicate a possible miscarriage.

    (ii) The uterine size is compatible with the duration of pregnancy. A guide to the expected size of the uterus is given by:

        (a) bimanual examination – the uterus is the size of a hen's egg at 7 weeks, an orange at 10 weeks, and a grapefruit at 12 weeks

        (b) abdominal palpation: the fundus reaches the symphysis pubis at 12 weeks and the umbilicus at 24 weeks.

    (iii) The external cervical os is closed on speculum examination.

(2) *Inevitable miscarriage*

    (i) This represents a spontaneous miscarriage that cannot be arrested.

    (ii) The bleeding is heavier, followed by lower abdominal cramps that are more persistent.

    (iii) The external cervical os is open 0.5 cm or more, and the products of conception may be found in the vagina or protruding from the cervical canal.

    (iv) Symptoms and signs of pregnancy such as amenorrhoea, nausea, vomiting, breast enlargement, tenderness, tingling, areolar pigmentation, and frequency of micturition will disappear.

(3) *Incomplete miscarriage*

    (i) Parts of the fetus or placental material are retained in the uterus.

    (ii) The bleeding remains heavy and the cramps persist, even following the passage of clots and the products of conception.

(4) *Complete miscarriage*

    (i) All the fetal and placental material has been expelled from the uterus.

    (ii) The bleeding and cramps stop after the conceptus has been passed and the signs of pregnancy disappear.

    (iii) The cervical os is closed.

(5) *Silent miscarriage (missed abortion)*

    (i) An early pregnancy fetal demise in which all the products of conception are retained.

    (ii) Cramps and bleeding are replaced by an asymptomatic brownish vaginal discharge.

(iii) The uterus is small and irregular, and ultrasound fails to detect fetal heart motion.

(iv) Infection and disseminated intravascular coagulation (DIC) may occur.

(6) Gain i.v. access and send blood for FBC and G&S if the bleeding is heavy. Note the rhesus antibody status.

(7) Perform a quantitative serum beta-HCG to confirm the pregnancy, and as a baseline for subsequent serial testing to monitor for a continued pregnancy or fetal demise.

(8) Arrange a pelvic ultrasound to rule out an ectopic pregnancy and to assess fetal size and viability.

MANAGEMENT

(1) Commence an infusion of normal saline.

(2) Remove the products of conception with sponge forceps if they are blocking the cervical canal, to help relieve pain, bradycardia and hypotension. Send them for histology to exclude a hydatidiform mole.

(3) Refer patients with a threatened miscarriage to the EPEU (Early Pregnancy Evaluation Unit) or similar for ongoing counselling and management.

(4) Admit all other patients under the Gynaecology team for surgical or non-surgical management of uterine evacuation for an inevitable, incomplete or silent miscarriage.

(5) Give rhesus-negative mothers anti-D immunoglobulin 250 units i.m. within 72 hours up to 20 weeks of pregnancy and 500 units i.m. after 20 weeks (625 IU i.m. in Australia).

> ✓ **Tip:** miscarriage can be associated with significant psychological sequelae and an empathic approach to medical care and the provision of external counselling are essential.

INDUCED SEPTIC ABORTION

DIAGNOSIS AND MANAGEMENT

(1) This is usually the result of criminal abortion or occasionally therapeutic uterine evacuation.

(2) There is rapidly spreading pelvic infection, with salpingitis, peritonitis, pelvic and pulmonary thrombophlebitis, which can lead to septicaemia, DIC, shock and death.

(3) The patient presents unwell with fever, abdominal pain, foul-smelling vaginal discharge and bleeding. The patient will develop hypotension, oliguria, confusion and ultimately coma if untreated.

(4) Give the patient high-flow oxygen by face mask.

(5) Gain i.v. access, send blood for FBC, coagulation profile, U&Es, LFTs, blood sugar, two sets of blood cultures and G&S for rhesus D antibodies. Start rapid normal saline i.v.

(6) Commence gentamicin 5 mg/kg i.v., ampicillin 2 g i.v. and metronidazole 500 mg i.v., and refer the patient urgently to the Gynaecology team for evacuation of the uterine contents or emergency hysterectomy.

CONDITIONS IN LATE PREGNANCY

Ideally, all patients over 18–20 weeks pregnant should be sent straight to the labour ward. Occasionally, they are too unstable or there is not time to get them there. Thus the following conditions may be seen, all requiring prompt obstetric help.

TERMINOLOGY

Two terms are easy to confuse in obstetric practice:

Gravida is the number of times a woman has been pregnant, with twins counting as one. A first pregnancy is a primigravida.

Parity is defined as the number of times a woman has given birth to a fetus with a gestational age of 24 weeks or more.

ANTEPARTUM HAEMORRHAGE

DIAGNOSIS AND MANAGEMENT

(1) Vaginal bleeding after 24 weeks gestation can be a life-threatening emergency, particularly if associated with placenta praevia, placental abruption or uterine rupture.

(2) *Placenta praevia*

(i) This is classically associated with painless vaginal bleeding and uterine hypotonia, although mild abdominal cramping pain may occur if a small abruption coexists.

(ii) Abdominal examination confirms a 'soft' uterus with a high presenting part.

    (iii) The fetal condition is usually good and obstetric management is generally conservative.

(3) *Placental abruption*
    (i) This is commonly associated with dietary deficiency, pre-eclampsia, essential hypertension and a history of previous abruption.
    (ii) Patients present with severe lower abdominal pain and vaginal bleeding if the abruption is 'revealed'. Examination shows a hard 'woody' uterus, which is painful to palpate.
    (iii) There is a high incidence of fetal demise prior to delivery.

(4) *Never* perform a vaginal or speculum examination in the Emergency Department on patients with suspected antepartum haemorrhage, as this may precipitate torrential vaginal haemorrhage.
    (i) Such examinations should only be performed by an experienced obstetrician in an operating theatre prepared for urgent caesarean section.

(5) Give oxygen, place the patient in the left lateral position, insert two large-bore i.v. cannulae and send blood for FBC and coagulation profile, and cross-match 4 units. Start an i.v. infusion if the patient is hypotensive or shocked.

(6) Give non-sensitized rhesus-negative mothers anti-D immunoglobulin 500 units i.m. (625 IU i.m. in Australia).

(7) Request an ultrasound to differentiate the potential causes of antepartum haemorrhage. It can localize the placental position and determine the presence and size of a concealed abruption bleed.

(8) Refer the patient immediately to the Obstetric team.

PRE-ECLAMPSIA AND ECLAMPSIA

DIAGNOSIS AND MANAGEMENT

(1) Patients with pre-eclampsia classically have peripheral oedema, proteinuria and hypertension.

(2) The hypertension is defined by:
    (i) A systolic blood pressure greater than 140 mmHg and diastolic blood pressure greater than 90 mmHg in the third trimester of pregnancy.

Or:
    (ii) A rise in blood pressure of more than 25 mmHg systolic or

15 mmHg diastolic compared with early pregnancy (booking) blood pressure.

(3) Fulminant pre-eclampsia is associated with:
  (i) Headache, visual symptoms.
  (ii) Nausea, vomiting and abdominal pain.
  (iii) Irritability and hyper-reflexia.

(4) Complications of pre-eclampsia include:
  (i) HELLP syndrome – haemolysis, elevated liver enzymes and low platelets.
  (ii) Disseminated intravascular coagulation.
  (iii) Oliguria.
  (iv) Eclampsia (true seizures).

(5) Call the senior ED doctor and Obstetric team urgently. Give oxygen, gain i.v. access and send blood for FBC, U&Es, LFTs, blood sugar, coagulation profile and uric acid. Commence a normal saline infusion.

(6) Catheterize the patient. Place a wedge under the right hip, or nurse in the left lateral position.

(7) Magnesium sulphate is the drug of choice for eclampsia and for seizure prophylaxis in pre-eclampsia:
  (i) Give an initial dose of magnesium 4 g (16 mmol) i.v. over 5–10 min, then commence an infusion of magnesium 1 g/h (4 mmol/h) for at least 24 hours.
  (ii) Treat recurrent seizures with a further bolus of magnesium 2 g (8 mmol) i.v.

(8) Give diazepam 0.1–0.2 mg/kg i.v. if seizures persist.

(9) Treat severe hypertension with hydralazine 5 mg i.v. bolus every 20 min (to a maximum cumulative dose of 20 mg) or labetalol 20 mg i.v. bolus escalating to 40 mg bolus every 10 min (to a maximum cumulative dose of 300 mg).
  (i) Aim for a diastolic blood pressure of 90–100 mmHg to reduce the risk of cerebrovascular accident and further seizures.

(10) The only definitive treatment of eclampsia is delivery, once seizures are controlled, hypoxia is corrected and treatment of the severe hypertension is under way.

EMERGENCY DELIVERY

MANAGEMENT

(1) Call the Obstetric team and Paediatric or Neonatal team immediately.

(2) Allow the mother to lie or sit semi-upright, and give her 50% nitrous oxide with oxygen (Entonox™) during the first half of the contractions.

(3) A mediolateral episiotomy may be needed in primiparous women.

(4) Ask the mother to pant and thus to stop pushing as the head crowns, usually with the occiput upwards, which is followed by rotation (restitution) of the head.

(5) The next contraction delivers the anterior shoulder by gentle downward traction on the head, which is followed by the posterior shoulder and trunk.

(6) Then deliver the baby by lifting the head and trunk up and over the symphysis pubis, to lie on the mother's abdomen.

(7) Cut the cord immediately if it is wound tightly around the baby's neck. Otherwise clamp off or tie with two 2/0 silk ties after delivery, and divide.

(8) Aspirate mucus from the baby's nose and mouth, and keep the baby warm by wrapping it in a blanket. Be prepared to intubate if there is apnoea.

(9) Avoid the temptation to pull on the cord in the routine management of the third stage of labour, for fear of causing uterine inversion.

  (i) Try gentle abdominal massage to stimulate a uterine contraction, or give oxytocin 5 units with ergometrine (Syntometrine™) 500 μg (1 mL) i.m. This helps prevent post-partum haemorrhage and aids delivery of the placenta.

(10) Encourage the mother to commence suckling her baby immediately, as this will naturally stimulate uterine contraction, help to expel the placenta and reduce the risk of haemorrhage.

TRAUMA IN LATE PREGNANCY

The best treatment for the fetus is to rapidly stabilize the mother. Treatment priorities for trauma in a pregnant patient are the same as for the non-pregnant patient.

MANAGEMENT

(1) Follow the immediate management guidelines as for multiple injuries (see p. 204), but note the following additional considerations:

  (i) Tilt the supine, third trimester patient laterally using a wedge or pillow under the right hip, and manually displace the gravid uterus upwards and to the left to minimize impaired venous return from inferior vena caval compression.

(ii) Protect the airway from the increased risk of gastric regurgitation and pulmonary aspiration.

(iii) Larger amounts of blood may be lost before obvious signs of hypovolaemia such as tachycardia, hypotension and tachypnoea occur, as both maternal blood volume and cardiac output increase in pregnancy.

   (a) common mistakes are failure to recognize shock despite normal vital signs, and failure to treat aggressively with crystalloids.

(iv) Observe and monitor by cardiotocograph (CTG) all pregnant women with even minor trauma, and a viable fetus (of more than 24 weeks gestation).

   (a) fetal distress without signs of maternal shock occurs readily, as blood is shunted preferentially away from the uterus to maintain the maternal circulation following blood loss.

(v) Arrange ultrasound, which is indispensable in the evaluation of the pregnant patient. It evaluates both the mother and the fetus and is highly sensitive for detecting free intraperitoneal fluid (blood) following blunt trauma.

(vi) Diagnostic peritoneal lavage is rarely ever used now to detect haemoperitoneum following blunt trauma, as it is invasive and yet does not provide information about the volume or site of bleeding.

   (a) use a supra-umbilical approach with the mini-laparotomy technique, after first inserting a nasogastric tube and urethral catheter. The same diagnostic criteria apply as for non-pregnant patients (see p. 228).

(vii) Retroperitoneal bleeding with pelvic fracture after blunt trauma may be massive from the engorged pelvic veins.

(2) Assess the fetus during the secondary survey after initial resuscitation of the mother.

(i) Examine fundal height, uterine tenderness, fetal movement, fetal heart rate and strength of contractions.

(ii) Use a fetal stethoscope, Doppler ultrasound or cardiotocograph to assess the fetal heart rate. Fetal distress is indicated by:

   (a) bradycardia less than 110 beats/min (normal 120–160 beats/min)

(b) loss of fetal heart acceleration to fetal movement, or late deceleration after uterine contractions.

(3) Important causes of fetal distress or fetal death in trauma include maternal hypovolaemia, placental abruption and uterine rupture.

(i) Signs of placental abruption vary from vaginal bleeding, abdominal pain, tenderness, increasing fundal height and premature contractions, to maternal shock.

(ii) Signs of traumatic uterine rupture, which occurs more commonly in the second half of pregnancy, range from abdominal pain, to maternal shock or a separately palpable uterus and fetus.

(4) Arrange continuous fetal monitoring with cardiotocograph for a minimum of 6 hours, even after apparently minor maternal trauma.

(5) Give all rhesus-negative mothers anti-D immunoglobulin 500 units i.m. (625 IU i.m. in Australia).

(6) Call the Obstetric team to review and admit all pregnant trauma cases. Call the Paediatric team in addition if the fetus is over 24–26 weeks gestation and immediate delivery is indicated.

(7) Emergency caesarean section may even still be performed within 5 min of maternal cardiac arrest to maximize the chance of fetal survival and to improve any chance of maternal survival (see below).

CARDIOPULMONARY RESUSCITATION IN LATE PREGNANCY

DIAGNOSIS

(1) Causes of cardiac arrest in late pregnancy include uteroplacental bleeding, cerebrovascular haemorrhage, pulmonary embolus, amniotic fluid embolus and cardiac disease.

(2) Impaired venous return from inferior vena caval compression by the gravid uterus, with the patient supine, renders resuscitation ineffectual unless deliberately minimized.

(3) Rapidly gain i.v. access.

MANAGEMENT

(1) Key interventions to prevent cardiac arrest in pregnancy:

(i) Tilt the patient laterally using a wedge or pillow under the right side, and displace the uterus by lifting it manually upwards and to the left off the great vessels.

(ii) Give 100% oxygen and administer a fluid bolus.

(2) Modifications to basic life support (BLS) in pregnancy:

(i) Apply cricoid pressure whenever administering positive-pressure ventilation as there is increased risk of regurgitation and pulmonary aspiration.

(ii) Place hands higher on the chest wall, slightly above the centre of the sternum. Effective external chest compression is more difficult due to flared ribs, raised diaphragm, breast enlargement, and inferior vena caval compression.

(iii) Remember, defibrillation shocks are not a risk to the fetus.

(3) Modifications to advanced life support (ALS):

(i) Hypoxaemia is common due to reduced functional residual capacity and increased oxygen demand.

(ii) Intubation is more difficult during pregnancy secondary to physical factors outlined in (2)(ii) above. Be prepared to use an endotracheal tube that is 0.5–1.0 mm smaller in diameter than expected, as the airway is often narrower secondary to laryngeal oedema.

(iii) Do not use the femoral veins for venous access. Drugs administered via this route may not reach the maternal heart until after the fetus has been delivered.

(iv) Continue to use all the recommended resuscitation procedures and drugs for circulatory support.

(4) Consider immediate caesarean section if the resuscitation is not rapidly successful, having called the Obstetric and Paediatric teams on the arrival of the patient.

(i) Ideally, surgical intervention should be within 5 min of cardiac arrest for optimum maternal and neonatal survival.

(ii) Continue cardiopulmonary resuscitation throughout the procedure and afterwards until a stable rhythm with a sustained cardiac output is obtained.

WOMEN'S MEDICINE CRISES

POST-COITAL CONTRACEPTION

Occasionally, patients present for emergency contraceptive measures after unprotected intercourse. There are two possibilities:

(1) *Post-coital pill*

This may be used up to 72 hours after unprotected intercourse. Taking the dose as soon as possible increases the efficacy.

(2) *Intrauterine contraceptive device (IUCD)*

  (i) A copper device may be used up to 5 days after unprotected intercourse and is more effective than hormonal methods of emergency contraception.

  (ii) Test for sexually transmitted diseases on IUCD insertion and consider a single dose of azithromycin 1 g orally prophylactically in the casual sexual encounter, if the patient is worried.

POST-COITAL ('MORNING AFTER') PILL

(1) Give levonorgestrel 1.5 mg as a single dose.

  (i) Do not prescribe in women with severe liver disease or active acute porphyria.

  (ii) Give 2.25 mg levonorgestrel (1.5 mg taken immediately and 750 μg taken 12 hours later) in patients taking enzyme-inducing drugs such as carbamazepine, rifampicin, phenytoin and phenobarbitone (phenobarbital).

(2) Give a replacement dose with an antiemetic if vomiting occurs within 3 hours, such as domperidone 20 mg orally or 60 mg p.r.

(3) Explain to the patient that:

  (i) Her next period may be early or late.

  (ii) A barrier method of contraception should be used until her next period.

  (iii) There is an increased risk of ectopic pregnancy and she should seek medical advice immediately if abdominal pain occurs.

(4) Refer all patients for follow-up to their GP or a Family Planning clinic to check that:

  (i) The pregnancy test is negative 3–4 weeks later.

  (ii) There is no ectopic pregnancy.

  (iii) The patient receives proper contraceptive advice for the future.

MISSED ORAL CONTRACEPTIVE PILL

Usually a frantic call on the telephone requests advice on what to do following a missed oral contraceptive pill. The critical time for loss of contraceptive protection is at the beginning or end of the menstrual cycle, due to extension of the 'pill-free' interval.

(1) Patients on the *combined* oral contraceptive pill:
   (i) *Up to 12 hours late:* Take the missed pill and carry on as usual.
   (ii) *Over 12 hours late*
      (a) continue normal pill taking, but for the next 7 days either abstain from sex or use an alternative barrier method of contraception such as the condom
      (b) start the next packet immediately the present one is over, if these 7 days run beyond the end of the packet; i.e. no gap between packets
         – this will mean that no period may occur until the end of two packets, but this is not dangerous
      (c) miss out the seven inactive pills if the everyday pills are the ones being taken
      (d) emergency contraception is recommended if more than two pills are missed from the first seven tablets in a packet.
(2) Patients on the *progestogen-only* pill:
   Over 3 hours late, continue normal pill taking, but abstain from sex or use an alternative barrier method of contraception for the next 7 days.

DOMESTIC VIOLENCE TO FEMALES

DIAGNOSIS
(1) A similar management approach is applicable to both sexes, including in the elderly.
(2) Domestic violence affects women of every class, race and religion. It may commence at times of acute stress such as unemployment, first pregnancy or separation.
(3) The victim may present with injury, abdominal pain, substance abuse, attempted suicide, rape, or with multiple somatic complaints.
(4) Victims may delay attending, and may be evasive and embarrassed. Their partner may answer for them or act unconcerned.

MANAGEMENT
(1) Ensure privacy by interviewing alone without the partner. Ask gently but directly about the possibility of violence, which may initially be denied.
(2) Record all injuries, measuring bruises or lacerations with a ruler, and institute any urgent treatment to save life.
(3) Enquire about any additional risk of physical or sexual abuse to

other members of the household, particularly children (see p. 375).

(4) Offer admission if it is unsafe for the patient to return home or if acute psychiatric illness is present, e.g. depression.

(5) Call the duty social worker. However, if in the meantime the patient wishes to return home, give written contact numbers, including:

(i) GP.

(ii) Social worker.

(iii) Local police.

(iv) Local domestic violence 24-hour specialist helplines.

FEMALE RAPE

Follow a standard procedure in all cases of alleged rape in which the patient requests or accepts police involvement.

MANAGEMENT

(1) Be accompanied by a senior female nurse escort at all times.

(2) Record a careful history of exactly what occurred and when, and a description of the assailant.

(3) Institute any urgent treatment to save life, e.g. cross-match and starting a transfusion for haemorrhage.

(4) Contact the police and inform the duty police surgeon. The police surgeon will perform the forensic examination with the patient's consent. This is aimed at meticulously collecting evidence regarding:

(i) Proof of sexual contact.

(ii) Lack of consent.

(iii) Identification of the assailant.

(5) Meanwhile, examine the patient for associated injuries, measuring bruises or lacerations with a ruler. Request informed, written consent to keep all clothing for forensic analysis.

(i) Ask the patient to undress on a sheet to collect any debris.

(ii) Wear gloves and wrap each garment in a brown paper bag fastened with tape and labelled with the patient's name, the date, the nature of the sample, and the name of the person taking the sample.

(6) Request a senior gynaecology doctor to perform the examination of the external genitalia and vagina if the duty police surgeon is unavailable.

(7) Check whether the police have been able to arrange for a designated sexual offences unit to attend (usually non-uniformed women police officers who have received special training).

(8) Call the duty social worker or give the patient written contact telephone numbers/addresses if a social worker is not available immediately.

(9) Offer admission to the patient if indicated and discuss the following issues:

   (i) The post-coital pill to prevent pregnancy.

   (ii) The need to exclude a sexually transmitted disease or to provide prophylactic treatment and follow-up.

   (iii) Specialist counselling from various external organizations based in most regional centres, e.g. rape crisis lines.

(10) Provide written aftercare instructions with details of all the tests performed, treatments provided, and other arrangements made, as the patient's memory at this time of intense stress will not be reliable.

FURTHER READING

American Heart Association (2005) Guidelines for cardiopulmonary resuscitation and emergency cardiovascular care. Part 10.8: Cardiac arrest associated with pregnancy. *Circulation* **112**:IV-150–53.

American Heart Association http://www.circulationaha.org/ (CPR and ECC guidelines 2005).

European Resuscitation Council (2005) European Resuscitation Council guidelines for resuscitation. Section 7: Cardiac arrest in special circumstances. *Resuscitation* **67** (**Suppl 1**):S135–70.

European Resuscitation Council. http://www.erc.edu/ (ERC guidelines and resuscitation practice).

National Blood Authority. http://www.nba.gov.au/PDF/glines_anti_d.pdf/ (Guidelines on the prophylactic use of Rh D immunoglobulin (anti-D) in obstetrics 2003).

National Institute for Health and Clinical Excellence http://www.nice.org.uk/ (antenatal care and emergencies).

Resuscitation Council UK. http://www.resus.org.uk/ (Resuscitation guidelines 2005).

Royal College of Obstetricians and Gynaecologists. http://www.rcog.org.uk/ (anti-D rhesus prophylaxis).

ENT EMERGENCIES

TRAUMATIC CONDITIONS OF THE EAR

SUBPERICHONDRIAL HAEMATOMA

DIAGNOSIS
(1) Blunt trauma to the ear causes bleeding between the perichondrium and auricular cartilage, known as a subperichondrial haematoma.
(2) This will lead to a 'cauliflower ear' deformity from proliferative fibrosis if left untreated.

MANAGEMENT
(1) Refer the patient with a large and extensive bleed directly to the ENT team for immediate surgical drainage.
(2) Otherwise, aspirate small clots under local anaesthesia, and apply firm pressure by packing around the interstices of the ear with cotton-wool under a turban dressing.
    (i) Refer the patient to the next ENT clinic, because the bleeding may recur.
(3) Give the patient flucloxacillin 500 mg orally q.d.s. for 5 days to protect against perichondritis.

WOUNDS OF THE AURICLE

MANAGEMENT
(1) Perform minimal debridement of devitalized tissue under local anaesthesia.
(2) Refer the patient to the ENT team or plastic surgeons if there are extensive lacerations or skin loss leaving exposed cartilage.
(3) Otherwise, appose the edges of the cartilage with 5/0 absorbable suture such as polydioxanone or polyglactin through the perichondrium.
(4) Suture the skin with 6/0 non-absorbable monofilament nylon or polypropylene and apply a firm dressing. Remove the sutures after 5 days.
(5) Give the patient flucloxacillin 500 mg orally q.d.s. for 5 days to protect against perichondritis, and administer tetanus prophylaxis.

FOREIGN BODY IN THE EXTERNAL EAR

DIAGNOSIS AND MANAGEMENT

(1) A foreign body in the external ear causes pain, deafness and discharge if left.

(2) Attempt gentle removal if the foreign body is superficial, with an angled probe or alligator forceps.

(3) Do not attempt any further manoeuvres if the object is not freed instantly, or if the patient is uncooperative, as the object may be pushed in further causing extreme pain and eardrum damage.

  (i) Refer the patient to the next ENT clinic.

PERFORATED EARDRUM

DIAGNOSIS

(1) The eardrum may be perforated by direct injury from a sharp object, such as a hairpin, or indirectly by pressure from a slap, blast injury, scuba diving, or from a fracture of the base of the skull (see below).

(2) There is pain, conductive deafness and sometimes bleeding.

(3) Suspect inner ear involvement if there is tinnitus, vertigo or complete hearing loss.

MANAGEMENT

(1) Refer the patient immediately to the ENT team if inner ear damage is suspected.

(2) Otherwise, do not put anything into the ear or attempt to clean it out. Advise the patient to keep water out of the ear canal.

(3) Give an antibiotic such as amoxicillin 500 mg orally t.d.s., and refer the patient to the next ENT clinic.

BASAL SKULL FRACTURE

Most basal skull fractures (see also p. 238) involve the temporal bone. Fractures may be divided into tympanic bone fractures, longitudinal fractures and transverse fractures.

DIAGNOSIS

(1) The temporal bone forms the glenoid fossa of the temporomandibular joint, and is damaged if the mandibular condyle is driven upwards into the middle ear or external auditory

canal, causing bleeding or laceration of the canal.

(2) Alternatively, a longitudinal fracture of the temporal bone will tear the eardrum and cause dislocation of the ossicular chain, with conductive deafness, haemotympanum and CSF leakage.

(i) Occasionally, delayed facial nerve damage is seen.

(3) A transverse fracture of the temporal bone results in complete sensorineural deafness associated with tinnitus, vertigo and nystagmus.

(i) Facial nerve palsy is more common than with longitudinal fractures.

(4) Do not insert an auriscope to examine obvious bleeding from the external auditory meatus, because infection may be introduced.

(5) Remember that basal skull fracture can be a clinical diagnosis. X-rays may have to wait until the patient is stable and other injuries to the head, neck and chest have been assessed fully.

(i) Request an immediate CT head scan if the patient has been stabilized.

(ii) Lateral skull X-ray showing intracranial air or a fluid level in the sphenoid sinus is suggestive of basal skull fracture, when CT is unavailable.

MANAGEMENT

(1) Admit the patient under the Surgical team for head injury care and advice from the Neurosurgical unit or ENT specialist.

NON-TRAUMATIC CONDITIONS OF THE EAR

All these conditions present with pain and/or hearing loss.

OTITIS EXTERNA

DIAGNOSIS

(1) A bacterial or fungal infection is usually responsible, often following repeated use of cotton-wool buds, or exposure to water ('swimmer's ear').

(2) There is pain, desquamation of skin, and on otoscopy an oedematous, narrowed ear canal, often containing debris and discharge.

MANAGEMENT

(1) Attempt aural toilet using a cotton wick or fine aspiration tube on suction to gently remove the debris, although pain may preclude this.

(2) Insert a Merocel™ wick to maintain external ear canal patency. Add a proprietary anti-infective and steroid preparation such as Otosporin™, Sofradex™ or Locorten-Vioform™ three drops 2–4 times daily into the external auditory canal, or onto the wick.

(3) Refer the patient to the ENT clinic for formal aural toilet.

(4) Refer the patient directly to the ENT team if the otitis externa is severe with painful occlusion of the external ear canal.

FURUNCULOSIS OF THE EXTERNAL EAR

DIAGNOSIS

(1) A furuncle may develop in the outer part of the external auditory canal causing extreme pain.

(2) Movement of the pinna and introduction of a speculum exacerbate the pain. Deafness is minimal.

(3) Remember to test the urine for sugar.

MANAGEMENT

(1) Insert a wick soaked in 10% ichthammol in glycerin to encourage discharge of the pus, start flucloxacillin 500 mg orally q.d.s. and give an analgesic such as paracetamol 500 mg and codeine phosphate 8 mg two tablets orally q.d.s.

(2) Refer the patient to the ENT clinic for follow-up.

ACUTE OTITIS MEDIA

DIAGNOSIS

(1) This is common in children, due to viral or bacterial infection such as pneumococcus, *Moraxella* or *Haemophilus influenzae*, which is now rapidly decreasing in children under 6 years with HiB immunization.

(2) There is intense earache, variable fever, conductive deafness, and on examination of the eardrum in the early stages there is loss of the light reflex and injected vessels are seen around the malleus.

(3) As the infection progresses, a bulging, immobile drum is seen, which may perforate, discharging pus.

MANAGEMENT

(1) Most cases settle spontaneously with regular analgesia such as paracetamol 15 mg/kg orally q.d.s. or ibuprofen 10 mg/kg orally t.d.s.

(2) The role of antibiotics is contentious. If systemically unwell, or no better by 72 hours give amoxicillin 250–500 mg orally t.d.s. for 5 days with the analgesia.

    (i) Give erythromycin 250–500 mg orally q.d.s. for 5 days if the patient is allergic to penicillin.

MASTOIDITIS

DIAGNOSIS AND MANAGEMENT

(1) There is extension of infection from acute otitis media into the mastoid air-cell system.

(2) The patient is ill and feverish, with local redness and tenderness over the mastoid, and the pinna is pushed down and forwards.

(3) Complications include cranial nerve palsy, meningitis and subperiosteal abscess.

(4) Refer the patient immediately to the ENT team for X-ray, CT scan and parenteral antibiotics.

VERTIGO

DIAGNOSIS

(1) Two main groups occur:

    (i) *Peripheral vertigo* (85%).

    This is due to lesions in the vestibular nerve and inner ear, such as acute labyrinthitis, vestibular neuronitis, Ménière's disease with accompanying sensorineural deafness and tinnitus, benign paroxysmal positional vertigo, otosclerosis, cholesteatoma or ototoxic drugs such as gentamicin and rapid, high-dose frusemide (furosemide).

    (ii) *Central vertigo* (15%).

    This is due to lesions in the CNS, such as a vertebrobasilar TIA, a cerebellar or brainstem stroke, cerebellopontine angle tumour, demyelination, vertebrobasilar migraine, or alcohol and drug toxicity.

(2) Peripheral vertigo is associated with nystagmus, deafness, nausea, vomiting and sweating, whereas central vertigo is usually dominated by associated neurological signs.

MANAGEMENT
(1) Give patients with incapacitating vertigo diazepam 0.1 mg/kg i.v.
    or midazolam 0.05–0.1 mg/kg i.v. as symptomatic treatment, and
    rest until the vertigo has gone.
    (i) Alternatively, give prochlorperazine 12.5 mg i.m. but beware
        that it may cause dystonia including akathisia – an unpleasant,
        intolerable sense of restlessness.
(2) Refer patients with peripheral causes of vertigo that do not settle to
    the ENT team, and with central causes of vertigo to the Medical
    team.

FACIAL NERVE PALSY

DIAGNOSIS
(1) Lower motor neurone paralysis.
    (i) There is weakness of the whole side of the face, including the
        forehead muscles.
    (ii) Causes include:
        (a) Bell's palsy with an abrupt onset sometimes associated with
            postauricular pain, hyperacusis and abnormal taste in the
            anterior two thirds of the tongue
        (b) trauma to the temporal bone or a facial laceration in the
            parotid area
        (c) tumours, such as an acoustic neuroma or parotid malignancy
        (d) infection, such as acute otitis media, chronic otitis media
            with cholesteatoma or geniculate herpes zoster, the Ramsay
            Hunt syndrome
        (e) miscellaneous, including Guillain–Barré syndrome,
            sarcoidosis, diabetes and hypertension.
(2) Upper motor neurone paralysis.
    (i) There is weakness of the lower facial muscles sparing the
        forehead, often associated with other neurological signs such as
        hemiplegia.
    (ii) The cause is usually a stroke.
(3) Examine the external auditory canal, eardrum, parotid region and
    make a full neurological assessment.

MANAGEMENT
(1) Refer all acute cases with associated signs immediately to the
    medical, surgical or ENT team according to the likely aetiology.

(2) Give prednisolone 50 mg orally once daily plus aciclovir 400 mg orally 5 times a day in a patient with Bell's palsy if seen within 3 days of onset. Add hypromellose artificial tears, tape or pad the eye closed at night, and refer to the next ENT clinic.

TRAUMATIC CONDITIONS OF THE NOSE

FRACTURED NOSE

DIAGNOSIS

(1) This injury is usually obvious following a direct blow, causing swelling, deformity and epistaxis.
(2) Exclude a more serious facial bone fracture, e.g. with cerebrospinal rhinorrhoea from cribiform plate damage (see p. 439).
(3) Look carefully for a septal haematoma which, if left, leads to necrosis of the nasal cartilage and septal collapse.
  (i) The nasal passage is blocked by a dull-red swelling replacing the septum, associated with marked nasal obstruction.
(4) Do *not* take an X-ray as this will not alter the clinical management.

MANAGEMENT

(1) Refer any patient with a grossly deformed or compound fracture, or a septal haematoma to the ENT team.
  (i) Refer more serious facial bone fractures to the maxillofacial surgery team.
(2) Otherwise, refer the patient to the ENT clinic within the next 5–10 days, if the patient requests operative treatment to straighten the nose for cosmetic reasons.

FOREIGN BODY IN THE NOSE

DIAGNOSIS AND MANAGEMENT

(1) This may be quite asymptomatic, or it may lead to a serosanguinous, offensive, unilateral nasal discharge.
(2) Attempt removal with a bent probe or pair of forceps if the object is easily accessible in the anterior part of the nose, after the patient has vigorously blown the nose (which may dislodge the object anyway).
(3) However, refer immediately to the ENT team if removal is difficult, or a child is uncooperative.

(i) Sudden posterior dislodgement with inhalation of the foreign body into the airway is a real danger.

NON-TRAUMATIC CONDITIONS OF THE NOSE

EPISTAXIS

DIAGNOSIS

(1) This is usually spontaneous in children, occurring from vessels in Little's area on the anterior part of the septum, possibly precipitated by rhinitis or minor trauma such as picking.
(2) The bleeding occurs posterior to Little's area in adults and may be associated with a bleeding diathesis, including anticoagulant drugs.
(3) Bleeding originates higher in the posterior part of the nose in the elderly from arteriosclerotic vessels, and rapidly leads to haemorrhagic shock if profuse.
(4) Send blood for FBC, clotting study and G&S in any patient with profuse bleeding. Establish an i.v. infusion with normal saline 10 mL/kg, before the patient becomes hypotensive, and restore the circulation.
   (i) Call the senior ED doctor immediately in these cases.

MANAGEMENT

(1) Bleeding from Little's area:
   (i) Pinch the anterior part of the nose for 10 minutes with the patient sitting forward until the bleeding stops. Forbid the patient to pick, blow, or sniff through the nose to prevent recurrence of the epistaxis.
   (ii) Identify with suction or by swabbing if a bleeding point persists, and anaesthetize the area with a cotton-wool pledget soaked in 4% lignocaine (lidocaine) with adrenaline (epinephrine).
   (iii) Cauterize the bleeding point with a silver nitrate stick touched onto the area for 10 seconds. Avoid overzealous application or cauterization of both sides of the septum, as these will lead to septal necrosis.
(2) Persistent anterior bleeding and failed cautery:
   (i) *Anterior nasal tamponade*
   Insert an epistaxis balloon catheter or nasal Merocel™ tampon,

both of which are much easier to insert than formal packing.

(ii) *Anterior nasal pack*

    (a) cover the patient and yourself with protective drapes when no nasal tamponade device is available, and wear a face mask and goggles

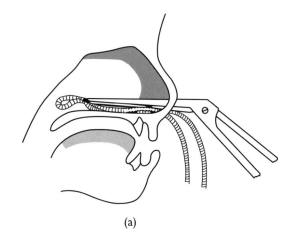

(a)

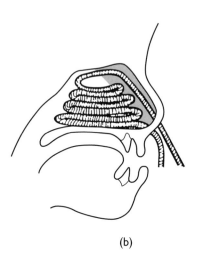

(b)

Figure 12.1 Anterior nasal packing

(a) Introducing the first loop horizontally along the floor of the nose, and (b) building the layers horizontally upwards until pack is in place.

(b) apply further local anaesthetic with cotton-wool pledgets soaked in 4% lignocaine (lidocaine) with adrenaline (epinephrine) (maximum dose 12 mL or approximately 500 mg lignocaine (lidocaine) with adrenaline (epinephrine) in a 65-kg patient, i.e. 7 mg/kg)

(c) use 2-cm petroleum-jelly gauze or a calcium alginate (Kaltostat™) 2 g pack

(d) insert successive layers horizontally along the floor of the nose using Tilley's nasal dressing forceps

(e) remember in adults the nose extends 6.5–7.5 cm backwards to the posterior choanae (see Fig. 12.1).

(iii) Give the patient amoxicillin 500 mg orally t.d.s. and refer to the ENT team for admission and removal of the pack within 48 hours.

(3) Severe posterior bleeding:

(i) *Anterior and posterior nasal tamponade*
Attempt to stem posterior nasal bleeding by inserting a double epistaxis-balloon device, with separate balloons for anterior plus posterior tamponade. Tape securely to the cheek.

(ii) Use a Foley urethral catheter if tamponade is unavailable, and insert far back along the floor of the nose, inflate the retaining balloon with air, and pull the catheter forwards to occlude the back of the nose. Tape the catheter securely to the cheek to prevent it slipping backwards.

(a) then insert an anterior nasal pack as described previously

(b) occasionally both sides of the nose require packing to stop the bleeding.

(iii) Refer the patient immediately to the ENT team for admission.

TRAUMATIC CONDITIONS OF THE THROAT

See *Section VII* Surgical Emergencies under Neck Injuries.

NON-TRAUMATIC CONDITIONS OF THE THROAT

TONSILLITIS

DIAGNOSIS AND MANAGEMENT

(1) This is more frequently viral than bacterial, but differentiating the two clinically is difficult.
   (i) Fever above 100°F (38°C), tender cervical adenopathy, tonsillar exudate and absence of cough suggest beta-haemolytic *Streptococcus*, particularly in older children.
   (ii) Glandular fever (EBV) may present with a grey, exudative tonsillitis in late adolescence.
(2) There is fever, fetor, sore throat and dysphagia. A febrile convulsion may be precipitated in a child under 5 years old.
(3) Give an antipyretic analgesic, and consider penicillin V 250–500 mg orally q.d.s. for 10 days, particularly when systemically unwell, immunosuppressed or there is peritonsillar cellulitis.
(4) Return the patient to the care of their GP.

QUINSY (PERITONSILLAR ABSCESS)

DIAGNOSIS AND MANAGEMENT

(1) This may follow tonsillitis and is more common in adults.
(2) There is a worsening of the illness, with high temperature, muffled voice, dysphagia, referred earache and trismus.
(3) Examination shows unilateral swelling of the soft palate, with displacement of the tonsil downwards and medially, and deviation of the uvula to the unaffected side.
(4) Give benzylpenicillin 1.2 g i.v. q.d.s. and metronidazole 500 mg i.v. t.d.s. Refer the patient immediately to the ENT team for operative drainage.

FOREIGN BODY IN THE PHARYNX

DIAGNOSIS

(1) Fish or meat bones are the most common objects to cause symptoms.
(2) Usually, a fish bone will impact in the tonsil, base of the tongue, or posterior pharyngeal wall.

(i) Depress the tongue to visualize the tonsil, or use a laryngeal mirror to see the back of the tongue and posterior pharynx.

(3) Request a lateral soft-tissue X-ray of the neck if no bone is seen despite symptoms.

(i) Calcification of superimposed hyoid, thyroid, cricoid and laryngeal cartilages may cause confusion in the diagnosis.

MANAGEMENT

(1) Refer the patient immediately to the ENT team for oesophagoscopy if oesophageal impaction is suspected from dysphagia, excessive salivation, local tenderness or pain.

(2) Otherwise, attempt to remove a fish bone from the tonsil or the back of the tongue using Tilley's curved forceps.

(i) Refer the patient immediately to the ENT team if this fails in a patient with pain or who is salivating excessively.

(3) Alternatively, the pharyngeal mucosa may only have been scratched. If symptoms are minimal, prescribe an antibiotic such as amoxicillin 500 mg orally t.d.s. and ask the patient to return in 24 hours for review.

SWALLOWED FOREIGN BODY

DIAGNOSIS

(1) Coins are the most common objects swallowed by pre-school children, although small children swallow almost anything, and the elderly may swallow their dentures.

(2) Oesophageal impaction, usually around the cricopharyngeus at the level of C6, causes dysphagia, excessive salivation, local tenderness or retrosternal pain, but may be totally asymptomatic.

(3) Button batteries pose a particular risk, as they may cause local mucosal perforation or corrosive effects with later stenosis.

(4) Occasionally, airway obstruction occurs from upper oesophageal impaction, or the object may in fact have been inhaled, not swallowed (see p. 358).

(5) Request X-rays of the neck and chest to look for oesophageal impaction.

(i) Include anteroposterior (AP) and lateral views to avoid missing a radio-opaque object super-imposed over the skeletal or cardiac shadows on the AP view, and to differentiate tracheal lodgement.

(6) Request an abdominal X-ray in button-battery ingestion, or for symptoms such as abdominal pain, distension or gastrointestinal bleeding.

MANAGEMENT

(1) Refer the following patients immediately to the ENT team:
   (i) Airway obstruction or foreign body inhalation.
   (ii) Oesophageal impaction suspected clinically.
   (iii) Oesophageal lodgement seen on X-ray or inferred from pre-vertebral soft-tissue swelling, soft-tissue gas, or air in the upper oesophagus.
   (iv) Button battery seen in the oesophagus or stomach.

(2) Allow the patient home, if the patient is asymptomatic, and neck and chest X-rays are normal.
   (i) Reassure the parents that most objects will pass spontaneously.
   (ii) Request immediate review if symptoms develop.
   (iii) Consider a repeat abdominal X-ray after 4 days in button-battery ingestion if it has not been passed in the stools.
   (iv) Otherwise, repeat X-rays are required only if the patient develops symptoms.

STRIDOR

See p. 356 in *Section X* Paediatric Emergencies.

FURTHER READING

Cochrane Collaboration.
http://www.cochrane.org/reviews/en/topics/60.html/ (Cochrane review topics: Ear, nose and throat disorders).

Drotts D, Vinson D (1999) Prochlorperazine induces akathisia in emergency patients. *Ann Emerg Med* **34:**469-75.

OPHTHALMIC EMERGENCIES

Ophthalmic emergencies may be grouped into traumatic or non-traumatic, and subdivided according to whether the eyelids are affected, or if the eye is red, painful, or has diminished visual acuity.

VISUAL ACUITY

Always record visual acuity, with distance glasses if they are worn, at the start of every eye examination before any drops or dyes have been introduced.

Acuity is measured by reading a Snellen chart at a distance of 6 metres.

Each eye is tested separately, and the lowest line that can be read accurately is recorded. Normal vision is 6/6.

Ask patients with refractive errors who have left their glasses at home to look through a pinhole to optimize their visual acuity.

TOPICAL OPHTHALMIC PREPARATIONS

The following preparations are referred to in the text:
- Antibiotic drops: 0.5% chloramphenicol solution, two drops every 2–3 hours.
- Antibiotic ointment: 1% chloramphenicol ointment, one application to the lower lid conjunctival sac every 4 hours, or at night (if drops are used during the day).
- Local anaesthetic: 1% amethocaine (tetracaine) solution or 0.4% oxybuprocaine solution, one or more drops as required.
  - The patient must then wear a protective eye pad for 1–2 hours until corneal sensitivity returns
  - Never allow the patient to take the drops home.
- Fluorescein corneal stain: fluorescein sodium strips, or 2% fluorescein solution (do not use with soft contact lenses).
- Short-acting mydriatic and cycloplegic dilating drops to examine the fundus: 1% tropicamide, two drops repeated after 15 minutes if necessary (do not use in patients with narrow anterior chambers, to avoid precipitating glaucoma).

- Cycloplegic to paralyse the ciliary body: 1% cyclopentolate two drops lasts 6–24 hours and 1% homatropine two drops lasts 1–2 days.
- Miotic to constrict the pupil or reverse a mydriatic: 2% pilocarpine one or two drops.

> **Warning:** steroid preparations should *not* be used except by an experienced ophthalmologist. Any condition diagnosed that needs steroid drops also needs an ophthalmic opinion first.

TRAUMATIC CONDITIONS OF THE EYE

PERIORBITAL HAEMATOMA ('BLACK EYE')

DIAGNOSIS AND MANAGEMENT

(1) This is caused by a direct blow. If bilateral, suspect local trauma to the nose or a basal skull fracture (see p. 238).

(2) Always perform a thorough stepwise assessment:
  (i) Check that the patient can see, if necessary by opening the eyelids manually, and record the visual acuity.
  (ii) Check the eyeball for damage. Examine the cornea for abrasions, the anterior chamber for hyphaema, the pupil size and reactions, and the sclera for perforation. Also check for the presence of a red reflex through the pupil and a normal fundus.
  (iii) Refer any abnormal findings suggestive of one of the above complications immediately to the ophthalmology team.
  (iv) Palpate to see whether the bony margin of the orbit is intact.
  (v) Test that the eye movements are full and the eyeball is not tethered, suggesting a 'blow-out' fracture of the orbital floor (see p. 438).

(3) Request appropriate facial X-rays if a 'blow-out' or a malar fracture is suspected, and refer the patient to the Maxillofacial Surgery team.

(4) Otherwise, give the patient an analgesic such as paracetamol 500 mg and codeine phosphate 8 mg two tablets q.d.s. and chloramphenicol eye ointment if the eye is shut.

(5) Review the patient within 48 hours when the swelling has decreased to re-confirm the absence of significant ocular damage.

SUBCONJUNCTIVAL HAEMATOMA

DIAGNOSIS AND MANAGEMENT

Two types are recognized – spontaneous and traumatic.

(1) *Spontaneous*

    (i) This may arise from coughing or from atherosclerotic vessels, particularly in the elderly, and is occasionally associated with hypertension or a bleeding diathesis.

    (ii) Measure the blood pressure and reassure the patient that the subconjunctival blood will disperse within 2 weeks. No treatment is needed.

(2) *Traumatic*

    (i) This may be due to a surface conjunctival foreign body, or a more serious penetrating foreign body or bulging scleral perforation. Gentle digital assessment may reveal reduced eyeball tone in penetration of the globe.

    (ii) Refer all patients immediately to the Ophthalmology team if a serious cause is suspected.

    (iii) Consider a basal skull fracture if the posterior margin cannot be seen. Refer this patient to the Neurosurgical team (see p. 238).

    (iv) Otherwise, minor cases require reassurance only.

EYELID LACERATION

DIAGNOSIS AND MANAGEMENT

(1) Refer the patient directly to the Ophthalmology or Plastic Surgery team if the laceration involves the tarsal plate, upper eyelid, lid margin, or the medial canthus and the lacrimal apparatus.

(2) Otherwise, suture the eyelid under local anaesthesia using fine 6/0 non-absorbable monofilament nylon or polypropylene sutures. Remove after 4 days.

EYELID BURN

DIAGNOSIS AND MANAGEMENT

(1) Examine the eye carefully for evidence of corneal or scleral damage before oedema makes the examination impossible, although the

blink reflex usually protects the globe.

(2) Give the patient antibiotic drops, analgesia and tetanus prophylaxis, and refer immediately to the Ophthalmology team.

CHEMICAL BURNS TO THE EYE

DIAGNOSIS AND MANAGEMENT

(1) Alkalis are more deeply penetrating and dangerous than acids, and include common agents such as cement, plaster powder, and oven and drain cleaners.

(2) The mainstay of treatment is immediate, copious, prolonged irrigation with normal saline from an i.v. giving set. Instil local anaesthetic drops to open the eye initially.

(3) Give additional analgesia if necessary with morphine 5 mg i.v. plus an antiemetic such as metoclopramide 10 mg i.v.

(4) Take care to irrigate all corners of the eye and to evert the upper eyelids to remove any particulate matter, and to irrigate the superior fornix of the conjunctiva.

(5) Refer the patient immediately to the Ophthalmology team, unless fluorescein staining reveals no corneal damage and the surrounding conjunctiva appears normal and is pain-free, i.e. no injury is apparent.

CONJUNCTIVAL FOREIGN BODY

DIAGNOSIS AND MANAGEMENT

(1) Usually a piece of grit blows into the eye causing pain, redness and watering, and is easily seen on direct vision.

(2) Remove with a moistened cotton-wool bud after instilling local anaesthetic. Provide an eye pad to be worn for 1–2 hours until the return of normal sensation.

(3) The object may have impacted on the upper subtarsal conjunctiva if nothing is seen immediately. The eye will be red and painful to blink, and fluorescein staining will reveal multiple linear corneal abrasions.

(4) Evert the upper eyelid.
   (i) Stand behind the patient to evert the upper lid, supporting the head against your body.
   (ii) Instruct the patient to look downwards, pull the upper lid eyelashes down and then up and over the tarsal plate, which is

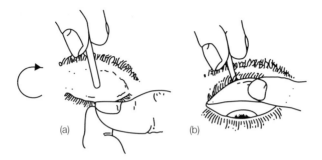

Figure 13.1 Eversion of the upper eyelid

(a) Lifting the tarsal plate up and over, and (b) demonstrating the underside of the upper eyelid (subtarsal conjunctiva).

     held depressed by a glass rod or orange stick (see Fig. 13.1).
(iii) Remove the foreign body with a moistened cotton-wool bud.

(5) Give the patient antibiotic drops for 2 days if fluorescein shows signs of corneal abrasion.

(6) Always consider the possibility of intraocular penetration, with any high velocity injury, e.g. by a metal fragment from drilling or a stone from mowing (see p. 422).

CORNEAL FOREIGN BODY

DIAGNOSIS AND MANAGEMENT

(1) The foreign body may be obvious, or revealed by fluorescein staining.

(2) Instil local anaesthetic drops and attempt removal of the foreign body with a moistened cotton-wool bud or the bevel of a hypodermic needle, introduced from the side.

(3) However, leave deep or recalcitrant foreign bodies, and those with an extensive rust ring alone. Refer the patient to the Ophthalmology team to avoid causing further damage during attempted removal.

(4) As local anaesthetic was used, pad the eye for 1–2 hours until the return of normal sensation. Treat any corneal epithelial defect demonstrated on fluorescein staining as for a corneal abrasion (see below p. 421).

(5) Review the patient within 2 days to exclude infection, but ask them to return earlier if pain increases or vision deteriorates.

(i)   Refer the patient immediately to the Ophthalmology team if there is then evidence of an infected corneal ulcer.

CORNEAL ABRASION

DIAGNOSIS AND MANAGEMENT

(1)   Corneal abrasion is due to a foreign body or to direct injury from a finger, stick, or a piece of paper.

(2)   There is intense pain, watering and blepharospasm. Local anaesthetic drops may be needed before the eye can be opened properly.

(3)   Use fluorescein staining to reveal the damage. Give the patient 0.5% chloramphenicol eye drops and mydriatic drops, and review within 2 days.

(4)   An eye pad is no longer recommended, other than for 1–2 hours following local anaesthetic use.

(5)   The cornea should be fully recovered by 2 days, but refer the patient to the ophthalmology team if there is delayed healing or a recurrence.

FLASH BURN (ARC EYE)

DIAGNOSIS AND MANAGEMENT

(1)   Exposure to ultraviolet light from welding without using protective goggles, or from a sun lamp, causes a superficial keratitis.

(2)   There is intense pain, watering and blepharospasm occurring after a few hours. Fluorescein staining reveals a pitted corneal surface due to a superficial punctate keratitis.

(3)   Instil local anaesthetic drops and mydriatic/cycloplegic drops. Double-pad the eyes shut until the return of normal sensation and the blepharospasm settles.

(4)   Give an analgesic such as paracetamol 500 mg and codeine phosphate 8 mg two tablets q.d.s. Recovery occurs within 12–24 hours.

BLUNT TRAUMA TO THE EYE

DIAGNOSIS AND MANAGEMENT

(1)   Always consider injury to the eye in any trauma to the face. Eye examination must not be omitted just because other injuries appear more dramatic, or periorbital oedema obscures the eye.

(2) Blunt trauma may cause a sequence of injuries from the front to the back of the eye. Systematically exclude each one:

(i) Periorbital haematoma or subconjunctival haemorrhage.

(ii) Corneal abrasion or laceration.

(iii) Bleeding into the anterior chamber, called hyphaema. This may be microscopic or macroscopic with formation of a fluid level.

(iv) A fixed pupil or torn iris, known as traumatic mydriasis and iridodialysis, respectively.

(v) A dislocated lens or subsequent traumatic cataract.

(vi) Vitreous haemorrhage, causing a dull or absent red reflex and obscuring the fundus.

(vii) A retinal tear, with retinal detachment seen as a dark, wrinkled, ballooned area diametrically opposite any resultant visual field defect.

(viii) Retinal oedema (*commotio retinae*) seen as whitish areas of oedema, usually associated with haemorrhage.

(ix) Optic nerve damage, causing blindness with no direct pupillary response to light.

(x) Ruptured globe, with marked visual loss, a soft eye, and shallow anterior chamber.

(xi) Retrobulbar haematoma, with pain, proptosis and a fixed, dilated pupil.

(xii) Orbital fracture, usually a 'blow-out' fracture of the orbital floor (see p. 438).

(3) Refer a patient with any of the complications above from (ii) through to (xi) directly to the Ophthalmology team. Do not allow the patient home in the meantime, but arrange for them to lie quietly and semi-upright, pending expert assessment.

(i) Ideally, pad both eyes and give appropriate analgesia.

(ii) Protect a suspected ruptured globe with an eye shield, not an eye pad.

PENETRATING TRAUMA TO THE EYE

DIAGNOSIS AND MANAGEMENT

(1) Penetrating trauma is usually obvious, although on occasions it may be difficult to recognize initially and must be thought of after a high-velocity mechanism injury such as drilling or mowing.

(2) Look for the following injuries:

(i) Corneal laceration, often with prolapse of the iris into the defect.

(ii) Scleral perforation with chemosis or bulging local haemorrhage. This must be differentiated from a trivial subconjunctival bleed.

(iii) Collapse of the anterior chamber, hyphaema or vitreous haemorrhage, pupil irregularity and lens dislocation.

(3) Intraocular foreign body:

(i) This is usually a metal fragment from using a hammer and chisel, metal drill or grinding wheel.

(ii) Sudden sharp pain is followed by localized redness, or the outside of the eye may appear deceptively normal and the incident forgotten.

(iii) Examine carefully for a puncture wound, and use an ophthalmoscope to inspect the inner eye, although a traumatic cataract may preclude this.

(iv) X-ray the orbit if there is the remotest possibility of penetration. Request two soft-tissue films, with the eye looking up and down, to identify a radiodense intraocular foreign body.

(a) request a CT of the orbit if the X-ray is negative, but suspicion remains high.

(4) Instil antibiotic eye drops (not ointment), protect the eye from further damage with an eye shield, and give tetanus prophylaxis.

(i) Provide analgesia if required, e.g. morphine 5 mg i.v. with an antiemetic such as metoclopramide 10 mg i.v.

(ii) Give gentamicin 5 mg/kg i.v. plus ceftriaxone or cefotaxime 1 g i.v.

(5) Refer all cases of documented penetrating injury to the eye and actual or suspected intraocular foreign bodies immediately to the ophthalmology team.

CONDITIONS AFFECTING THE EYELIDS

BLEPHARITIS

DIAGNOSIS AND MANAGEMENT

(1) Blepharitis is an infection of the eyelid margin, causing red, itchy, crusted lids, which may become chronic with an allergic element.

Styes and chalazions are commonly associated.

(2) Prescribe antibiotic ointment, but refer the patient to the Ophthalmology clinic for follow-up if this condition becomes persistent or recurrent.

EXTERNAL STYE (HORDEOLUM)

DIAGNOSIS AND MANAGEMENT

(1) This is due to an infection of a lash follicle pointing on the lid margin.

(2) Give the patient antibiotic ointment and remove any protruding eyelash. Warm bathing may help.

INTERNAL STYE

DIAGNOSIS AND MANAGEMENT

(1) This is an infected Meibomian gland within the tarsal plate. It does not discharge as easily as an external stye, and it may leave a residual Meibomian cyst.

(2) Alternatively, it may point and discharge inwards through the tarsal plate, causing conjunctivitis and discharge.

(3) Commence flucloxacillin 500 mg orally q.d.s. and refer the patient to the Ophthalmology clinic. Warm bathing is unhelpful.

MEIBOMIAN CYST (CHALAZION)

DIAGNOSIS AND MANAGEMENT

(1) This feels like a hard pip within the tarsal plate, usually from chronic inflammation causing granuloma formation.

(2) Refer the patient to the Ophthalmology clinic for incision and curettage.

DACRYOCYSTITIS

DIAGNOSIS AND MANAGEMENT

(1) Dacryocystitis is inflammation of the lacrimal sac in the inner canthus of the lower eyelid. Dacryoadenitis is inflammation of the lacrimal gland in the outer upper eyelid.

(2) There is a localized, tender, red swelling and watering of the eye due to the blocked lacrimal duct.

(3) Start a systemic antibiotic such as flucloxacillin 500 mg orally q.d.s. after sending a swab of any exuding pus.

(4) Refer the patient to the next Ophthalmology clinic.

ORBITAL CELLULITIS

DIAGNOSIS AND MANAGEMENT

(1) This condition follows sinusitis or a periorbital injury, with intense pain, swelling, reduced eye movements and exophthalmos.

    (i) Infection may be preseptal 'periorbital cellulitis', or post-septal and true 'orbital cellulitis'.

(2) There is generalized malaise, a raised temperature, and a discharging, congested eye. Adjacent sinuses are tender when associated with the infection.

(3) Take blood for FBC and two sets of blood cultures and give flucloxacillin 2 g i.v. plus ceftriaxone 1 g i.v. or cefotaxime 1 g i.v.

(4) Refer the patient immediately to the ophthalmology team, and obtain a CT scan and ENT opinion if the paranasal sinuses are involved.

(5) Complications, particularly in children, can occur within hours, including central retinal vein occlusion, optic nerve compression, cavernous sinus thrombosis and meningitis.

BASAL CELL CARCINOMA (RODENT ULCER)

DIAGNOSIS AND MANAGEMENT

(1) Basal cell carcinoma is the commonest malignancy of the eyelid, more frequent on the lower lid and following prolonged exposure to sunlight.

(2) An early, opalescent pink papule with surface telangiectasia progresses slowly to an ulcerated nodule with a pearly, rounded edge that is locally invasive.

(3) Refer the patient to the next Ophthalmology clinic for treatment by excision, curettage, cryotherapy or radiotherapy in the elderly.

OPHTHALMIC SHINGLES (HERPES ZOSTER OPHTHALMICUS)

DIAGNOSIS AND MANAGEMENT

(1) This presents as a vesicular rash over the distribution of the ophthalmic division of the trigeminal (Vth) cranial nerve. Pain and

tingling often precede the rash.

(2) The patient is usually unwell and in pain. The eye may be involved, resulting in blepharitis, conjunctivitis, keratitis, uveitis, secondary glaucoma, ophthalmoplegia or optic neuritis.

(3) Treatment of the varied ocular problems is awkward, as eyelid swelling makes topical therapy difficult and pain may be incapacitating.

(4) Start aciclovir 800 mg orally five times daily with 3% aciclovir ophthalmic ointment or famciclovir 250 mg orally t.d.s. to decrease pain, corneal damage and uveitis.

(5) Refer the patient to the Ophthalmology team for inpatient care.

THE PAINFUL, RED EYE

There are five important causes to consider:
- Acute conjunctivitis
- Acute episcleritis and scleritis
- Acute keratitis
- Acute iritis
- Acute glaucoma

ACUTE CONJUNCTIVITIS

DIAGNOSIS

(1) The causes are:
   (i) Allergic.
   (ii) Bacterial, e.g. staphylococci, pneumococci, *Haemophilus* or gonococci.
   (iii) Viral, particularly adenovirus or enterovirus.
   (iv) Chlamydial.

(2) There is generalized conjunctival injection, with gritty discomfort, mild photophobia and variable discharge. Vision should be normal.

MANAGEMENT

(1) Advise the patient to clean away the discharge with moist cotton-wool balls, and avoid irritating cosmetics and eye lotions.

(2) Allergic conjunctivitis responds to NSAID, sodium cromoglycate, or steroid eye drops, but the latter should only be prescribed by an

ophthalmologist.
    (i)   Initially prevent secondary bacterial infection with antibiotic drops and refer the patient to the Ophthalmology clinic.
(3) Viral conjunctivitis, due to the adenovirus ('pink eye') or enterovirus, is highly contagious and person-to-person spread is rapid unless scrupulous care is taken with hand washing.
    (i)   Give antibiotic drops and ointment to prevent secondary bacterial infection.
    (ii) Refer the patient to the next Ophthalmology clinic for a definitive diagnosis and to monitor for the development of keratitis.
(4) Bacterial conjunctivitis requires frequent antibiotic drops, as often as hourly in severe cases, and ointment at night. Refer the patient to the Ophthalmology clinic if the infection does not settle.
(5) Chlamydial conjunctivitis usually occurs in young adults, causing chronic bilateral conjunctivitis with mucopurulent discharge. The cornea may be involved (keratitis).
    (i)   The diagnosis is difficult but should be suspected when conventional antibiotic therapy fails.
    (ii) Associated urethritis or salpingitis may suggest the aetiology.
    (iii) Take special swabs for antigen detection, polymerase chain reaction (PCR) or culture, and treat with azithromycin 1 g orally.
    (iv) Discuss with the patient the need to attend a Genitourinary Medicine clinic (Special Clinic) for further contact screening and treatment.

ACUTE EPISCLERITIS AND SCLERITIS

DIAGNOSIS
(1) Episcleritis is localized inflammation beneath the conjunctiva adjacent to the sclera that resolves spontaneously in 1–2 weeks.
(2) Scleritis is a more painful inflammation of the sclera itself. Rheumatoid arthritis, SLE and other systemic illnesses such as sarcoid and TB may be associated.
(3) The eye is locally red in episcleritis, and diffusely red and sore with reflex watering but no discharge in scleritis. Progression to eyeball perforation may occur in scleritis.
(4) Send blood for FBC, ESR, rheumatoid factor, ANA and DNA antibodies. Commence a non-steroidal anti-inflammatory agent

such as ibuprofen 200–400 mg orally t.d.s. or naproxen 250 mg orally t.d.s.

MANAGEMENT

(1) Refer the patient to the ophthalmology team for definitive treatment, including steroid eye drops.

ACUTE KERATITIS

DIAGNOSIS

(1) There are many possible causes of inflammation of the cornea, including viruses such as herpes simplex virus (HSV) and the adenovirus, bacterial infection of a corneal ulcer, abrasion, exposure, or wearing contact lenses.

(2) The main distinguishing feature from conjunctivitis is the prominent pain, with diminution of vision if there is a central ulcer or a hypopyon (pus in the anterior chamber).

(3) Use fluorescein staining to demonstrate a marginal or central ulcer, or the typically branching, dendritic ulcer of herpes simplex.

MANAGEMENT

(1) Commence antibiotic drops or 3% aciclovir ointment five times daily for herpes simplex ulceration. Refer the patient immediately to the ophthalmology team.

(2) Steroid eye drops are absolutely forbidden.

ACUTE IRITIS

DIAGNOSIS

(1) Although most are idiopathic, iritis is occasionally due to exogenous infection from a perforating wound or corneal ulcer.

(2) Otherwise, ill-understood endogenous mechanisms, some linked with HLA-B27 and seronegative arthropathy, may be causally related such as ankylosing spondylitis, Reiter's syndrome, ulcerative colitis, Crohn's disease, and Still's disease.

    (i) Rarer causes still include sarcoidosis, toxoplasmosis, Behçet's, TB and herpes zoster ophthalmicus.

(3) There is circumcorneal ciliary injection, constant pain, photophobia and impaired vision. The pupil contracts, and tiny aggregates of cells, known as keratic precipitates (KPs) may be seen

on the inner surface of the cornea.

(4)   Pus forms in the anterior chamber causing a hypopyon in severe cases, and the iris may adhere to the anterior lens surface causing posterior synechiae.

MANAGEMENT

(1)   Refer the patient immediately to the ophthalmology team for treatment with steroid drops and a cycloplegic such as homatropine.

(2)   Attacks may become recurrent and progress to secondary glaucoma.

ACUTE GLAUCOMA

DIAGNOSIS

(1)   Glaucoma is associated with a narrowed anterior chamber with obstruction to the outflow of aqueous humour.

(2)   It is more common in middle-aged or elderly hypermetropes (long-sighted people), and is precipitated by pupillary dilation.

(3)   There is severe throbbing, boring pain accompanied by headache, nausea, vomiting and prostration.

  (i)   Vision is reduced with haloes around lights, and the cornea becomes hazy with a fixed, semi-dilated oval pupil. On gentle palpation the eye feels hard.

MANAGEMENT

This is an ocular emergency requiring urgent referral to the Ophthalmology team. On their advice commence:

(1)   Miotic drops such as pilocarpine every 5 minutes for up to 1 hour.

(2)   Acetazolamide 500 mg slowly i.v. then 250 mg i.v. or orally t.d.s. – but contraindicated in sulphonamide allergy.

(3)   An antiemetic such as metoclopramide 10 mg i.v. and analgesia such as morphine up to 2.5 mg i.v. for severe pain.

SUDDEN LOSS OF VISION IN THE UNINFLAMED EYE

Conditions to be considered include:

- ● Central retinal artery occlusion
- ● Central retinal vein occlusion

- Vitreous haemorrhage
- Retinal detachment
- Optic neuritis

CENTRAL RETINAL ARTERY OCCLUSION

DIAGNOSIS

(1) This condition is most common in the elderly arteriosclerotic patient, but it may occur due to emboli or in association with temporal arteritis.

(2) There is sudden blindness associated with a relative afferent pupillary defect (RAPD), known as a Marcus Gunn pupil:
   (i) A swinging light directed into one eye then briskly into the other produces apparent dilation of the pupil in the affected eye, as the relaxing consensual reflex in the good eye is dominant.
   (ii) It is an excellent sign of a unilateral or asymmetrical optic nerve or retinal lesion.

(3) The fundus is milky white, the optic disc is pale and swollen, and a cherry-red spot develops at the macula in 1–2 days.

MANAGEMENT

(1) Commence acetazolamide 500 mg slowly i.v. to reduce intraocular pressure.

(2) Give gentle pulsed ocular massage with sustained pressure on the globe for 5–10 seconds, followed by sudden release repeated for 10–15 minutes.

(3) Refer the patient urgently to the Ophthalmology team, as treatment within 1–2 hours including anterior chamber paracentesis may restore the retinal circulation.

(4) When there is a prodromal history of headache, scalp tenderness and malaise, consider temporal arteritis causing anterior ischaemic optic neuropathy with optic disc oedema.
   (i) Measure an ESR and, if raised, give the patient prednisolone 60 mg orally to prevent the other eye becoming involved (see p. 78).

CENTRAL RETINAL VEIN OCCLUSION

DIAGNOSIS

(1) This condition is most common in elderly patients with atherosclerosis, hypertension and simple glaucoma. Diabetes and hyperviscosity also predispose to this.

(2) Visual loss is less abrupt but may be noticed suddenly. An RAPD (Marcus Gunn pupil) may be seen in extensive cases.

(3) The fundus shows congested veins with scattered flame haemorrhages and optic disc swelling.

MANAGEMENT

(1) There is no specific treatment, although predisposing conditions must be looked for.

(2) Refer the patient to the Ophthalmology clinic to monitor for the development of secondary acute glaucoma (some weeks later) from neovascularization.

VITREOUS HAEMORRHAGE

DIAGNOSIS

(1) This may be traumatic or spontaneous, associated with diabetes, various blood disorders, and chronic central or branch retinal vein occlusion.

(2) There is a reduced or absent red reflex and diminution in vision, preceded by a history of 'cobwebs' or 'floaters'.

MANAGEMENT

(1) Refer the patient to the Ophthalmology team to exclude retinal detachment and to look for other predisposing conditions.

(2) Vitrectomy may be necessary if the haemorrhage fails to clear.

RETINAL DETACHMENT

DIAGNOSIS

(1) This may be traumatic, or spontaneous in myopes (short-sighted people), or may follow a vitreous haemorrhage.

(2) There is peripheral visual loss, like a curtain, which may be profound if the macula is affected. A preceding history of sudden flashes of light or floaters is common.

(3) The retina is dark, wrinkled and ballooned, and the choroid may appear as a red tear, although peripheral detachments may not be seen.

   (i) An RAPD (Marcus Gunn pupil) only occurs if the detachment is large.

MANAGEMENT

(1) Refer the patient immediately to the Ophthalmology team for possible surgical repair.

OPTIC NEURITIS

DIAGNOSIS

(1) This may be idiopathic, post-viral or associated with demyelination from multiple sclerosis.

(2) There is more gradual loss of central, particularly colour vision, with pain on moving the eye, and an RAPD (Marcus Gunn pupil).

(3) There is papillitis if the optic disc is involved, which must be distinguished from papilloedema.

   (i) Papilloedema tends to be bilateral and pain-free with normal pupil responses. There is no visual loss, but an enlarged blind spot is found on field testing.

(4) Examine the patient for other signs of demyelination, but never inform him or her of your suspicions at this early stage.

MANAGEMENT

(1) Refer the patient to the Ophthalmology clinic.

FURTHER READING

Cochrane Collaboration.
http://www.cochrane.org/reviews/en/topics/63.html/ (Cochrane review topics: Eyes and vision).

Durkin SR, Casey TM (2005) Beware of the unilateral red eye: don't miss blinding uveitis. *Med J Aust* **182**:296-7.

MAXILLOFACIAL AND DENTAL EMERGENCIES

TRAUMATIC CONDITIONS OF THE FACE AND MOUTH

LACERATIONS

MANAGEMENT
(1) *Face*
   (i) Meticulously debride facial cuts under local anaesthesia, and suture using fine 5/0 non-absorbable monofilament nylon or polypropylene sutures, removed by 4 days.
(2) *Lips*
   (i) Use 3/0 or 4/0 absorbable sutures such as polydioxanone or polyglactin for intraoral lesions, and 5/0 non-absorbable monofilament nylon or polypropylene sutures for external lacerations.
   (ii) Refer the patient to the Oral Surgery team if the full thickness of the lip is lacerated vertically, breaching the vermilion border, to avoid cosmetic deformity from inexperienced repair.
(3) *Tongue*
   (i) Leave most lacerations unless they are larger than 1 cm or through the edge, or bleeding profusely. In these cases repair with an absorbable suture such as 3/0 polydioxanone or polyglactin.
   (ii) Advise regular mouthwash of warm saline.

TOOTH INJURIES

MANAGEMENT
(1) *Chipped tooth*
   (i) *Enamel or dentine damage:* the tooth will be sensitive but viable. Advise the patient to avoid hot and cold drinks and refer to the patient's own dentist within 24 hours.
   (ii) *Pulp space exposed:* the tooth may be bleeding from the pulp, and sensitive to light touch. Refer the patient immediately to the Oral Surgery team, as there is a risk of pulp infection or necrosis.
(2) *Displaced tooth*
   (i) Do not manipulate unless the tooth is about to fall out, in

which case it should be firmly replaced in its socket.

(ii) Refer the patient to a dental surgeon as soon as possible for immobilization of the tooth.

(3) *Avulsed permanent incisor tooth*

The best chance of successful re-implantation is by reposition of an avulsed tooth within 30 minutes outside its socket, or up to 2 hours if stored in saliva or milk.

(i) Transport the tooth in the buccal sulcus of the patient's own cheek, or in milk or saline if immediate re-implantation is not possible, when the patient is uncooperative or unconscious.

(ii) Handle the tooth by the crown only on arrival in the Emergency Department, rinse it in saline, and replace back into the socket with firm pressure. No analgesia is necessary.

(iii) Splint the tooth with aluminium foil, give the patient an antibiotic such as amoxicillin 500 mg orally t.d.s., and give tetanus prophylaxis.

(a) an avulsed tooth is considered a 'tetanus-prone' wound (see p. 323).

(iv) Refer the patient to a dental surgeon as soon as possible.

> **!** **Warning:** whenever a tooth or denture is found to be missing following trauma, perform an AP and lateral CXR to exclude inhalation into the lung, or AP and lateral neck X-rays to exclude obstruction in the upper oesophagus (see p. 413).

(4) *Bleeding tooth socket*

(i) This can be post-traumatic or post-extraction.

(ii) Clear out clots and arrest haemorrhage using a calcium alginate (Kaltostat™) dressing or gauze roll. Ask the patient to bite on it for 15–30 minutes.

(iii) Infiltrate with 1% lignocaine (lidocaine) with 1 in 200 000 adrenaline (epinephrine) if the bleeding persists, and close the mucosa over the socket using 3/0 absorbable polydioxanone or polyglactin sutures. Refer the patient to the Oral Surgery team if this fails.

(5) *Broken dentures*

(i) Always save these as they will be invaluable to the maxillofacial surgeon to aid in the fixation of jaw fractures, or if a splint is needed.

FRACTURED MANDIBLE

(1) This is due to a blow on the jaw causing a unilateral or frequently bilateral fracture. Occasionally, the temporomandibular joint may be dislocated or the condylar process driven back into the temporal bone, causing bleeding and deformity of the external auditory canal.

(2) Look for localized pain, particularly on attempted jaw movement and malocclusion. Inside the mouth, bruising or bleeding of the gum and discontinuity of the teeth are seen if there is a displaced fracture.

(3) Assess for numbness of the lower lip if the inferior dental nerve has been damaged in its course through the mandible.

(4) Request X-rays including an anteroposterior view, with a panoramic orthopantomogram (OPG) or lateral views of the mandible.

MANAGEMENT

(1) Clear the airway of any clots or debris, and ensure that the tongue or a portion of the mandible does not slip back and occlude the pharynx.

(2) Refer any unstable or grossly displaced injuries immediately to the Maxillofacial Surgery team.

(3) Otherwise, give the patient tetanus prophylaxis and antibiotics for an undisplaced fracture, as most fractures are compound into the mouth.

  (i) Give amoxicillin 500 mg and clavulanic acid 125 mg one tablet orally t.d.s. for 5 days.

(4) Refer the patient to the next Maxillofacial Surgery clinic.

DISLOCATED MANDIBLE

(1) Dislocation may occur spontaneously after yawning or it may follow a blow to the jaw. It may be unilateral or more commonly bilateral and may become recurrent.

(2) The mouth is stuck open and is painful.

(3) Ask about possible drug-induced dystonia to metoclopramide or phenothiazines on direct questioning, as this may mimic or even predispose to dislocation.

(i) Treat this with benzatropine 1–2 mg i.v. followed by 2 mg orally once daily for 3 days (see p. 330).

(4) Request an anteroposterior and lateral X-ray of the temporomandibular joints to exclude an associated fracture, unless the dislocation was spontaneous or recurrent.

MANAGEMENT

(1) Try to reduce without sedation in the absence of a fracture. Give diazepam 0.1–0.2 mg/kg i.v. or midazolam 0.05–0.1 mg/kg i.v. with full resuscitation facilities available if unsuccessful.

(2) Reduction of the dislocation:

(i) Stand in front of the patient and press firmly downwards applying pressure to the angle of the jaw, with your gauze-wrapped thumbs inside the mouth to distract the condyle, placing your fingers under the chin. Then push backwards to relocate the condyle in the fossa.

(ii) Reduce one side at a time in bilateral dislocations.

(iii) Repeat the X-ray to confirm reduction, and refer to the next Maxillofacial Surgery clinic. Advise the patient to avoid excessive mouth opening.

(iv) Apply a barrel bandage to discourage wide opening if the dislocation is recurrent or required diazepam or midazolam i.v.

FRACTURE OF THE ZYGOMATIC OR MALAR COMPLEX

DIAGNOSIS

(1) This injury is due to a direct blow to the cheek, which may fracture the zygomatic arch in isolation, or more usually causes a 'tripod' fracture through three structures:

(i) Superiorly through the zygomaticofrontal suture.

(ii) Laterally through the zygomatic arch or zygomaticotemporal suture.

(iii) Medially through the zygomaticomaxillary suture or the infraorbital foramen region.

(2) There is flattening of the malar process best seen from above (which may become masked by oedema), epistaxis, subconjunctival haemorrhage extending posteriorly, and infraorbital nerve paraesthesia.

(i) Jaw movement may be limited if the coronoid process obstructs under the zygomatic arch.

(3) Although these fractures are best diagnosed clinically, particularly by finding local bony tenderness, request facial X-rays including occipitomental views (OM 10° and OM 30°).

    (i) Look carefully for the fractures, comparing with the normal side.

    (ii) Or look for secondary evidence of injury, e.g. opacity of the maxillary antrum from bleeding into the maxillary sinus or overlying soft-tissue swelling.

    (iii) Request a CT scan for more extensive injuries, including an additional 'blow-out' fracture of the orbital floor.

MANAGEMENT

(1) Advise the patient *not* to blow his or her nose, as subcutaneous emphysema may develop if the paranasal sinuses are involved.

(2) Commence amoxicillin 500 mg orally t.d.s. (or erythromycin 500 mg orally q.d.s. if the patient is allergic) as most fractures are compound into the maxillary sinus, with an analgesic such as paracetamol 500 mg and codeine phosphate 8 mg two tablets orally q.d.s.

(3) Refer the patient to the Maxillofacial Surgery team within 24 hours for elevation of the depressed cheekbone within 7 days.

'BLOW-OUT' FRACTURE OF THE ORBITAL FLOOR

DIAGNOSIS

(1) This uncommon fracture is due to blunt trauma to the eye from a small object about the size of a squash ball, that drives the eyeball backwards and ruptures the weak bony floor of the orbit.

    (i) Orbital fat and occasionally the inferior rectus muscle herniate through the defect into the maxillary sinus.

(2) Exclude blunt trauma to the eye initially (see p. 421). The fracture itself causes enophthalmos, which may be masked by periorbital oedema, infraorbital nerve loss and diplopia with restricted upwards gaze due to trapping of the inferior rectus muscle or orbital fat.

(3) Request facial X-rays, although these rarely show the fracture itself. It can be inferred from an opaque maxillary sinus or a fluid level from bleeding, and a 'tear drop' soft-tissue opacity hanging from the roof of the sinus.

(4) Request a CT scan if there is doubt, as this demonstrates the fracture clearly.

MANAGEMENT
(1) Refer blunt eye damage immediately to the Ophthalmology team.
(2) Commence amoxicillin 500 mg orally t.d.s. and 1% chloramphenicol eye ointment 4-hourly.
(3) Refer the patient to the Maxillofacial Surgery team within 24 hours.

MIDDLE-THIRD OF FACE FRACTURES

DIAGNOSIS

These complicated fractures are usually bilateral and are divided into three groups:
(1) *Le Fort I*
    (i) This is due to a blow to the maxilla causing a horizontal fracture separating the alveolar bone and teeth from the maxilla.
    (ii) There is epistaxis and malocclusion, and crepitus may be elicited.
(2) *Le Fort II*
    (i) This is a pyramidal fracture extending up from a Le Fort I fracture to involve the nasal skeleton and the middle of the face. The middle of the face is thus 'stove in', elongating the face and causing malocclusion.
    (ii) The airway may be compromised and CSF may leak from the nose.
(3) *Le Fort III*
    (i) This dislocates the entire mid-facial skeleton from the base of the skull (craniofacial dysjunction).
    (ii) There is massive facial swelling and bruising, and often brisk pharyngeal bleeding that may cause haemorrhagic shock. The airway is again in danger.
(4) Remember that the blow to the face may have caused an additional cervical spine injury or head injury.
    (i) Request a lateral cervical spine X-ray and a head CT scan, which become the priority after airway stabilization.
    (ii) Delay any specific facial-view X-rays until all the other major injuries are stabilized and a cervical spine injury is excluded, unless a CT scan of the face is combined with the head CT scan.

MANAGEMENT
(1) Attend urgently to the airway.
  (i) Sometimes, if the face is stove in, manually lifting the whole segment forwards relieves the airway.
  (ii) Call immediately for senior ED doctor help if there is difficulty maintaining an adequate airway, and prepare for orotracheal intubation or even a cricothyrotomy.
(2) Refer all mid-face fractures immediately to the Maxillofacial Surgery team.

NON-TRAUMATIC CONDITIONS OF THE MOUTH

TOOTHACHE

DIAGNOSIS AND MANAGEMENT
(1) Toothache is usually due to inflammation of the pulp space in a carious tooth.
(2) Exclude a dental abscess (see below) and give the patient an analgesic such as paracetamol 500 mg and codeine phosphate 8 mg two tablets orally q.d.s.
(3) Return the patient to his or her own dentist.

DENTAL ABSCESS

DIAGNOSIS AND MANAGEMENT
(1) An apical or periapical abscess is an extension of a pulp space infection.
  (i) The tooth is tender on tapping, with associated soft-tissue swelling and continuous pain.
  (ii) There may be systemic malaise and fever.
(2) Refer the patient to the Oral Surgery team if severely ill, or the abscess is pointing extra-orally.
(3) Otherwise, commence an antibiotic such as amoxicillin 500 mg orally t.d.s. then give an analgesic (e.g. codeine phosphate 30–60 mg orally q.d.s.) and return the patient to his or her own dentist.

LUDWIG'S ANGINA

DIAGNOSIS AND MANAGEMENT
(1) This condition is a bilateral, fulminant, brawny cellulitis of the sublingual and submandibular areas, associated with poor dental hygiene or dental instrumentation.
(2) There is trismus, dysphagia, submandibular pain and swelling, and a risk of sudden respiratory obstruction from displacement of the tongue.
(3) Call immediately for senior ED doctor help, and prepare for orotracheal intubation or even a cricothyrotomy.
(4) Give benzylpenicillin 1.8 g i.v. and metronidazole 500 mg i.v. and admit the patient immediately under the ENT team for careful observation of the airway.
(5) Request a CT scan only if the airway is protected, or not considered at risk.

SUBMANDIBULAR SWELLINGS

DIAGNOSIS AND MANAGEMENT
Look for the following possible causes:
(1) *Submandibular stone*
    This intermittently blocks the submandibular duct, causing pain and swelling aggravated by food. The stone is palpable on bimanual examination in the floor of the mouth and is seen on X-ray. Refer the patient to the Oral Surgery team.
(2) *Submandibular abscess*
    The pain is constant with associated malaise, swelling in the angle of the jaw, and trismus. Refer the patient to the Oral Surgery team.
(3) *Dental abscess*
    This may point downwards from a molar tooth to the submandibular area. Treat with antibiotics and analgesia and refer to the Oral Surgery team.
(4) *Lymph node enlargement*
    The most common causes of cervical adenopathy in this area are tonsillitis and pharyngitis.
(5) *Mumps*
    This affects the parotids and is usually bilateral, but can affect the submandibular glands. Remember the association with orchitis. Give the patient paracetamol elixir, and reassure them.

(6) *Rare*

These include carcinoma, lymphoma, sarcoid, TB, osteomyelitis, and a bony cyst or fibrous dysplasia. Refer to the appropriate specialty team.

FURTHER READING

Cochrane Collaboration.
http://www.cochrane.org/reviews/en/topics/84.html/ (Cochrane review topics: Oral health).

PSYCHIATRIC EMERGENCIES

DELIBERATE SELF-HARM

DIAGNOSIS

(1) The most common method of deliberate self-harm is by acute poisoning.

    (i) This may be admitted freely, or may be evident from finding a suicide note or an empty bottle beside the patient.

    (ii) The possibility should also be considered in any unconscious or confused patient, or in patients with unexplained metabolic, respiratory or cardiac problems (see p. 148).

(2) Other more violent methods of deliberate self-harm include cutting the wrists or throat, shooting, hanging, suffocation, gassing, jumping from a height, and drowning.

(3) Perform a formal psychiatric assessment when the patient has made a full recovery, is alert and orientated and all necessary medical therapy is completed. This will help determine the further management of the patient.

    (i) Assessment of current suicidal intent.
    Enquire specifically about:

        (a) present suicidal thoughts

        (b) previous deliberate self-harm

        (c) evidence of a pre-meditated act without the intention of being found.

    (ii) Determine other high-risk factors for completed suicide:

        (a) mental illness including depression and schizophrenia; severe anxiety

        (b) violent self-harm attempt, such as jumping, hanging or shooting

        (c) previous self-harm attempt

        (d) chronic alcohol abuse, drug dependence, unemployment, homelessness

        (e) older, single, urban, lonely male

        (f) chronic, painful or terminal physical illness

        (g) puerperium.

    (iii) Record a general mental state examination:

        (a) general appearance, behaviour, attitudes

        (b) speech including pressure of speech, neologisms

        (c) mood and affect, appropriateness

        (d) thought processes for content and form

    (e) perception including delusions and hallucinations
       (especially auditory)
    (f) cognition (see Table 1.5 on p. 60)
    (g) insight and judgement
    (h) impulsivity.

MANAGEMENT

(1) Perform the necessary investigations and resuscitative procedures to save life, and refer the patient directly to the medical, surgical or orthopaedic team if there is serious illness or injury.

(2) A medically unimportant acute poisoning, including a patient intoxicated with alcohol, may have been a serious self-harm attempt.

    (i) Admit the patient for 24 hours, possibly to the Emergency Department's own observation ward.

(3) Then refer any patient considered to have a continuing suicide risk or mental illness behaviour immediately to the psychiatric team.

(4) Alternatively, make a Psychiatric outpatient appointment for the patient if there is no current suicidal intent, no high-risk factor for completed suicide, and a normal mental state examination.

(5) Refer problems with a domestic or social basis to the Social Work team.

(6) Inform the GP by fax and letter in all cases, if the patient is allowed home. The patient should ideally be accompanied by a relative or friend when they go.

THE VIOLENT PATIENT

DIAGNOSIS

(1) Much violence encountered by staff in the Emergency Department will be the result of alcohol intoxication, either by the patient or by their relatives or friends, who may be irritated and angry at having to wait if the department is busy.

(2) Other causes for violent behaviour include:

    (i) Hypoglycaemia, including as the patient recovers from a hypoglycaemic episode after i.v. dextrose administration.

    (ii) Hypoxia.

    (iii) Post-ictal state.

(iv) Other organic confusional state (see p. 58).

(v) Drugs, including amphetamines, LSD and cocaine.

(vi) Withdrawal syndromes from alcohol or barbiturates.

(vii) Mental illness especially mania and paranoid schizophrenia, personality disorder.

MANAGEMENT

(1) Explain what is happening at all times, reassure the patient, and avoid confrontation. Never turn your back on a patient or allow them between you and the cubicle door.

(2) Attempt verbal restraint by defining acceptable and unacceptable behaviour and their likely consequences. Speak firmly with courtesy and respect.

(3) Consider physical restraint if verbal restraint fails.

(i) Call the police or security guards, and await adequate numbers, ideally five or six people, as a 'show of force'.

(ii) Never try to restrain a patient single-handedly, particularly if they have a weapon.

(iii) Conversely, never remove physical restraints until a full evaluation has been made and help is standing by.

(4) Consider chemical restraint if physical restraint fails.

(i) Give diazepam 5–10 mg i.v. or midazolam 5–10 mg i.v. for rapid control. This may be supplemented with haloperidol or droperidol 5–10 mg i.m. or slowly i.v.

(ii) Such treatment may be given without consent under common law in an emergency if the patient is a danger to others or themselves.

(iii) Monitor every sedated patient in a resuscitation area until the risks of respiratory depression and hypotension have passed.

(iv) Complete a full physical examination, looking for evidence of organic disease (see p. 59).

(5) Record exact details of events and the necessary action taken in the notes.

(6) Admit the patient under the Medical or Psychiatric team if further treatment is indicated.

(7) Debrief staff in the Emergency Department, and consider immediate support for staff injury or intimidation.

(i) Plan future strategies for violence prevention and management.

ALCOHOL AND DRUG DEPENDENCY AND ABUSE

ALCOHOL AND DRUG WITHDRAWAL

DIAGNOSIS AND MANAGEMENT

(1) Patients may be seen who are dependent on or abuse the following classes of drugs:

(i) Alcohol.

(ii) Opiates.

(iii) Stimulants including amphetamines and cocaine.

(iv) Sedatives including benzodiazepines and barbiturates.

(v) Miscellaneous substances including cannabis, LSD and solvents.

(2) Abrupt withdrawal of many of these drugs causes acute symptoms.

(i) Alcohol withdrawal causes agitation, irritability, tremor and seizures, then delirium tremens (see p. 64).

(a) give a benzodiazepine i.v. or orally if symptoms are distressing

(b) seek help for the patient from an expert Addiction unit.

(ii) Opiate withdrawal causes restlessness, excitability, muscle cramps, diarrhoea, tachycardia and sweating – known as 'cold turkey'.

(a) give a benzodiazepine i.v. or orally if symptoms are distressing

(b) seek help for the patient from an expert Addiction unit.

(iii) Benzodiazepine withdrawal causes a rebound increase in tension, anxiety and apprehension, with anorexia, insomnia and epileptic seizures.

(a) seek help for the patient from an expert Addiction unit.

(iv) Barbiturate withdrawal causes hallucinations and epileptic seizures.

(a) seek help for the patient from an expert Addiction unit.

PROBLEM DRINKING

DIAGNOSIS

(1) Alcohol misuse is related to many Emergency Department presentations, from falls, collapse, head injury and assault to non-specific gastrointestinal problems, psychiatric problems and the repeat attender.

(2) Ask the patient directly if they drink alcohol, how much on a regular daily basis, and whether their attendance is related to alcohol.

(3) Or use a validated screening questionnaire such as the CAGE (see Table 15.1).

(4) Alternatively, alcohol-dependent patients may themselves request help or be brought in by concerned others to stop drinking.

Table 15.1 CAGE screening questionnaire for alcohol abuse

C	Have you ever felt you should **C**ut down on your drinking?
A	Have people **A**nnoyed you by criticising your drinking?
G	Have you ever felt bad or **G**uilty about your drinking?
E	Have you ever had a drink as an **E**ye-opener first thing in the morning to steady your nerves or help get rid of a hangover?

Yes to two or more indicates probable chronic alcohol abuse or dependence.

MANAGEMENT

(1) Refer the patient immediately to the Psychiatric team if there is actual suicidal depression or total inability to cope at home.

(2) Otherwise, refer the patient to the appropriate hospital or community clinic for Outpatient assessment.

  (i) Or refer to the Social Work department or a special Alcohol Health Worker for a brief intervention programme, including advice and management on alcohol-related harm to health.

(3) Meanwhile, give the patient the telephone numbers of local support organizations to contact, such as Alcoholics Anonymous and Al-Anon. These provide help and advice to both the problem drinker and their family and friends.

(4) Always write to or fax the GP to enlist their help and support.

OPIATE AND INTRAVENOUS DRUG ADDICTION

MANAGEMENT

(1) Admit opiate and intravenous drug-addicted patients under the Medical team in the usual way, when they develop the following particular medical emergency complications:

  (i) Acute poisoning (see p. 148).

  (ii) Cellulitis and abscesses.

  (iii) Pulmonary and cerebral infections.

    (iv) Septicaemia.

    (v) Bacterial endocarditis.

    (vi) Hepatitis B, C or D, and, increasingly, HIV infection.

(2) Otherwise, when a regular opiate user needs admission to the Emergency Department observation ward, perhaps following an orthopaedic or minor operative procedure:

    (i) Give salicylate or paracetamol for mild or moderate pain, and methadone orally or i.m. for severe pain.

    (ii) Give the patient diazepam 5–10 mg orally if signs of opiate withdrawal occur, repeated as required.

(3) Refer patients wishing to stop their habit and seeking help to:

    (i) A drug dependency clinic.

    (ii) A drug dependency 24-hour emergency organization such as Narcotics Anonymous.

    (iii) The Social Work department.

    (iv) The patient's own GP.

> (!) **Warning:** if a patient should demand a controlled drug, explain that it is actually an offence for a doctor to administer or authorize the supply of a drug of addiction, except in the treatment of an organic disease or injury, unless licensed to do so.

BENZODIAZEPINE, BARBITURATE AND SOLVENT ADDICTION

MANAGEMENT

(1) Patients who are addicted to these groups of drugs all require referral to specialist clinics to coordinate their withdrawal regimen. Help and advice is available from:

    (i) Psychiatric outpatient clinics.

    (ii) A local Drug Dependency organization including self-help groups.

    (iii) The Social Work department.

    (iv) The patient's own GP.

INVOLUNTARY DETENTION

(1) It is rarely necessary to detain a patient against his or her will in or through the Emergency Department under the prevailing local Mental Health Act (MHA).

    (i) Always request the help and advice of the Psychiatric team in such circumstances. It is unusual to have to act in their absence.

(2) Generic criteria that must be fulfilled for instigating involuntary assessment include:

    (i) The person appears to have a mental illness that requires immediate assessment at an authorized mental health service.

    (ii) There is a risk the person may cause harm to self or another, or might suffer serious mental or physical deterioration.

    (iii) Plus there is no less restrictive way of ensuring the patient is assessed.

    (iv) And the person is lacking the capacity to consent to be assessed or has unreasonably refused to be assessed.

(3) Various broad types of order or Section for regulated (compulsory) admission exist according to the MHA policy in use locally.

    (i) Make sure you know details of the local policy, which varies from country to country, and state to state.

    (ii) Most include an emergency 24-hour to 3-day detention order signed by the police or a medical practitioner.

    (iii) Or a 3-day, or 21-day, or 28-day or longer detention period may be applied for by an authorized person or nearest relative and supported by a medical recommendation.

(4) All regulated patients admitted involuntarily are then subject to mandatory psychiatric review according to the local MHA legislation.

(5) Make sure you also know who can sign which order, when the order lapses, and what it allows the medical practitioner to do.

    (i) In particular, make sure you understand the distinction between involuntary detention for assessment, and administering emergency treatment without consent under common law.

FURTHER READING

ACEP Policies Subcommittee (2006) Clinical policy. Critical issues in the diagnosis and management of the adult psychiatric patient in the emergency department. *Ann Emerg Med* **47**:79–86.

Crawford MJ, Patton R, Touquet R *et al.* (2004) Screening and referral for brief intervention of alcohol-misusing patients in an emergency department: A pragmatic randomised controlled trial. *Lancet* **364**:1334–9.

Eddey D, Mason S (2004) Mental health and the law: the Australasian and UK perspectives. In: Cameron P, Jelinek G, Kelly A-M *et al. Textbook of Adult Emergency Medicine*, 2nd edn, pp. 660–67. Churchill Livingstone, Edinburgh.

Touquet R, Brown A (2006) Alcohol misuse – Positive response. Alcohol Health Work for every acute hospital saves money and reduces repeat attendances. *Emerg Med Australas* **18**:103–7.

ADMINISTRATIVE AND LEGAL ISSUES

EXCELLENT HABITS OF THE GOOD EMERGENCY DEPARTMENT DOCTOR

THE EXCELLENT EMERGENCY DEPARTMENT (ED) DOCTOR

The excellent ED doctor cultivates the following good habits:
- Listens to the patient
- Continually refines a possible diagnosis when assessing a patient ('rules in'), and the differential diagnoses ('rules out'), never trivializing, so starting with potentially the most severe conditions
- Seeks advice and avoids getting out of depth by asking for help
- Treats all patients with dignity and compassion
- Makes sure the patient and relatives know at all times what is happening, and why, and what any apparent waits are for
- Maintains a collective sense of teamwork, by considering all ED colleagues as equals whether medical, nursing, allied health, or administrative
- Consistently makes exemplary ED medical records (see below)
- Communicates whenever possible with the GP (see below p. 456)
- Adopts effective risk management techniques (see below p. 456)
- Knows how to break bad news with empathy (see below p. 458)

EMERGENCY DEPARTMENT MEDICAL RECORDS

Record accurate and concise information for every patient examined in the department. Details will obviously vary according to the nature and layout of each department's records. Computerization of the medical record mandates the same high standards of recording.

(1) Ensure all the boxes at the top of the page have been filled in (usually by the reception staff) to identify the patient fully.

(2) Start by printing your own name and designation, and the date and time you commenced seeing the patient.

(3) Write legibly throughout. Other members of staff will be reading your notes, which will be meaningless if they are illegible.

(4) Record all the positive clinical findings in the history and examination, and relevant negative findings.

(5) Avoid the use of abbreviations, except for unambiguous, approved examples, such as BP. Digits should be named not numbered, and 'left' and 'right' should be written in full.

(6) Make detailed notes in assault or motor vehicle crash attendances from the patient's recall of events, or from a witness. Document the exact size of bruises or lacerations measured with a ruler.

    (i) Statements may subsequently be required by the police or a solicitor, and could be requested months or even years later, so you cannot rely on your memory.

    (ii) A photograph is an invaluable record and may save a detailed description. Access to a suitable digital camera is ideal, provided that written and signed consent to take the photo is obtained from the patient.

    (iii) Keep the consent and the photo in the medical record.

(7) Record your diagnosis and differential diagnosis.

(8) Record any investigations performed, and put down the results, including your own interpretation of the ECG or X-ray.

(9) Record whether you discussed the case with a senior ED doctor, their name and grade, the time, and exactly what they advised.

(10) Detail your proposed treatment plan, printing drug names and quantities.

(11) Document any verbal or written instructions or advice given to the patient.

(12) Record the disposition of the patient.

    (i) Record on the notes to whom clinical responsibility has been transferred if you hand the patient over to another ED doctor at the end of your shift.

    (ii) Record the name and seniority of the doctor concerned if you refer to an Inpatient team, and the time the patient was referred.

    (iii) Record the clinic name and the consultant if possible when a patient is referred to Outpatients.

    (iv) Write the ward and the consultant under whom the patient was admitted on the record when a patient is admitted.

    (v) Attach a copy onto the Emergency Department record of any discharge letter to the GP, if the patient is referred back to their own doctor.

    (a) computerization of the medical record now enables a printed letter to be generated for every patient.

(13) Sign your name clearly at the end of the record, and print your name and initials underneath for future identification.

> ✓ **Tip:** Most of the above points may appear obvious, but they are essential to the quality and continuity of the medical care of the patient, and underpin good risk management practice.

COMMUNICATING WITH THE GENERAL PRACTITIONER

Communicate whenever possible with the general practitioner (GP).

(1) Ring the GP to clarify current management, including medications and allergies when the patient is unsure, or for a recent past history in complex or atypical presentations.

(2) Write a letter, keeping a copy in the patient's medical record, if:
  (i) The GP writes a referral letter to you.
  (ii) You do any tests, including bloods, urinalysis, ECG or X-ray, even if they are normal.
  (iii) You make a new diagnosis.
  (iv) You start new medication, or change or stop an existing treatment regimen.
  (v) You refer the patient back to the GP for further care and review, including removing sutures or changing dressings.
  (vi) You refer the patient to Outpatients.
  (vii) The patient is admitted, or a patient is brought in dead (or dies in the department).

(3) Fax the letter, and give the patient a copy to deliver by hand.
  (i) Assume it is likely to be opened and read, so fax, post or email *only* letters containing sensitive information, and when you have any doubt about the reliability or capacity of the patient to transfer the letter on.

RISK MANAGEMENT AND INCIDENT REPORTING

The five mainstays of effective risk management include credentialling of medical staff, incident monitoring and tracking, complaints monitoring and tracking, infection control, and documentation in the medical record.

Whether any or all of these activities are adopted at your hospital, you can begin by empowering yourself.

(1) Know the types of Emergency Department situations that lead to incidents and claims, or to an ED doctor requiring medicolegal assistance from a medical defence organization (MDO). These include:

    (i) Failure to correctly diagnose the patient's medical condition.

    (ii) Delay in diagnosis.

    (iii) Failure to treat the patient.

    (iv) Dissatisfaction with treatment.

    (v) Dissatisfaction with the medical practitioner's conduct.

    (vi) Medicolegal assistance:

        (a) regarding death of a patient

        (b) for a medical report regarding diagnosis and treatment.

(2) Some of the common reasons Emergency Department presentations are reported as incidents to an MDO are for the following failures:

    (i) Failure to diagnose:

        (a) myocardial infarction

        (b) cerebral haemorrhage, particularly subarachnoid

        (c) appendicitis

        (d) torsion of the testis

        (e) All other fractures, e.g. scaphoid, phalanx, neck of femur, talus, calcaneus, etc.

    (ii) Failure to diagnose or treat appropriately:

        (a) tendon/nerve injury, particularly lacerations to the hand or foot

        (b) wounds/wound infections, particularly inadequate debridement and cleaning

        (c) foreign body, including glass and intraocular

        (d) spinal fracture.

    (iii) Made medication error.

(3) Therefore, adopt the following strategies to minimise your medicolegal risk:

    (i) Always ask more senior ED staff for advice when you are unsure.

    (ii) Never stereotype a patient, trivialize their complaint, or jump to an easy conclusion.

    (iii) Follow the guidelines above for good ED record keeping.

    (iv) Learn to be an excellent communicator – with the patient, your medical colleagues, nursing staff, and with the GP.

(v) Be a team player and use the supports available to you.

(4) Notify the senior ED doctor and contact your MDO immediately if an incident occurs that you believe could turn into a complaint or claim. Include the following situations:

(i) Missed or delayed diagnosis.

(ii) Adverse outcome.

(iii) Communication breakdown.

(iv) Angry or disgruntled patient.

(v) 'Gut feeling' that something is not quite right.

(5) Your initial reaction to the incident may help ameliorate the likelihood of a claim being lodged or pursued. Make sure you:

(i) Talk the problem through with the patient in lay-person's language.

(ii) Express regret and empathy for the adverse outcome.

(iii) Be honest, open and concerned – not defensive.

(iv) Continue to liaise with the medical team to ensure proper follow-up.

(v) Document meticulously, but *never* backdate, alter, or delete a medical record.

(vi) Contact your MDO early.

BREAKING BAD NEWS

(1) Breaking bad news to a relative concerning critical illness, injury or sudden death, especially when unexpected after trauma or cardiac arrest, must be done in the privacy of a quiet relatives' room.

(2) Be accompanied by an experienced nurse and/or social worker. Introduce yourself, identify the patient's nearest relative, and sit by them.

(3) Come to the point avoiding any pre-amble or euphemisms. Use the words 'dead' or 'death' or 'critically ill' early on, followed by a brief account of events.

(4) Be prepared to touch or hold the relative's hand and do not be afraid to show concern or empathy yourself. Allow a period of silence, avoiding platitudes or false sympathy, but encourage and answer any questions.

(5) Understand that the relative's reaction may vary from numbed silence, disbelief, acute distress to anger, denial and guilt.

(6) Indicate that the nurse or social worker can stay with them.

(7) Encourage the relative, when ready to do so, to see and touch the

body for cases involving death, and to say goodbye to their loved one alone.

(8) Ask whether the relative wishes the hospital chaplain or bereavement counsellor to be contacted. Avoid giving sedative drugs, which will only postpone acceptance of what has happened.

(9) Telephone or fax the GP and inform the coroner as appropriate.

(10) Retain the property of the patient, whatever its condition, for collection by the next of kin in accordance with his or her wishes. Avoid presenting the property in a plastic bin bag.

(11) Finally, appreciate the stress and anxiety caused to yourself and the nursing team following an unsuccessful or critical resuscitation.

    (i) Try to meet together briefly to talk over events and express your own feelings and emotions.

    (ii) Thank everyone for their efforts, particularly the nurse who dealt with the relatives and the nurses who were left to lay out the body in the case of sudden death.

TRIAGE

(1) All patients presenting to an Emergency Department should be sorted or triaged on arrival, usually by an experienced, specially trained ED nurse in order to direct resources to the more seriously ill first.

    (i) The triage nurse allocates an acuity category from the relevant National Triage Scale following assessment of current physiological disturbance and the risk of serious underlying illness or injury.

(2) The triage category answers the question: 'This patient should wait for medical assessment and treatment no longer than...', an ideal time period embodied in the treatment acuity (see Tables 16.1 and 16.2).

(3) Children and patients who are in pain may be up-triaged to a more acute category to facilitate expeditious care. Psychiatric patients are triaged according to a Mental Health Triage Scale.

(4) A patient's triage category underpins sentinel ED performance indicators, such as waiting times (by triage category), admission rates, and 'did not wait' (DNW) rates, and aids the prediction of optimal staffing levels, resources, space, and budget requirements.

Table 16.1 UK national triage scale

Designation	Treatment acuity	Numeric code
Immediate resuscitation	Immediately	1
Very urgent	Within 10 min	2
Urgent	Within 60 min	3
Standard	Within 120 min	4
Non-urgent	Within 240 min	5

Table 16.2 Australasian triage scale

Designation	Treatment acuity	Numeric code
Resuscitation	Immediately	1
Emergency	Within 10 min	2
Urgent	Within 30 min	3
Semi-urgent	Within 60 min	4
Non-urgent	Within 120 min	5

CONSENT, COMPETENCE AND REFUSAL OF TREATMENT

CONSENT AND COMPETENCE

(1) Consent may be implied, verbal, or written. However, to be valid it must be informed, specific, freely given, and cover what is actually done, and the patient should legally be capable of giving it.

(2) Patients over the age of 16 years in many circumstances, and 18 years in most, may sign or withhold their own informed consent. This may be done under common law principles or as set out in local legislation, provided they are deemed competent to do so.

(3) *Competence* requires that a patient understands what is proposed, the options involved, the treatment and the risks of treatment or lack of it, and the possible outcomes.

  (i) Thus competence incorporates the elements of comprehension, appreciation, reasoning and choice.

(4) Therefore, explain the details of the proposed procedure, and warn of any possible complications. The patient must understand the implications and nature of the treatment proposed, or of not accepting the treatment.

(5) The doctor should proceed even if consent was not obtained in cases of emergency to save life.

(6) Patients under the age of 16 years may even be able to consent for treatment provided they have the ability to understand what is proposed, although for major treatment it is appropriate to seek consent from the parent or guardian (or teacher in an emergency).

    (i) It is again appropriate to proceed to life-saving treatment of a minor even if the parent or guardian refuses, such as a blood transfusion in a Jehovah's Witness minor. Contact the hospital administration, the Paediatric team and at least commence application for a court order.

(7) Conversely, medical information should not then be supplied to others, including parents, without permission.

REFUSAL OF TREATMENT AND DISCHARGE AGAINST MEDICAL ADVICE

(1) Patients who refuse admission to hospital and/or a recommended treatment plan may be permitted to discharge themselves against advice, provided they are competent and informed – that is they understand fully the consequences of their actions.

(2) Make meticulous notes of exactly what was said to the patient, and their response, demonstrating that they understood the issues.

    (i) They may sign the appropriate form, accepting responsibility for their own action. However, it is more important to document clearly in long-hand in the medical notes exactly what they understood.

(3) Record if the patient refuses to sign any form, or disappears before a form is signed, and have this countersigned by a witness, such as a senior nurse or a second doctor.

(4) Patients who are not deemed competent, that is with conditions that preclude comprehension of the nature and implications of the treatment proposed, may be given emergency treatment without consent, to save life or to prevent serious damage to health.

(5) Similarly, patients suffering from a mental illness may be involuntarily detained against their will under the relevant Mental Health Act, if they are a danger to themselves or others (see p. 450).

    (i) They may receive treatment under common law if there is the overriding principle of best care by the treating doctor.

THE POLICE, CORONER AND ATTENDING COURT

The police are involved within the Emergency Department in a number of ways.

POLICE REQUEST FOR PATIENT INFORMATION

(1) All medical information concerning the care of a patient in the Emergency Department is confidential and must not be divulged without the patient's written consent, except on behalf of a coroner (or procurator fiscal in Scotland).

(2) Traffic police investigating a crash may be told the name, address and age of any patient involved, and a brief description of the injury, and in particular whether the crash is likely to prove fatal or whether the patient is to be admitted or sent home.

(3) A doctor may disclose information to a senior police officer concerning patients suspected of being involved in a serious arrestable offence, such as murder, rape, child abuse, armed robbery, or terrorist activity, thereby acting in the public interest for the safety of the lives of others.

    (i) Obtain the advice of the senior ED doctor or hospital administration whenever there is any doubt as to the appropriateness of releasing non-clinical information to the police.

POLICE REQUEST TO INTERVIEW A PATIENT

(1) Grant permission if the patient is medically in a fit state to be seen, after informing the patient.

(2) The doctor may suggest a time limit.

POLICE REQUEST FOR AN ALCOHOL BREATH TEST OR BLOOD SAMPLE

(1) The doctor should first give the police permission to perform these, provided the patient's clinical condition will not be adversely affected.

(2) Permission cannot be granted in certain circumstances: if the patient is unconscious, critically ill, or incapable of cooperating, possibly due to a facial injury. Local legislation may still permit a blood alcohol sample to be drawn.

(3) Inform the patient that you have allowed the police to be involved if permission is granted, and write in the ED record that in your opinion the patient was fit to be seen at the time.

(4) The police medical officer or police surgeon then takes the sample, using all their own equipment, and will not involve the hospital facilities at any stage.

(i) Alternatively, local legislation may dictate that the ED doctor draws the blood sample.

REQUEST FOR A POLICE MEDICAL STATEMENT

(1) The purpose of this statement is to act as a record to be read out in court without necessitating the doctor being present.

(i) The patient must first provide written consent before you may disclose confidential medical information.

(ii) Use any pre-printed forms supplied by the police.

(iii) State your full name, age, contact address and telephone number, medical qualifications, job status, your employing health authority and duration of that employment.

(iv) State the date you were on duty in the Emergency Department, the hospital's name, and the time you examined the patient.

(v) Continue with the full name, age, sex, occupation and address of the patient. Record the time and date of any subsequent attendances in the Emergency Department.

(vi) Recount the history (as told to you) without making personal inferences. Record the physical findings noted using language a non-medical person can understand.

(vii) State where possible the actual size of abrasions, bruises and lacerations. Make a comment as to whether the injuries found are consistent with the use of a particular weapon or implement as suggested by the patient's history.

(viii) List all the investigations performed, such as X-rays and laboratory tests, and their results, including relevant negatives.

(ix) State the treatment given, including sutures and their number, and record the time the patient spent in hospital or attending Outpatients.

(x) Finally, end the report where possible with a rough prognosis. Sign the report where indicated on each separate page.

(2) Always keep a photocopy of your report, and note the name and number of the police officer requesting the statement, and his or her police station.

THE CORONER

(1) Inform the coroner (procurator fiscal in Scotland) of all sudden or unexpected deaths, and deaths involving homicide, suicide, an accident or injury, drowning, poisoning, surgery, abortion, infancy, neglect, negligence, or patients in police custody or held in a mental hospital.

(2) Thus, virtually all patients brought in dead are reported to the coroner.

(3) Any patient actually dying in the department should also be reported. This should be done whatever the time of day or night if there are any suspicious circumstances, by contacting the local police station (the police are very often involved anyway).

(4) Therefore, the Emergency Department doctor is rarely in a position to sign a death certificate.

(i) However, try to contact the patient's own doctor when death clearly occurs as a direct result of a known illness, to see if that doctor is able to sign the certificate.

ATTENDING AN INQUEST

An inquest takes place in the coroner's court. Although it is purely a fact-finding inquiry, not a trial, there is usually a mix of 'inquisitorial' and 'adversarial' legal approaches. It is held in public, and the press may be present.

(1) The coroner's office will inform you of the date, time and place of the inquest. Make sure you tell your MDO that you have been asked to attend.

(2) Arrive punctually and dress suitably.
   (i) Legal representation may be arranged for you by your MDO if, on discussion with them, they consider it appropriate.

(3) Take the medical notes and a copy of your statement with you. Read both thoroughly beforehand several times so you have the facts readily available.

(4) Take the oath or affirmation, then the coroner will go through your statement with you and ask questions.

(5) Your replies should be concise, clear and factual. Indicate whether they are based on hearsay.

(6) You may be examined following this, by any 'properly interested persons' or usually their lawyer. You are not obliged to answer any questions that may incriminate you.

(7) The coroner's officer will pay you the appropriate witness fee and expenses after the inquest.

(8) Follow the same preparation for a civil negligence trial, where although using hearsay is admissible, the rules of evidence are based 'on the balance of probabilities'. Make sure your MDO has been involved throughout.
   (i) Attending a criminal trial is rare. Evidence must be 'beyond all reasonable doubt'. MDO representation is absolutely essential.

RETRIEVAL AND INTER-HOSPITAL TRANSFER

(1) Retrieval is the transport of a sick or injured patient by specially trained staff from a lesser-equipped (sending) hospital to a higher-level (receiving) hospital for further care.

(2) The sending doctor should speak directly to the receiving hospital doctor or retrieval specialist using a dedicated, single-point-contact coordinated communication system.

(3) The decision to transfer, the risks involved, the benefits expected, and the patient preparation are agreed on.
   (i) The sending doctor commences usual required care, such as two i.v. cannulae, nasogastric tube, indwelling catheter,

fracture splinting, and advanced airway/respiratory/ cardiovascular procedures, according to their ability.

(4) A transfer letter, photocopy of notes and forms, lab results, X-rays, ECGs, etc. are prepared for the retrieval team/receiving hospital.

(5) Road transport is suitable for short distances, and helicopters for longer ones.

(i) Helicopters and small aircraft require expert crew and landing areas, incur high costs, need dedicated equipment, and involve flight physiology considerations such as altitude hypoxia and trapped gas expansion (e.g. in a pneumothorax).

(6) Retrieval equipment must be compact, portable, light, robust and reliable, and have adequate battery capacity. Special ventilators, monitors, suction equipment, alarms, defibrillator, mattress, and an equipment frame 'bridge' are essential.

(7) Retrieval staff will spend time assessing, stabilizing and packaging the patient at the sending hospital, pre-empting any potential complications prior to transfer. It is not a time to rush.

(8) The aim is to improve the level of care at each stage, particularly during high-risk times such as loading and unloading during the inter-hospital travel.

MASS CASUALTY DISASTER AND THE MAJOR INCIDENT

(1) Each hospital will have its own plan for coping with large numbers of casualties, known as a Major Disaster Plan, Majax Plan or Medical Displan.

(i) This should be linked to regional and state plans for mass casualty situations in any location, however remote.

(2) Portions of the major disaster plan pertinent to individual members of staff are frequently summarized on documents known as Action Cards.

(i) Those concerned with the medical and nursing staff within the Emergency Department should be distributed to, and read by, all new members of staff.

(3) All new ED doctors must also make certain that the switchboard has a reliable contact telephone number for the purpose of an emergency call-out. In addition, make sure you:

(i) Know the call-out procedure, the different states of alert, and the significance of being the designated hospital or the supporting hospital.

(ii) Understand your role within the department, which senior doctor you are responsible to, and from whom you should receive advice.

(iii) Can operate any equipment reserved for a major incident, including that used by the mobile Medical team.

(iv) Are familiar with the special stationery and records used in a major incident, including the significance of the triage labels and where to find details of any pre-hospital care given, particularly drugs and fluids.

(v) Know where to obtain social and psychological support following the incident to minimize the potential for post-traumatic stress.

(4) Some incidents pose an additional danger to staff themselves from chemical, nuclear, biological, or radiological (CNBR) hazards.

(i) *Chemical and biological hazards*

(a) chemical contamination may occur following an industrial accident or deliberate release. Chemicals likely to be used in a deliberate release may be broadly divided into:

– nerve agents, such as sarin and VX, that act by interfering with activation of the parasympathetic nervous system, resulting in excessive secretions, arrhythmias, seizures and death

– vesicant agents, such as mustard gas and Lewisite, that cause blistering similar to large thermal burns

– choking agents, such as chlorine and phosgene, that cause irritation and injury to lungs, eyes and skin

– blood agents, such as hydrogen cyanide and other cyanogens, that inhibit cytochrome oxidase and prevent cellular oxygen use, resulting in rapid onset of convulsions, respiratory arrest and death

(b) biological contamination may be from bacteria such as the plague; viruses such as smallpox; spores such as anthrax; fungi such as *Fusarium*; or toxins such as ricin

– effects from contamination with biological agents may take days or even weeks to manifest

(c) the fire brigade is responsible for identifying toxic chemical spillage and for decontaminating on site, usually with large volumes of water

(d) designated isolation and decontamination areas and protective equipment and clothing or personal protective equipment (PPE) are used by staff. Practise putting them on and wearing them *before* a major event occurs

(e) exclude patient hypothermia from wet protective blankets in all cases, and adopt standard resuscitation procedures without delaying for the arrival of specific antidotes, either at the scene 'hot zone' or in the post-decontamination 'cold zone'

(f) most patients require admission for a period of observation, even if asymptomatic. Inhalation injury and absorption through skin, e.g. of phenol, may cause delayed toxic effects, which should be anticipated in advance.

(ii) *Radiological or nuclear hazards*

Ionizing radiation particles include alpha, beta and gamma particles, X-rays and neutrons (indirectly ionizing). Two types of radiation-induced injury can occur:

(a) external irradiation, where the patient has been exposed to radiation from an external source, such as a nuclear blast. Patients who have been externally irradiated are not radioactive and do not require decontamination

(b) contact with radiological materials, where the patient has become contaminated externally, internally, or both, with radioactive particles. These particles continue to emit ionizing radiation (alpha, beta or gamma) leading to cellular radiation injury if not removed
– these patients require formal decontamination

(c) patients requiring urgent treatment are taken to the nearest major Emergency Department

(d) Emergency Department staff attending these patients will be assigned to a pre-determined isolation and decontamination area. Make sure to wear caps, masks, theatre clothes, aprons, double gloves, and boots, which again you should be familiar with in advance

(e) advice and help are usually given by a radiation physicist or by contacting the local National Arrangements for Incidents involving Radioactivity (NAIR) staff or police.

FURTHER READING

Brentnall E, Galvin M, Parker H (2004) Consent and competence: The Australasian and UK perspectives. In: Cameron P, Jelinek G, Kelly A-M, *et al. Textbook of Adult Emergency Medicine*, 2nd edn, pp. 674–80. Churchill Livingstone, Edinburgh.

Health Protection Agency. http://www.phls.co.uk/ (CNBR hazards).

MDU. http://www.the-mdu.com/gp/services/publications/ order_publication/index.asp/ (advisory and risk management publications).

United Medical Protection. http://www.unitedmp.com.au/0/0.13/Home.htm/ (legal issues in medical practice).

Young S, Parker H (2004) The Coroner: The Australasian and UK perspectives. In: Cameron P, Jelinek G, Kelly A-M, *et al. Textbook of Adult Emergency Medicine*, 2nd edn, pp. 667–74. Churchill Livingstone, Edinburgh.

Glossary

AAA	abdominal aortic aneurysm
ABG	arterial blood gas
AC	alternating current
ACE	angiotensin-converting enzyme
ACS	acute coronary syndromes
ACTH	adrenocorticotrophic hormone
AED	automatic external defibrillator
AF	atrial fibrillation
AIDS	acquired immune deficiency syndrome
ALS	advanced life support
ALT	alanine aminotransferase
AMPLE	allergies, medications, past history, last meal, events preceding present injury
ANA	antinuclear antibody
AP	anteroposterior
APTT	activated partial thromboplastin time
ATLS	Advanced Trauma Life Support
ATN	acute tubular necrosis
AV	atrioventricular
b.d.	bis die (twice daily)
BLS	basic life support
BNF	British National Formulary
BP	blood pressure
BSA	body surface area
C1/C7	first and seventh cervical vertebrae
C7/T1	seventh cervical and first thoracic vertebrae
CABG	coronary artery bypass graft
CAD	coronary artery disease
CAGE	cut down, annoyed, guilty, eye-opener
CAP	community-acquired pneumonia
CCU	coronary care unit
CD4+	cluster designation (of antigen) 4+

CDAD	*Clostridium difficile* antibiotic-related diarrhoea
CDC	Centers for Disease Control and Prevention
CHS	classic heat stroke
CK	creatine kinase
CK-MB	creatine kinase MB isoenzymes
Cl	chloride
CLD	chronic lung disease
CMV	cytomegalovirus
CNBR	chemical, nuclear, biological, radiological
CNS	central nervous system
CO_2	carbon dioxide
COPD	chronic obstructive pulmonary disease
CPAP	continuous positive airways pressure
CPR	cardiopulmonary resuscitation
CPU	chest pain unit
CRF	chronic renal failure
CRP	C-reactive protein
CSF	cerebrospinal fluid
CSM	carotid sinus massage
CT	computerized (axial) tomography
CTG	cardiotocograph
cTnI	cardiac troponin I
cTnT	cardiac troponin T
CTPA	computerized tomography pulmonary angiogram
CVA	cerebrovascular accident
CVP	central venous pressure
CXR	chest X-ray
D&C	dilation and curettage
DC	direct current
DCI	decompression illness
DHF	dengue haemorrhagic fever
DIC	disseminated intravascular coagulation
DKA	diabetic ketoacidosis
DNA	deoxyribonucleic acid
DNW	did not wait
DPL	diagnostic peritoneal lavage
DU	duodenal ulcer
DVT	deep vein thrombosis
EBV	Epstein–Barr virus
ECG	electrocardiogram

ED	emergency department
EEG	electroencephalograph
EHS	exertion heat stroke
ELFTs	electrolytes and liver function tests
EMD	electromechanical dissociation
EMST	Early Management of Severe Trauma
ENT	ear, nose and throat
EPEU	early pregnancy evaluation unit
ERPC	evacuation of retained products of conception
ESR.	erythrocyte sedimentation rate
EST	exercise stress test
ET	endotracheal
FAST	focused assessment by sonography for trauma/focused abdominal sonogram for trauma
FBC	full blood count
FEV_1	forced expiratory volume in 1 second
FiO_2	fractional inspired oxygen concentration
G&S	group and save (blood)
GA	general anaesthesia
GCS	Glasgow Coma Scale
GFR	glomerular filtration rate
GI	gastrointestinal
GP	general practitioner
GTN	glyceryl trinitrate
GU	gastric ulcer
h	hour
H_1/H_2	histamine type 1 and type 2
Hb	haemoglobin
HBIG	hepatitis B immune globulin
HBO	hyperbaric oxygen
HBsAg	hepatitis B surface antigen
HCG	human chorionic gonadotrophin
HCO_3	bicarbonate
HELLP	haemolysis, elevated liver enzymes, low platelets
HHNS	hyperglycaemic, hyperosmolar non-ketotic syndrome
HIV	human immunodeficiency virus
HLA	human leucocyte antigen
HSV	herpes simplex virus
HTIG	human tetanus immunoglobulin
HUS	haemolytic-uraemic syndrome

i.m.	intramuscular
i.o.	intraosseous
i.v.	intravenous
ICC	intercostal catheter
ICS	intercostal space
ICU	intensive care unit
IDC	in-dwelling catheter
Ig	immunoglobulin
ILCOR	International Liaison Committee on Resuscitation
INR	international normalised ratio (of prothrombin time)
ITP	idiopathic thrombocytopenic purpura
IU	international units
IUCD	intrauterine contraceptive device
IVP	intravenous pyelogram
J	joule
JVP	jugular venous pressure
K	potassium
KCl	potassium chloride
kPa	kilopascal
KUB	kidneys, ureters, bladder
LBBB	left bundle branch block
LFTs	liver function tests
LMW	low-molecular-weight
LP	lumbar puncture
LSD	lysergic acid diethylamide
MAP	mean arterial pressure
MAST	military antishock trousers
MCP	metacarpophalangeal
MDI	metered-dose inhaler
MDO	medical defence organisation
mEq/L	milliequivalents per litre
MHA	Mental Health Act
MI	myocardial infarction
mmHg	millimetres of mercury
cmHg	centimetres of mercury
MMSE	Mini-Mental State Examination
MSU	mid-stream urine
MTP	metatarsophalangeal
Mu	megaunit
Na	sodium

NAA	nucleic acid amplification
NAC	*N*-acetylcysteine
NAI	non-accidental injury
NAIR	National Arrangements for Incidents involving Radioactivity
NAPCAN	National Association for Prevention of Child Abuse and Neglect
NGT	nasogastric tube
NIV	non-invasive ventilation
NPA	nasopharyngeal aspirate
NSAID	non-steroidal anti-inflammatory drug
NSPCC	National Society for the Prevention of Cruelty to Children
NSTEMI	non-ST elevation myocardial infarction
NTS	nose/throat swab
NZ	New Zealand
O&G	obstetrics and gynaecology
OM	occipitomental
OPG	orthopantomogram
p.r.	per rectum
$PaCO_2$	partial pressure of carbon dioxide (arterial)
PaO_2	partial pressure of oxygen (arterial)
PCI	percutaneous coronary intervention (coronary angioplasty)
PCP	*Pneumocystis carinii* pneumonia
PCR	polymerase chain reaction
PCV	packed cell volume
PE	pulmonary embolus
PEA	pulseless electrical activity
PEF	peak expiratory flow
PGL	persistent generalized lymphadenopathy
pH	negative logarithm of the hydrogen ion concentration
PID	pelvic inflammatory disease
PMR	polymyalgia rheumatica
PND	paroxysmal nocturnal dyspnoea
PPE	personal protective equipment
PTA	post-traumatic amnesia
PTI	prothrombin index
q.d.s.	quater in die sumendus (four times daily)
RAPD	relative afferent pupil defect (Marcus Gunn pupil)
RBBB	right bundle branch block
RNA	ribonucleic acid
ROSC	return of spontaneous circulation

r-PA	recombinant plasminogen activator
RSI	rapid sequence induction
rt-PA	recombinant tissue-type plasminogen activator
s	second
s.c.	subcutaneous
SaO_2	oxygen saturation
SARS	severe acute respiratory syndrome
SCIWORA	spinal cord injury without radiological abnormality
SIADH	syndrome of inappropriate ADH secretion
SIDS	sudden infant death syndrome
SJS	Stevens–Johnson syndrome
SLE	systemic lupus erythematosus
SLR	straight-leg raising
SNP	sodium nitroprusside
STD	sexually transmitted disease
STEMI	ST elevation myocardial infarction
SVT	supraventricular tachycardia
t.d.s.	ter in die sumendus (three times daily)
TA	transabdominal
TB	tuberculosis
TCA	tricyclic antidepressant
TEN	toxic epidermal necrolysis
TIA	transient ischaemic attack
TNK	tenecteplase
TTP	thrombotic thrombocytopenic purpura
TURP	transurethral resection of the prostate
TV	transvaginal
u	unit
U&Es	urea and electrolytes
UA	unstable angina
UF	unfractionated (heparin)
UTI	urinary tract infection
V/Q	ventilation perfusion (lung scan)
VDK	venom detection kit
VEB	ventricular ectopic beat (extrasystole)
VF	ventricular fibrillation
VT	ventricular tachycardia
VTE	venous thromboembolism
WBI	whole bowel irrigation
WCC	white cell count

APPENDIX: CRITICAL-CARE AREAS DRUG INFUSION GUIDELINE

These infusion guidelines were developed for use in critical care areas only. Most require close monitoring with titration to response, and are thus *inappropriate* for general ward areas. All calculations assume an adult weight of 70–80 kg. Paediatric resuscitation drug doses are available in Figure 10.1 and Table 10.4 in *Section X Paediatric Emergencies*.

Other paediatric doses are available in any paediatric formulary.

Readers are strongly advised to *re-check all doses* with another medical person before commencing therapy.

Drug	Loading dose	Paediatric infusion range (< 30 kg)	Dilution		Concentration	Adult dose (70–80 kg)	
			Infusion pump (IP)	Syringe driver		Dose per hour	Volume per hour
Adrenaline (epinephrine)	According to condition 1–100 µg/kg	0.05–1.0 µg/kg/min	6 mg in 100 mL DS	3 mg in 50 mL DS	60 µg/mL	2–20 µg/min	2–20 mL/h
Aminophylline [b]Standard	5.0 mg/kg in 100 mL DS over 20 min by IP	0.5–0.9 mg/kg/h	1000 mg in 500 mL DS	—	2 mg/mL	0.5–0.9 mg/kg/h	17.5–30 mL/h
[a]Transport	5.0 mg/kg in 100 mL DS over 20 min by IP	0.5–0.9 mg/kg/h	500 mg in 100 mL DS	250 mg in 50 mL DS	5 mg/mL	0.5–0.9 mg/kg/h	7–13 mL/h
Amiodarone [b]Standard	2–5 mg/kg in 100 mL DW over 30 min by IP	5–15 µg/kg/min	600 mg in 500 mL DW glass bottle. Discard at 12 h	—	1.2 mg/mL	20–60 mg/h (max. 15 mg/kg/24h)	17–52 mL/h
[a]Transport	2–5 mg/kg in 100 mL DW over 30 min by IP	5–15 µg/kg/min	300 mg in 100 mL DW	150 mg in 50 mL DW	3 mg/mL	20–60 mg/h (max. 15 mg/kg/24h)	7.5–22 mL/h
Clonazepam	1.0–2.0 mg	5–10 µg/kg/h	10 mg in 100 mL DS	5 mg in 50 mL DS	0.1 mg/mL	0.35–0.7 mg/h	3.5–7.0 mL/h
Dobutamine	—	2–30 µg/kg/min	250 mg in 100 mL DS	125 mg in 50 mL DS	2.5 mg/mL	2–30 µg/kg/min	2–30 mL/h
Dopamine	—	Renal: 0.5–2.5 µg/kg/min Inotrope: 5–20 µg/kg/min	200 mg in 100 mL DS	100 mg in 50 mL DS	2 mg/mL	Renal: 0.5–2.5 µg/kg/min Inotrope: 5–20 µg/kg/min	Renal: 1–5 mL/h Inotrope: 10–40 mL/h
Fentanyl	1–5 µg/kg	1–10 µg/kg/h	1000 µg in 100 mL DS	500 µg in 50 mL DS	10 µg/mL	50–200 µg/h	5–20 mL/h

Glyceryl trinitrate (GTN)							
bStandard	—	1–10 µg/kg/min	200 mg in 500 mL DW. Use glass bottle/low-absorption set	—	400 µg/mL	0.4–8 mg/h	1–20 mL/h
aTransport	—	1–10 µg/kg/min	50 mg in 100 mL DW	25 mg in 50 mL DW	500 µg/mL	0.5–10 mg/h	1–20 mL/h
Insulin (short-acting)	2–20 units	0.03–0.3 units/kg/h	100 units in 100 mL NS	50 units in 50 mL NS	1 unit/mL	2–20 units/h	2–20 mL/h
Isoprenaline							
Low dose	50–100 µg increments	0.5–7.5 µg/min	1 mg in 100 mL DS	0.5 mg in 50 mL DS	10 µg/mL	0.5–7.5 µg/min	2–30 mL/h
High dose	—	0.05–1.0 µg/kg/min	6 mg in 100 mL DS	3 mg in 50 mL DS	60 µg/mL	2–20 µg/min	2–20 mL/h
Ketamine	IV: 1–2 mg/kg IM: 5–10 mg/kg	5–20 µg/kg/min	1000 mg in 100 mL DS	500 mg in 50 mL DS	10 mg/mL	0.3–1.2 mg/kg/h	2–10 mL/h
Lignocaine (lidocaine)							
bStandard	1–2 mg/kg	15–50 µg/kg/min	Pre-mixed: 2 g in 500 mL DW	Pre-mixed: 2 g in 500 mL DW	4 mg/mL	*8 mg/min **4 mg/min ***2 mg/min	*120 mL/h for 20 min **60 mL/h for 60 min ***30 mL/h for 24 h
aTransport	1–2 mg/kg	15–50 µg/kg/min	2 g in 100 mL DW	1 g in 50 mL DW	20 mg/mL	*8 mg/min **4 mg/min ***2 mg/min	*24 mL/h for 20 min **12 mL/h for 60 min ***6 mL/h for 24 h

Drug	Loading dose	Paediatric infusion range (< 30 kg)	Dilution		Concentration	Adult dose (70–80 kg)	
			Infusion pump (IP)	Syringe driver		Dose per hour	Volume per hour
Magnesium sulphate 49.3% solution in 5 mL = 10 mmol = 2.47 g	0.15–0.3 mmol/kg = 10–20 mmol (adult) Dilute in 50 mL DS Infuse: 2 min (VT) to 20 min (pre-eclampsia)	0.05–0.1 mmol/kg/h	40 mmol in 100 mL DS	20 mmol in 50 mL DS	0.4 mmol/mL or 0.1 g/mL	2–8 mmol/h 0.5–2.0 g/h	5–20 mL/h
Methyl prednisolone *Spinal injury*	30 mg/kg over 30 min by IP	5.4 mg/kg/h	4 g in 100 mL. Reconstitute in water BP. Dilute in DS	2 g in 50 mL. Reconstitute in water BP. Dilute in DS	40 mg/mL	5.4 mg/kg/h for 23 h	10 mL/h (70 kg)
Midazolam	0.05–0.1 mg/kg in 1–2.5 mg increments	10–100 µg/kg/h	50 mg in 100 mL DS	25 mg in 50 mL DS	0.5 mg/mL	2.5–10 mg/h	5–20 mL/h
Morphine	2.5–15 mg in 2.5 mg increments	10–50 µg/kg/h	100 mg in 100 mL DS	50 mg in 50 mL DS	1 mg/mL	2–10 mg/h	2–10 mL/h
Naloxone	0.4–2.0 mg (max. 10 mg)	10 µg/kg/h	4 mg in 100 mL DS	2 mg in 50 mL DS	40 µg/mL	0.5–1.0 mg/h	12.5–25 mL/h
Nimodipine	—	6–30 µg/kg/h	10 mg in 50 mL dispensed	10 mg in 50 mL dispensed	0.2 mg/mL	0.4–2.0 mg/h. Titrate to maintain MAP	Start 2 mL/h. Increase 2 mL/h every hour to max. of 10 mL/h
Noradrenaline (norepinephrine)	—	0.05–1.0 µg/kg/min	6 mg in 100 mL DS	3 mg in 50 mL DS	60 µg/mL	2–20 µg/min	2–20 mL/h
Octreotide	50–200 µg	3–5 µg/kg/h	1000 µg in 100 mL DS	500 µg in 50 mL DS	10 µg/mL	25–100 µg/h	2.5–10 mL/h

Phenobarbitone (phenobarbital)	15–25 mg/kg in 100 mL DS over 20–30 min (max. 50 mg/min) by IP	—	—	—	—	—	—
Phenytoin	15–18 mg/kg in 100 mL NS over 20–30 min (max. 50 mg/min) by IP	—	—	—	—	—	—
Procainamide	10 mg/kg (max. 1000 mg) in 100 mL DW over 30 min by IP	20–80 µg/kg/min	1000 mg in 100 mL DW	500 mg in 50 mg DW	10 mg/mL	2–6 mg/min	12–36 mL/h
Propofol	Sedation: 0.5–1.0 mg/kg Induction: 2–3 mg/kg	1–10 mg/kg/h	—	500 mg in 50 mL (dispensed as 20-mL and 50-mL amps, both with 10 mg/mL)	10 mg/mL	Sedation 1–2 mg/kg/h Anaesthesia 5–10 mg/kg/h	Sedation 7–15 mL/h Anaesthesia 35–70 mL/h
rt-PA (alteplase)	15-mg bolus (15 ml)	—	100 mg in 100 ml water BP	—	1 mg/ml	(a) 15-mg bolus (b) 0.75 mg/kg (max 50 mg) over 30 min (c) 0.5 mg/kg (max 35 mg) over 60 min	
r-PA (reteplase)	10-U bolus in 2 min. After 30 min, second 10-U bolus in 2 min	—	2 vials/prefilled syringes/reconstitution devices and needles				

Drug	Loading dose	Paediatric infusion range (< 30 kg)	Dilution			Adult dose (70–80 kg)		
			Infusion pump (IP)	Syringe driver	Concentration	Dose per hour	Volume per hour	
Salbutamol (asthma)	5–10 µg/kg in 100 ml DS over 10 min	1.0–5.0 µg/kg/min	6 mg in 100 ml DS	3 mg in 50 ml DS	60 µg/ml	5–50 µg/min	5–50 ml/h	
Salbutamol (obstetric)	5–10 µg/kg in 100 ml DS over 10 min	0.2–1.0 µg/kg/min	6 mg in 100 ml DS	3 mg in 50 ml DS	60 µg/ml	10–50 µg/min	10–50 ml/h	
Sodium nitroprusside	—	0.05–10 µg/kg/min	100 mg in 500 mL DW in glass bottle. Protect from light. Discard at 24 h	—	Min 200 µg/mL Max 800 µg/min	0.05–10 µg/kg/min (max. 1.5 mg/kg/24h)	1–210 mL/h 500 mL/24h	
Streptokinase *AMI*	1.5 million units in 100 mL NS over 45 min by IP	—	—	—	15 000 units/mL	2.5 mL/min	150 mL/h	
PE, DVT, etc.	250 000 units in 100 mL NS over 30 min by IP	1500–2000 units/kg/h	500 000 units in 100 mL NS	—	5000 units/mL	100 000 units/h	20 mL/h	
Thiopentone (thiopental)	3–6 mg/kg (0.5 mg/kg in shock)	1–5 mg/kg/h	2500 mg in 100 mL water BP. Protect from light	1250 mg in 50 mL water BP. Protect from light	25 mg/mL	75–350 mg/h	3–15 mL/h	

Drug	Loading dose	Paediatric infusion range (< 30 kg)	Dilution Infusion pump (IP)	Syringe driver	Concentration	Adult dose (70–80 kg) Dose per hour	Volume per hour
Vecuronium	0.1 mg/kg	0.05–0.1 mg/kg/h	100 mg in 100 mL. Reconstitute in water BP. Dilute in DS	50 mg in 50 mL. Reconstitute in water BP. Dilute in DS	1.0 mg/mL	4–8 mg/h	4–8 mL/h

AMI, acute myocardial infarct; DS, dextrose saline, or any isotonic crystalloid; DVT, deep vein thrombosis; DW, 5% dextrose in water; IM, intramuscular; IP, infusion pump; IV, intravenous; MAP, mean arterial pressure; NS, normal saline; PE, pulmonary embolus; VT, ventricular tachycardia; water BP, water for injection.

[b]Standard: use in Emergency department.

[a]Transport: use for retrievals/interhospital transfers.

Reproduced by kind permission of Dr CT Myers, Senior Staff Specialist, Department of Emergency Medicine, Royal Darwin Hospital, Darwin. 2006.

Index